Kinship and Demographic Behavior in the Past

International Studies in Population

Volume 7

The International Union for the Scientific Study of Population (IUSSP)

The IUSSP is an international association of researchers, teachers, policy makers and others from diverse disciplines set up to advance the field of demography and promote scientific exchange. It also seeks to foster relations between persons engaged in the study of demography and population trends in all countries of the world and to disseminate knowledge about their determinants and consequences. The members of the IUSSP scientific group responsible for this book were chosen for their scientific expertise. This book was reviewed by a group other than the authors. While the IUSSP endeavors to assure the accuracy and objectivity of its scientific work, the conclusions and interpretations in IUSSP publications are those of the authors.

International Studies in Population (ISIP) is the outcome of an agreement concluded by IUSSP and Springer in 2004. The joint series covers the broad range of work carried out by IUSSP and includes material presented at seminars organized by the IUSSP. The scientific directions of the IUSSP are set by the IUSSP Council elected by the membership and composed of:

John Cleland (UK), President
Peter McDonald (Australia), Vice-President
Nico van Nimwegen (Netherlands), Secretary General and Treasurer

Elizabeth Annan-Yao (Ivory Coast)	Hoda Rashad (Egypt)
Graziella Caselli (Italy)	Catherine Rollet (France)
John Casterline (USA)	Yasuhiko Saito (Japan)
Maria Coleta de Oliveira (Brazil)	Zeba Sathar (Pakistan)
Thomas Kingston Le Grand (Canada)	Zeng Yi (China)

Kinship and Demographic Behavior in the Past

Edited by

TOMMY BENGTSSON
Lund University, Sweden

GERALDINE P. MINEAU
University of Utah, U.S.A.

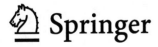 Springer

Tommy Bengtsson
Centre for Economic Demography
and Department of Economic History
Lund University
Sweden

Geraldine P. Mineau
Department of Oncological Sciences
and Huntsman Cancer Institute
University of Utah
USA

ISBN 978-90-481-2374-2 (PB)
ISBN 978-1-4020-6732-7 (HB)   e-ISBN 978-1-4020-6733-4

Library of Congress Control Number: 2009922602

Printed on acid-free paper.

9 8 7 6 5 4 3 2 1

springer.com

Preface

The International Union for the Scientific Study of Population's Panel on Historical Demography applies a historical perspective, such as the importance of kinship networks for demographic outcomes later in life, to promote work of contemporary relevance. Connections over time, whether across generations or different segments of the life course, are an area of convergent interest among multiple disciplines. Specific topics of common interest are the influence of conditions earlier in life on outcomes later in life, intergenerational associations in social, economic, and demographic outcomes, socioeconomic differences in health status and demographic outcomes, and the influence of industrialization and modernization on such patterns and relationships. Historical population databases, currently under expansion in a variety of locations around the world, provide longitudinal data on individuals across multiple generations and are especially amenable to the examination of such issues. Through a series of workshops scientists at the forefront of research on these issues were brought together in order to instigate a new wave of comparative work.

Kinship and Demographic Behavior in the Past is intended to extend the discussions that occurred at two seminars, cosponsored by the International Union for the Scientific Study of Population, to a broader community of population scientists. Experts from many disciplines have come together in this volume to highlight the convergence of research by demographers, economic historians, historians, anthropologists, sociologists, and geneticists. The contributors use longitudinal databases from different cultures to study families that existed in the past and focus on the role that family and kin groups played in both early and later life events. Our hope is that these contributions will be shared across the disciplines represented here and promote intergenerational research that is crucial in understanding demographic processes.

Acknowledgments

The present set of papers, focusing on the study of kinship, is selected from two seminars, cosponsored by the Scientific Committee on Historical Demography of the International Union for the Scientific Study of Population. The first seminar, in Paris in the fall of 2004, was organized in close collaboration with l'Institut National d'Études Démographiques (INED), l'École des Hautes Études en Sciences Sociales (EHESS), and the Centre for Economic Demography at Lund University. The organizing committee included Tommy Bengtsson (Lund University), James Z. Lee (University of Michigan), Geraldine P. Mineau (University of Utah), and Paul-André Rosental (EHESS/INED). The second seminar, in Salt Lake City in the fall of 2005, was organized and funded in collaboration with the Huntsman Cancer Institute at the University of Utah and the George S. and Dolores Doré Eccles Foundation of Utah, with Geraldine P. Mineau and James Z. Lee as organizers. We are most grateful to the institutions above for their generous support of the two seminars. We also owe a great debt to Madeleine Jarl at the Centre for Economic Demography, Lund University and Ellen Wilson at Huntsman Cancer Institute, University of Utah for assistance in editing this volume and, finally, to Cameron Campbell, Martin Dribe, and Frans van Poppel for providing comments on the introduction.

TOMMY BENGTSSON   GERALDINE P. MINEAU

Centre for Economic Demography and   *Department of Oncological Sciences and*
Department of Economic History,   *Huntsman Cancer Institute,*
Lund University, Sweden   *University of Utah, USA*

Contents

Introduction

Tommy Bengtsson[1] and Geraldine P. Mineau[2]

The historical demographic study of family structure and kinship has experienced tremendous change over the last 20 years. While the focus in the past has been on the family and the household, including coresident kin, considerable resources have recently been devoted to delineating nonresident kin. This has been done not only in societies where kinship was a major organizing principle by which social groups maintained the security and well-being of their members, but also in Western societies, where the state played part of this role.[1] The reason for the interest in family and kin networks also in Western societies is due to the fact that, while the state had the ultimate responsibility for the security and well-being of its citizens, this task was often devolved to families and employers, the state stepping in only if these agents failed.[2] Thus, for most of the time, and for the majority of the population, the family and the household, and sometimes also the nonresident kin, were instrumental in securing living standards for their members in both the West and the East.

Much of our understanding of past differences in family and kin systems between various parts of the world has been formed by a few classical studies— some based on national or regional aggregated data, others on local individual-level data. Malthus, and his predecessors, argued that major differences existed between

[1] Centre for Economic Demography and Department of Economic History,
Lund University, Sweden

[2] Department of Oncological Sciences and Huntsman Cancer Institute,
University of Utah, USA

[1] Paradoxically, while historical demographers, economic historians, and sociologists have expanded into analyses of kinship size and structure and thereby provided much more information on kin relations, anthropologists have moved away from the kinship concept (see Overing 2001).

[2] The Western state or the local community assisted, for example, children and elderly without relatives, the sick and the handicapped, and the utterly poor, accounting for only a fraction of the population. This seems to be the general pattern in Europe, exemplified by Sweden (Bengtsson 2004). Also in England, which had a more developed and wide-ranging welfare system, kin had strong obligations to take care of relatives (Wall 2002). For comparisons between the role of the state in the East and the West, see Lee, Bengtsson, and Campbell (2004).

T. Bengtsson and G.P. Mineau (eds.), *Kinship and Demographic Behavior in the Past.*
© Springer Science+Business Media B.V. 2009

Europe and Asia in the way families and households were formed and sustained with marriage being early and universal in Asia, but late and with a considerable degree of celibacy in Europe (Malthus 1803). Early marriage in Asia is associated with vertically integrated families with more than two generations living in the same household, while late marriage in Europe is associated with nuclear families and few coresiding kin. Malthus (1803) argued that the Asian system promotes population growth since fertility was not restricted by changes in age at marriage and proportions marrying. By contrast, the European system has been claimed to have promoted economic growth, a result of savings for the establishment of new households (Macfarlane 1978).[3]

Le Play (1895), using information from family studies across Europe, identified differences within Europe as well as changes over time. Le Play argued that the large patriarchal family, once dominant all over Europe, was being replaced by nuclear families in Western Europe, while remaining in Eastern Europe (Kertzer 2001). This view, also held by American sociologists (Goode 1963), was challenged by Laslett who argued that the nuclear family system dominated not only Britain, but also the rest of Western Europe far back in history (Laslett 1965). Hajnal contrasted the European with the non-European marriage systems, as Malthus did, but showed a distinctive difference also between Eastern and Western Europe, putting the dividing line between St. Petersburg and Trieste (Hajnal 1965). He later retreated from this by making further divisions within Western Europe (Hajnal 1983). Goody (1983) expanded the analyses, adding other features that differentiated the European family systems from the rest of the world by including other aspects of family formation and family life, such as polygamy and child abandonment.

The largely Malthusian division of Europe into two parts by Hajnal (1965) is mainly based on aggregated data. Later studies have confirmed his results, provided that the information used is derived from an aggregated level (Plakans and Wetherell 2005). Local studies based on individual-level data, however, show a great deal of heterogeneity (Plakans and Wetherell 2005; Reher 1998; Ruggles 1994; Smith 1993). It is therefore no surprise that a recent attempt by Alan Thornton (2005) to formulate a new synthesis has caused a lively debate (Caldwell 2006; Probert 2006; Ruggles 2006; Smith 2006).

The expansion of historical studies on the family to include kinship started by identifying kin and other networks in which nuclear families, usually Western, were engaged in various forms of mutual assistance and collaboration (Hareven 2001). The effect of coresiding kin on the well-being of children—"helpers-in-the-nest"—is one example of such an approach. Kin networks as a way of organizing

---

[3] Today, the largely Malthusian view of the Asian demographic system as promoting population growth has been challenged foremost by Lee and Wang Feng (1999). By analyzing the mortality response to food price changes, Bengtsson et al. (2004) have also shown that the pressure on resources did not differ much between populations in Asia (China and Japan) and Europe (Italy, Belgium and Sweden).

care for aging parents is another. Other studies have focused on the importance of kin for organizing migration and creating employment opportunities (Anderson 1971; Hareven 1982). Thus, rather than disrupting kinship ties, migration could strengthen them. Analyses of shifts in family and kin relations over long time periods have also made it possible to question some generalizations, such as that the more modern the society becomes, the less kin matter (Sabean 1998).

Much of the early work on nonresident kin was devoted to developing methods of how best to make use of the information available to reconstruct kinship (Plakans 1984). The problem with incomplete data led to the use of theoretical models, originally developed for forecasting kin size and kin structure on modern survey data. While these models vary in their complexity, they basically describe kin relations as an outcome of demographic events (Smith and Oeppen 1993). These models provide investigators with the ability, either analytically, or through simulations, to study the demographic processes underlying kin relations.[4] The outcome depends to a considerable extent on underlying assumptions, which are often difficult to verify. Historians have therefore made use of complementary information to improve our measures and understanding of kin relations (Ruggles 1993; Smith and Oeppen 1993; Post et al. 1997). Just as the methods of family reconstitutions were developed in the 1960s, methods for reconstructing kin structures have in recent years been developed, thereby adding a new dimension to previous studies of the role of the family for individual well-being (Sabean 1998, 3–4).

To map kinship structures and to identify the economic, social, and demographic implications of specific structures of familial and kin networks in the past, historical demographic databases have been expanded to include notarial archives, tax records, land registers and other similar registers, in addition to pedigree data that span generations and allow for reconstruction of networks of kin. This expansion of information on kin relations has two potentially very important implications. First, it may lead to a fundamental revision of our present knowledge of family and kin systems as providers of well-being for their members. Presently, much of our knowledge of the different systems continues to be based on either highly *aggregated* information, covering entire nations, or highly *detailed* information for local communities. Large new historical databases could provide more details as well as allow for more comparisons and new synthesis. Second, since the new databases contain information on several consecutive generations, these are also a valuable source for biological and genetic studies. These expanded databases provide more information on occupation, landholding, and other socioeconomic factors than are usually available in biological and genetic studies, which means that such studies can allow for the use of models mixing socioeconomic and biological factors. In addition, this allows for testing assumptions, common in biological and genetic studies, regarding the influence of socioeconomic factors and social mobility.

The availability of data at the household level, both in developing and developed countries, was important for the evolution of the "new" household economics

---

[4] The most well-known simulation model among historians is the CAMSIM model developed by Smith and Oeppen (1993).

theory aimed at explaining fertility, marriage, divorce, migration, health, and mortality (Becker 1965, 1981; for an overview, see Rosenzweig and Stark 1997). Special attention was given to strategies of smoothing consumption over the individual life cycle, such as securing consumption at old age, but also of smoothing consumption over the family life cycle by adding adult kin to the household. Another issue was how migration of kin can secure consumption in situations of short-term economic stress by diversifying sources of income. Such studies consider not only human and ethnic capital factors, but also kinship factors, whether pecuniary or nonpecuniary. The main focus of economists has, however, been contemporary societies, whether developed or developing, and not historical societies, despite increasing access to such data.

A dialogue has meanwhile developed between scholars of different disciplines regarding the role of kinship structure and its effects on demographic behavior and population dynamics. Interest has grown with respect to biological processes and theories, in terms of their association with demographic events within family groups. Convergent issues in genetics and demography have previously been addressed by a group of authors in Adams et al. (1990). A continued interest has been motivated by the fact that demography addresses phenomena central to biology (fertility and mortality).

Extended kinship networks are analyzed by geneticists to identify the presence of disease aggregation in families and to study the association of consanguinity with health outcomes. A variety of genes contributing to disease have been identified, including genes important for heart disease (Wang et al. 1996; Splawski et al. 2002; Mohler et al. 2004), specific cancers (Miki et al. 1994; Easton et al. 1997), neurological disorders (Charlier et al. 1998; Leppert and Singh 1999), and other diseases. Methodologies to ensure success in identifying human disease genes for complex disorders depend on the identification of large families of related individuals that have a predisposition to a specific disease (Carlson et al. 2004). Studies of health outcomes indicate that consanguinity of the parents can have an adverse effect on the health and mortality of offspring due to the expression of specific disease mutations inherited by both parents from a common ancestor (Bittles 2001).

Anthropologists, behavioral scientists, and evolutionary biologists traditionally study the sociocultural basis and consequences of kinship systems. Genetic and evolutionary theories, sometimes combined with social support theories, have been used to address mechanisms related to fertility, longevity, and nuptiality. The importance of genetic effects on fertility has been readdressed in recent research as operating through fecundity as well as motivation (Rodgers et al. 2001). Evolutionary reproductive ecology focuses on the adaptive mechanism of the grandmother hypothesis which investigates the relationship between grandmothers and increased offspring survival (Beise and Voland 2002; Hawkes 2003; Tymicki 2004). When describing the field of biodemography and its links to evolutionary concepts, Vaupel et al. (1998, 858) noted that

> If older individuals contribute to the reproductive success of younger, related individuals, then they promote the propagation of their genes. It is reproductive success that is optimized [through natural selection], not longevity. Deeper understanding of survival at older ages thus hinges on intensified research into the interactions between fertility and longevity.

A growing body of research investigates the influence of number of offspring and mother's age at last birth on postreproductive longevity of parents (Smith, Mineau, and Bean 2002; Hurt, Ronsmans, and Thomas 2006; Alter, Dribe, and van Poppel 2007).

The expanding availability and increasing quality and depth of information in historical databases creates a growing body of research synergies and discoveries that further attracts and stimulates interaction between disciplines. Longitudinal databases with individual and family-level information have been derived from linked censuses, family registries, family reconstitutions, population and events registers, and genealogies. These are valuable resources for studies of the social and demographic consequences of familial and kinship networks in the past and are being used to expand the scope of understanding demographic processes. Inclusion of morbidity and cause of death information is an important new development that enables investigators to address novel questions such as the presence of disease aggregation in families and the relationship between consanguinity and health outcomes. The addition of information on socioeconomic status, such as occupation or landholdings, has further enhanced the richness of such analyses. Using multigenerational, longitudinal databases, investigators can also address behavior and resources passed on from one generation to the next. This is not always the case for modern datasets.

The studies in the present volume make important contributions, both methodologically and substantially, to our understanding of the importance of kin in the past. They show that security and well-being of individuals was an issue that included not only yourself, your family and the household you belonged to, but larger networks in which kin was an important element. While earlier research to a large extent has focused on the family itself and on coresident kin, several of the contributions in this volume also take nonresident kin into account. Much work is needed before we can synthesize the results of local studies, comparative or not. Nevertheless, the studies represented in this volume contribute to this effort by showing details and circumstances of importance for well-being, and in particular for survival, in the past.

While many volumes are organized around demographic events (such as fertility, nuptiality, or mortality) or theoretical approaches, we have arranged the topics in this book in terms of the role that families and kinship played. It begins with investigations focused on the capacity of the family to provide well-being for its present members, progresses to analyses of the importance of well-being over the life course, and ends with a section of studies using family and kinship information as markers of genetic proximity that influence demographic behavior.

In the first section, the focus is on the immediate impact of family, household, and kin structures on well-being and demographic outcomes of its members. The studies include the analysis of individual-level data and familial factors related to marriage patterns; however, the studies' data resources differ in terms of the inclusion of multiple levels of analysis. Manfredini and Breschi in Chapter 1, as well as Van de Putte, Matthijs, and Vlietinck in Chapter 2, have a common focus on single European villages, the study of which derives from registry information on individuals and families. However, Manfredini and Breschi also have access to household information and can examine its role in marriage patterns. In Chapter 3, Campbell and Lee study a rural region of China that includes more levels of analysis with access to linked information on individuals, households, kinship groups, and communities. Their analysis is also broader in scope by examining fertility, mortality, and social attainment. These studies illustrate the variety of questions and complexity that can be addressed.

In the first chapter of this book, Manfredini and Breschi study a nineteenth-century rural community in Northern Italy, using tax records for measuring family wealth and a combination of vital records of births, deaths, marriages, and annual records of household composition to establish kin relationships. The two major social groups, the sharecroppers and the day laborers, show distinct differences as regards household size and structure, as well as age at marriage. The structure of the database allows the authors to analyze the different roles of kin for men and women of these two major social groups in the marriage process. They find large divergences between sharecroppers and day laborers. Sharecroppers strived to keep the labor of adult children within the family, but could only accommodate one married son in their household; thus, other brothers experienced lower marriage rates or permanent celibacy. The marriage patterns of the daughters of sharecroppers were closer to that of day laborers rather than sharecropping males; and for day laborers, only birth order mattered for the timing of marriage. Thus, social class, interacting with kin factors, had an ultimate effect on the marriage process.

Van de Putte, Matthijs, and Vlietinck, in Chapter 2, combine demographic records with information on wealth by making use of occupational information in their analyses of marriages in a Flemish village from the eighteenth to the twentieth century. Their database includes data from both parochial and civil registers. Their approach, however, differs radically from the one taken in the previous chapter since the focus is placed on familial health characteristics as the basis for marriage partner selection. The data allow the authors to study how health-related characteristics, measured as the level of infant and child mortality in the family of origin, influence the choice of marriage partners for various social groups. The authors find that, after controlling for structural causes, men and women born in high-mortality families find their marriage partners in high-mortality families. Although children of low-mortality families had a greater chance of marrying, the authors identify variations by social class.

Moving from Europe to China, Campbell and Lee in Chapter 3 make use of detailed and voluminous longitudinal, individual, and household level data from rural Liaoning in China during the eighteenth and nineteenth centuries. They compare the role of kin networks, communities, and households in determining individual social and demographic outcomes. The authors emphasize social organization and assess the importance of each level by examining the individual chances of attainment, fertility, marriage, and mortality. Results indicate that each level of organization was important, though the patterns of association varied by outcome. For example in terms of marriage prospects, every level appears to matter; for attainment of official position, however, descent groups within the same village were more important than variation between villages; and for mortality, the village was a much more important source of variation than the descent group. The authors then define "collective efficacy" (Sampson, Raudenbush, and Earls 1997) in terms of how homogeneous the villages are with respect to descent groups or kin networks. This allows them to examine whether villages with high collective efficacy generate favorable social and demographic outcomes.

The studies in the second part of the book include not only immediate effects of family, household, and kin structures on individual well-being and demographic outcomes, but also cohort and life-course effects. They include these broader perspectives in the analyses of demographic outcomes, such as migration, fertility, and mortality. While the models are different from the ones in the first section, the data are similar.

Van Poppel and van Gaalen, in Chapter 4, study how family and household factors such as socioeconomic position and remarriage mediate the effect of parental loss on child survival. The study covers children born between 1850 and 1922 in three provinces of the Netherlands. This allows the authors to analyze how the effects of such factors change over time and space, the latter by including both urban and rural areas. They divide the period into two subperiods, 1850–1879 and 1880–1922: the first with stable birth and death rates and the second with falling rates, thus covering the start of the demographic transition, as well as the situation immediately preceding it. The prerequisite for their approach is the use of continuous time information on living arrangements with socioeconomic data included, which has been registered for 0.5 percent of the Dutch population born during this period. This allows van Poppel and van Gaalen to analyze how changes take place in the role of the father versus the mother, the role of quasi-kin such as stepparents, and the role of social class, at least broadly speaking, as the economic and demographic context changes. They find that loss of mother is important for children of all social classes; and while the loss of the father is comparatively less important, his relative role increases with the age of the child and over time. Remarriage of fathers is, likewise, more important in early cohorts than in later ones. The effect of loss of mother is not limited to younger ages, but remains and has a social gradient for older children. Thus, mothers are needed for small children regardless of class, particularly in the early period before the infant and child mortality start to decline. Later in childhood, and in the later period, when mortality has started to decline, the role of the father becomes more important, as does social class.

In Chapter 5, Tymicki focuses on effects of kin on fertility in a rural population in Poland. Again, the study covers both the premodern and the early transitional stage when fertility rates start to decline. The area is characterized by small differences in wealth between households while the size of extended kinship varies substantially. This allows the author to study the influence of helpers, both in- and outside the household, on fertility by birth order, controlling for various other factors, such as the fate of the previously born child. The support for the hypothesis that kin help should be of crucial importance at higher parities is only weak and does not change regardless of whether the fertility regime is natural or controlled. An exception to this finding is the positive effect of grandparents and specifically the benefit of the maternal grandmother.

Kesztenbaum, in Chapter 6, studies the influence of familial experience of migration stability or nonstability on the migration decisions of individuals. The data used for this study are genealogies constructed from the TRA study of archival data on French families over one and a half centuries. The data have been linked with military registers and administrative records on tax inheritance. The focus is on men from the military registers and on measuring their spatial capital which is determined by observing their family territory. The concept of family territory is based on an inventory of places of residence of family members. Kesztenbaum explores the residential experience of both the parental family and the ancestral family. The chapter demonstrates the importance of a history of migration in a given family in determining the mobility of its members. This allows the author to analyze how men use the spatial capital they inherit from their family and Kesztenbaum finds that families are diversified: on the one hand, migration appears to be inherited as both the size and scope of family territory increases the probability of migration, while, on the other hand, locations do not appear to be inherited as many men migrate to places that do not belong to the spatial capital of their family.

The essay by Bengtsson and Broström, in Chapter 7, explores the role played by inheritance on longevity, using data from five rural parishes in Southern Sweden between 1829 and 1894, which was a period of continued high fertility but declining infant and child mortality. The data include demographic and economic information from parish registers as well as taxation records over the entire life course, which allows the authors to disentangle the effects of inherited, achieved, and external environmental factors on mortality in older ages. After controlling for other factors throughout the life course, they find that length of life of both parents has a persistent impact on mortality in older ages of their offspring. Socioeconomic differences are small or nonexistent, but conditions in early life (the disease load in year at birth) have a strong impact on males. Thus, while socioeconomic factors are important in certain instances, such as to overcome short-term economic stress, they have has no direct effects on longevity. Instead, other noneconomic inherited factors are of importance, as are external environmental factors.

In the last part of the book, kinship is not a variable of interest in itself but rather a marker of genetic proximity for demographic behavior. Egerbladh and Bittles, in Chapter 8, use consanguinity as a marker in their analyses of infertility and health; in Chapter 9, Gagnon, Mazan, Desjardins, and Smith use fertility as a biological marker for postreproductive longevity; Kerber, O'Brien, Smith, and Mineau, in Chapter 10, identify the role of specific disease history among both close and distant kin for longevity; and Tremblay, Vézina, Desjardins, and Houde, in Chapter 11, study the origins of the French population in Quebec and, specifically, founder effects.

In Chapter 8, Egerbladh and Bittles analyze marriages in Northern coastal Sweden from 1720 through 1899 by using data from the Demographic DataBase at Umeå University. These marriages were characterized in terms of consanguinity in order to determine how closely related the couples were, ranging from first to sixth cousin. Having classified marriages in terms of their kinship structure, the authors were able to study two questions: whether marriages of close relatives result in consanguinity-associated infertility, and whether there is an adverse effect on the health of the children of such marriages. The study is made even more interesting by the fact that marriage legislation changed during the study period, increasing the consanguineous marriages. They find no indication of differences in fertility among groups; however, infant and childhood mortality were higher among first-cousin progeny. The authors discuss the genetic interpretation of their findings and its probable effect on the prevalence of genetic disorders.

Gagnon, Mazan, Desjardins, and Smith, in Chapter 9, examine the issue of fertility as a biological marker on postreproductive longevity in a natural fertility population in the Saint Lawrence Valley in Canada. Their chapter discusses both evolutionary and social support theories in hypothesizing the link between reproduction and longevity. This population remained almost closed until the nineteenth century and thus does not have the typical heterogeneity in terms of particular historical circumstances of open populations. The entire population is expected to live under similar economic circumstances since this was a frontier area. Detailed information on demographic events and completeness of the recording of births and deaths makes it possible for the authors to study effects of age at first birth, menopause, and other factors on mortality in older ages. They focus their study on women who survive to at least age 60 and find some evidence that having their first child either at early ages or at late ages enhances female longevity. The French Canadian data support results that show that women with a large number of births or high parity have higher postreproductive mortality, thus reducing longevity. On the other hand, the longevity of husbands was less sensitive to parity and reproductive history. The authors support the hypothesis that women bearing their last child late in life had longer postreproductive lives, suggesting that late menopause is associated with an overall slower rate of aging. In addition, they compare their results with findings from another North American frontier population in Utah.

In Chapter 10, Kerber, O'Brien, Smith, and Mineau consider how the causes of death of individuals may be related to a family history of disease in both close and distant relatives. Specifically, they study the familial aggregation of cause of death in large pedigrees and the interplay between familial tendencies to die of specific causes and familial longevity. Using the Utah Population Database, the authors identify cohorts of family members born from 1830 through 1937 who survived to at least age 65. Using genealogy records that have been linked to state-issued death certificates, they classify the underlying cause of death to one of the 10 leading causes for the United States. The methodology they use to analyze these data combines demography and epidemiology; they calculate familial standardized mortality, population attributable risk, and familial excess longevity, and present results in terms of familial risk and time periods. These results indicate that family histories of cause-specific mortality greatly affect risk of death from the same cause. However, familial excess longevity is associated with decreased risks of almost all causes of death, suggesting that whatever factors link kin survival, an important component is the aggregation of longevity within the extended family.

The volume concludes with Tremblay, Vézina, Desjardins, and Houde who, in Chapter 11, study the origins and genealogical structure of the Quebec population. A founder effect is the long-term genetic consequence of a migration movement initiated by a relatively small group of individuals from a parent population, in this case France. Using the BALSAC population register, the BALSAC-RETRO genea-logical database, and the Early Quebec Population Register, they identified indi-viduals married in Quebec between 1945 and 1965 and whose parents were also married in Quebec, and trace these individuals, for the most part, back to the first settlers in the early seventeenth century. Using a genetic approach, they calculate the relatedness of individuals, i.e., whether or not they share a common ancestor. The analysis indicates that almost all Quebecois of French descent share at least one common ancestor and, in many cases, many more than one. They also investi-gate the differential contribution of French provinces in order to determine the pro-portion of the gene pool shared by the subjects, and find that the most common places of origin of the French founders are found in the western part of France, especially in the north. The authors conclude that the early founder effects remain strongly perceptible and discuss the implications of this effect in terms of heredi-tary diseases.

To conclude, studies of kinship have, as shown by this volume, stimulated new analytical approaches and produced findings that are among the most innovative and productive in population and social history in recent years. The importance of taking into account not only coresident but also nonresident kin has been demon-strated in the contributions to this volume. By beginning with individual-level data, rather than aggregate data, the authors are able to evaluate proposed mechanisms that link kinship and demographic processes. Given the empirical results already achieved, and the ability to integrate the kinship level within existing theoretical frameworks, it is likely that further theoretical development, concepts, and meas-urements referring to activities at the kinship level using historical datasets will develop in the near future. This will establish a new basis for our understanding of the large differences in past, and possibly present, family and kin structure.

References

Adams, J., A. Hermalin, D. Lam, and P. Smouse. 1990. *Convergent Issues in Genetics and Demography*. Oxford University Press, Oxford.

Alter, G., M. Dribe, and F. van Poppel. 2007. Widowhood, family size, and post-reproductive mortality: a comparative analysis of three populations in nineteenth-century Europe. *Demography* 44(4): 785–806.

Anderson, M.S. 1971. *Family Structure in Nineteenth-century Lancashire*. Cambridge University Press, Cambridge.

Becker, G. 1965. A theory of the allocation of time. *Economic Journal* 75(299): 493–517.

Becker, G. 1981. *A Treatise on the Family*. Harvard University Press, Cambridge, MA.

Beise, J. and E. Voland. 2002. A multilevel event history analysis of the effects of grandmothers on child mortality in a historical German population (Krummhörn, Ostfriesland, 1720–1847). *Demographic Research* 7: 470–94.

Bengtsson, T. 2004. Mortality and social class in four Scanian Parishes, 1766–1865, in T. Bengtsson, C. Campbell, J.Z. Lee et al. (eds.), *Life under pressure. Mortality and living standards in Europe and Asia 1700–1900*, MIT, Cambridge, MA., pp. 135–71.

Bittles, A.H. 2001. Consanguinity and its relevance to clinical genetics. *Clinical Genetics* 81: 91–8.

Caldwell, J.C. 2006. Book review of Reading History Sideways (Thornton 2005). *Journal of the Royal Anthropological Institute* 12: 222–3.

Carlson, C.S., M.A. Eberle, L. Kruglyak, and D.A. Nickerson. 2004. Mapping complex disease loci in whole-genome association studies. *Nature* 429(6990): 446–52.

Charlier, C., N.A. Singh, S.G. Ryan, T.B. Lewis, B.E. Reus, R.J. Leach, and M. Leppert. 1998. A pore mutation in a novel KQT-like potassium channel gene in an idiopathic epilepsy family. *Nature Genetics* 18(1): 53–5.

Easton, D.F., L. Steele, P. Fields, W. Ormiston, D. Averill, P.A. Daly, R. McManus, S.L. Neuhausen, D. Ford, R. Wooster, L.A. Cannon-Albright, M.R. Stratton, and D.E. Goldgar. 1997. Cancer risks in two large breast cancer families linked to BRCA2 on chromosome 13q12-13. *American Journal of Human Genetics* 61(1): 120–8.

Goode, W.J. 1963. *World Revolutions and Family Patterns*. Collier-Macmillan, New York.

Goody, J. 1983. *The Development of the Family and Marriage in Europe*. Cambridge University Press, Cambridge.

Hajnal, J. 1965. European marriage patterns in perspective, in D.V. Glass and D. Eversley (eds.), *Population in history*, Aldine, Chicago, IL, pp. 101–43.

Hajnal, J. 1983. Two kinds of pre-industrial household formation systems, in R. Wall, R. Robin, and P. Laslett (eds.), *Family forms in historic Europe*, Cambridge University Press, Cambridge, pp. 65–104.

Hareven, T.K. 1982. *Family Time and Industrial Time: The Relationship Between the Family and Work in a New England Industrial Community*. Cambridge University Press, New York.

Hareven, T.K. 2001. History of family and kinship, in N.J. Smelser and P.B. Baltes (eds.), *International encyclopedia of the social & behavioral sciences*, online version updated 2004, pp. 5291–8.

Hawkes, K. 2003. Grandmothers and the evolution of human longevity. *American Journal of Human Biology* 15: 380–400.

Hurt, L.S., C. Ronsmans, and S.L. Thomas. 2006. The effect of number of births on women's mortality: Systematic review of evidence for women who completed their childbearing. *Population Studies* 60: 55–71.

Kertzer, D. 2001. Family systems in Europe, in N.J. Smelser and P.B. Baltes (eds.), *International encyclopedia of the social & behavioral sciences*, online version updated 2004, pp. 5357–61.

Laslett, P. 1965. *The World We Have Lost*. Methuen, London.

Lee, J.Z., T. Bengtsson, and C. Campbell. 2004. Family and community, in T. Bengtsson, C. Campbell, J.Z. Lee et al. (eds.), *Life under pressure. Mortality and living standards in Europe and Asia 1700–1900*, MIT, Cambridge, MA, pp. 85–105.

Lee, J.Z. and Wang Feng. 1999. *One Quarter of Humanity. Malthusian Mythology and Chinese Realities, 1700–2000*. Harvard University Press, Cambridge, MA/London.

Le Play, F. 1895. *L'Organisation de la Famille Selon le Vrai Modèle Signalé par l'Historie*, 4th edition. Alfred Mame, Paris.

Leppert, M.F. and N. Singh. 1999. Susceptibility genes in human epilepsy. *Seminars in Neurology* 19(4): 397–405.

Macfarlane, A. 1978. *Origins of English Individualism: The Family, Property, and Social Transition*. Blackwell, Oxford.

Malthus, T.R. 1803. *An Essay on the Principle of Population*, 2nd edition, in Donald Winch (ed.), Cambridge University Press, Cambridge.

Miki, Y., J. Swensen, D. Shattuck-Eidens, P.A. Futreal, K. Harshman, S. Tavtigian, Q. Liu, C. Cochran, L.M. Bennett, W. Ding et al. 1994. A strong candidate for the breast and ovarian cancer susceptibility gene BRCA1. *Science* 266(5182): 66–71.

Mohler, P.J., I. Splawski, C. Napolitano, G. Bottelli, L. Sharpe, K. Timothy, S.G. Priori, M.T. Keating, and V. Bennett. 2004. A cardiac arrhythmia syndrome caused by loss of ankyrin-B function. *Proceedings of the National Academy of Science USA* 101(24): 9137–42.

Overing, J. 2001. Kinship in anthroplogy, in N.J. Smelser and P.B. Baltes (eds.), *International encyclopedia of the social & behavioral sciences*, online version updated 2004, pp. 8098–105.

Plakans, A. 1984. *Kinship in the Past: An Anthropology of European Family Life 1500–1900*. Oxford University Press, Oxford.

Plakans, A. and C. Wetherell. 2005. The Hajnal line and Eastern Europe, in T. Engelen and A. Wolf (eds.), *Marriage and the family in Eurasia: Perspectives on the Hajnal hypothesis*, Aksant Academic, Amsterdam, pp. 105–28.

Post, W., F. van Poppel, E. van Imhof, and E. Kruse. 1997. Reconstructing the extended kin-network in the Netherlands with genealogical data: Problems, methods and results. *Population Studies* 51(3): 263–78.

Probert, R.J. 2006. Book review of Reading history sideways (Thornton 2005). *International Journal of Law, Policy, and the Family* 20: 127–32.

Reher, S.D. 1998. Family ties in Western Europe: Persistent contrasts. *Population and Development Review* 24(2): 203–34.

Rodgers, J.L., H.-P. Kohler, K. Ohm Kyvik, and K. Christensen. 2001. Behavior genetic modeling of human fertility: Findings from a contemporary Danish twin registry. *Demography* 38: 29–42.

Rosenzweig, M.R. and O. Stark. 1997. *Handbook of Population and Family Economics*. Elsevier, Amsterdam.

Ruggles, S. 1993. Confessions of a microsimulator: problems in modeling the demography of kinship. *Historical Methods* 26(4): 161–9.

Ruggles, S. 1994. The transformation of American family structure. *The American Historical Review* 99(1): 103–28.

Ruggles, S. 2006. Book review of Reading History Sideways (Thornton 2005). *Population and Development Review* 32(1): 174–6.

Sabean, D.W. 1998. *Kinship in Neckarhausen, 1700–1870*. Cambridge University Press, Cambridge.

Sampson, R., S. Raudenbush, and F. Earls. 1997. Neighborhood and violent crime: A multilevel study of collective efficacy. *Science* 277(5328): 918–24.

Smith, D.S. 1993. The curious history of theorizing about the history of the Western nuclear family. *Social Science History* 17: 325–53.

Smith, D.S. 2006. Book review of Reading History Sideways (Thornton 2005). *International Review of Social History* 51(2): 301–4.

Smith, K.R., G.P. Mineau, and L.L. Bean. 2002. Fertility and post-reproductive longevity. *Social Biology* 49: 185–205.

Smith, J.E. and J. Oeppen. 1993. Estimating numbers of kin in historical England using demographic microsimulation, in D.S. Reher and R. Schofield (eds.), *Old and new methods in historical demography*, Clarendon, Oxford, pp. 280–317.

Splawski, I., K.W. Timothy et al. 2002. Variant of SCN5A sodium channel implicated in risk of cardiac arrhythmia. *Science* 297(5585): 1333–6.

Thornton, A. 2005. *Reading History Sideways: The Fallacy and Enduring Impact of the Developmental Paradigm on Family Life*. University of Chicago Press, Chicago, IL.

Tymicki, K. 2004. Kin influence on female reproductive behavior: The evidence from reconstitution of the Bejsce parish registers, 18th to 20th centuries, Poland. *American Journal of Human Biology* 16: 508–22.

Vaupel, J.W., J.R. Carey, K. Christensen, T.E. Johnson, A.I. Yashin, N.V. Holm, I.A. Iachine, V. Kannisto, A.A. Khazaeli, P. Liedo, V.D. Longo, Y. Zeng, K.G. Manton, and J.W. Curtsinger. 1998. Biodemographic trajectories of longevity. *Science* 280: 855–60.

Wall, R. 2002. Families in crisis and the English poor law as exemplified by the relief programme in the Essex parish of Ardleigh 1795–7, in *The Logic of Female Succession: Rethinking Patriarchy and Patrilineality in Global and Historical Perspective*. International Symposium 19, International Research Centre for Japanese Studies, Kyoto, pp. 101–27.

Wang, Q., M.E. Curran, I. Splawski, T.C. Burn, J.M. Millholland, T.J. VanRaay, J. Shen, K.W. Timothy, G.M. Vincent, T. de Jager, P.J. Schwartz, J.A. Towbin, A.J. Moss, D.L. Atkinson, G.M. Landes, T.D. Connors, and M.T. Keating 1996. Positional cloning of a novel potassium channel gene: KVLQT1 mutations cause cardiac arrhythmias. *Nature Genetics* 12(1): 17–23.

Part I
Family and Kin as Immediate Providers of Well-being for Its Members

Chapter 1
Marriage and the Kin Network: Evidence from a 19th-Century Italian Community

Matteo Manfredini[1] and Marco Breschi[2]

Abstract This chapter deals with the role and influence of kinship on the decision to marry in a rural population of mid nineteenth century Italy. The reason for this choice lies in the particular social structure of that community, where the two most important social groups, sharecroppers and day laborers, had almost antithetic marriage patterns and family formation systems. Our study demonstrates the key role of kin, especially coresident ones, in modifying the risk of marriage. This situation was particularly pronounced within the large and complex sharecropping households. Constrained by the absolute necessity to maintain not only a balance between farm size and household size but also an adequate supply of labor within the household, sharecroppers posed limits and restrictions on marriages of members, especially men. Gender, age, and marital status were chief factors determining who could marry and when. On the other hand, day laborers were less sensitive to household structure as their activity depended neither on the household labor force nor on the characteristics of the farm. In this case, the access to marriage, ruled only by birth order, was less controlled for both men and women. As for the role of kin outside the household, difficulties in the reconstruction of the entire kin network made the results less conclusive. However, it was only effective in modifying the risk of marriage for women living in sharecropping households. Large and deep-rooted networks of relations favored a woman's access to marriage, especially when a local man was involved, suggesting the use of marriage to establish and reinforce local family alliances.

Keywords remarriage, widowhood, 19th-century Italy, parish registers

1 Introduction

Marriage has been an interesting issue in many research fields due to its interdisciplinary nature. Anthropologists, geneticists, demographers, scholars of social sciences, and evolutionary biologists have often addressed their attention to marriage

[1]Department of Genetics Anthropology Evolution, University of Parma, Italy

[2]Department of Economics, Enterprise, Regulation, University of Sassari, Italy

and the mating pattern of human populations. The reason is clear: marriage is a social and cultural event with profound qualitative and quantitative consequences to the future population structure.

To study the quantitative effects of marriage on population structure means investigating marital fertility in relation to age, provenience, occupation, and other characteristics of spouses. Qualitative changes concern many facets of the mating structure, from sociocultural topics, such as social endogamy (Campbell and Lee 2003; Dribe and Lundh 2005; Moring 1996; Segalen 1991; van Leeuwen and Maas 2002), to more biologic issues connected to changes in the genetic structure of populations (Castro De Guerra, Arvelo, and Pinto-Cisternas 1999; Crow and Mange 1965; Lasker, Mascie-Taylor, and Coleman 1986; Madrigal and Ware 1999; Mascie-Taylor, Lasker, and Boyce 1987; Relethford 1992).[1]

The social nature of marriage requires that its biological and demographic effects be studied in relation to the cultural, economic, and traditional aspects of the population analyzed (Kertzer 2002; Tittarelli 1991). As we will explain further in this chapter, family ties and kin networks are definitely important factors. It is actually well known that marriage was so seldom an individual choice, and often a shared family decision (Barbagli 1984; Derosas 2002; Kertzer and Saller 1991), that Bourdieu (1962) claimed that, paradoxically, it was the family that got married, not the individual. This was definitely true in the Italian society of the nineteenth century, where cultural and socioeconomic specificities put household and family ties at the heart of peoples' everyday life choices. Studying the marriage pattern of a rural sharecropping community of Central Italy, Tittarelli concluded that "marital decisions were made by the family—by the head of household or the dominant conjugal nucleus—and they were based on the family's circumstances at that particular time, not on the wishes of the person involved" (Tittarelli 1991, 285). Yet, beyond general comments and descriptive analyses, little is known about the complex interrelationship between household composition and the chances of marriage of each single member.

This chapter aims at investigating, for a rural nineteenth century Italian community of Tuscany, to what extent the decision to get married could be affected and driven by the local kin network. To control for the intimate mechanisms of a household life cycle, the analysis will be carried out at both household and individual levels.

2 Theoretical Background

In historical studies of European families, the link between forms of coresidence and marriage pattern has been speculated upon for a long time. The stem family group, characterized by the permanence of one married son within the native household after marriage and by an impartible system of inheritance, was at the heart of Le Play's theory on family systems (Le Play 1871). He believed that this

---

[1] Many of the cited papers dealing with genetic issues make use of surname frequencies as a tool to evaluate consanguinity, genetic distance, similarity among populations, and migration.

family formation system represented the ancient and traditional pattern of living arrangements of European populations, antithetic to the more unstable and emerging nuclear family model produced by the transformations associated with industrialization. Although Hajnal (1965) reversed the paradigm, claiming that simple families and neolocalism were the earliest and most widespread features in Western European family history, the strong connection between marriage and forms of living arrangement was preserved. Hajnal claimed that in societies where a nuclear household system was dominant—namely all those countries west of a hypothetical line connecting Trieste to Leningrad—age at first marriage of men was higher because they had to wait until they reached an autonomous economic position. Some years later, Laslett revised this theoretic scheme on two key points. First, he put the figure of life cycle servants at the heart of the mechanism of the nuclear family formation system: in those populations, men left their parental home long before marriage, and, having gained economic independence, married and lived with the bride in their own house (Laslett 1977). Secondly, Laslett adopted a more complex model of European family formation by admitting the existence of four different patterns across Europe. The nuclear-based model was now limited to Northwestern populations, and it was not present in Eastern and Southern ones, Italy included (Laslett 1983). In those countries, a system characterized by the coresidence of many kin of different nuclei under the same roof and a patrilocal system of living arrangement after marriage was the norm (joint family system). Laslett concluded that this system, based on a large number of coresident kin, made the circulation of life cycle servants unnecessary, since households had sufficient labor force to be autonomous. He coined the term Mediterranean to define such a pattern, which was also typified by young female age at first marriage, quasi-universal marriage and a reduced age gap between the spouses. These latter features were based on the argument that a large number of kin living in complex households formed unique working units able to incorporate the newly-formed couple without waiting for their economic independence.

However, these schematic and synthetic models had to face much criticism for their failure to take into account the great variability of family systems existent in Europe (Barbagli 1984; Berkner and Mendels 1978; Herlihy and Klapisch-Zuber 1985; Kertzer 1991; Rowland 1983). Italy was explicitly one of the most studied countries in which the large number of family forms not matching the criteria indicated by Laslett and Hajnal induced many scholars to seek other interpretations and explanations linking family formation system, coresidential pattern, and age at marriage (Barbagli 1984, 1990; Doveri 1990; Kertzer 1991; Kertzer and Brettell 1987; Viazzo 2003). The common point was that rather than differentiating family systems according to geographic areas and territories (of Italy), those authors associated household structure, marriage pattern, and residence after marriage to socio-economic niches, thereby admitting the possible coexistence of multiple schemes of family formation in just one place and even within just one population (Corsini 2000; Kertzer 1991). This assumption implies that timing of and access to marriage, family formation pattern, and household structure were shaped not only by social norms and cultural habits, such as the form of living arrangement after marriage, but also by economic constraints, specific to each professional position and role. Thus, the differentiation does not emerge only at the geographic level, through the contrasting patterns of South (Da Molin 1990; Delille 1985) and North Italy, but also between the mountain villages and the populations of the plain (Viazzo and Albera 1990), the urban (Derosas 2002) and the rural contexts, and the divergent marriage patterns of day laborers and sharecroppers in the rural setting of Central Italy (Angeli and Bellettini 1979; Biagioli 1986; Doveri 1982).

More recently, the literature has stressed the narrowness of the household approach, urging a redefinition of the kin network in its broader sense (Das Gupta 1997; Kertzer, Hogan, and Karweit 1992; Levi 1990; Perrenoud 1998). In a recent study on a population sample of the city of Venice, Derosas (2002) definitely proved the great extent to which the decision to marry relied not only upon the family, but also upon the network of kin beyond the strict household boundaries. If this was true in a nuclear family system, the same mechanism was likely to be present in a rural context, where family ties were expected to be more important and more influential on individual choices. In a study recently published on the sharecropping society of the territory of Siena in Tuscany, Grilli (2005) pointed out and described the matrimonial strategy set up by many kindred families living and working on the same large farm.

Actually, in rural nineteenth-century Italy marriage was commonly used as a strategic event to establish family alliances and networks of mutual support in order to guarantee stability (both at the territorial and economic level), and to acquire a more central role in the social life of the community (Ehmer 2002; Tittarelli 1991). In this view, it would sound strange that the decision of the household head with regard to the possible marriage of a kinsman did not also take into consideration the local kin network in its totality. Furthermore, the existence of a large network of kin outside the household usually implied longer permanence in the village, and consequently a deeper knowledge of the community and its members. This fact would have made the search for the right spouse easier, at least in comparison to the most mobile sectors of the population.

3 The Community Studied: Casalguidi, 1820–1858

The parish territory of Casalguidi is included in what is today the province of Pistoia, but it was not far from Florence, only about 20 km. Throughout the period of analysis, 1819–1859, Casalguidi belonged to the Grand Duchy of Tuscany, sharing its destiny until the annexation to the Italian Kingdom in 1861.[2] People resided

---

[2]Casalguidi is one of the Italian populations studied within the international *EurAsian Project on Population and Family History* (EAP), collaborative research among teams from different countries across the world (Belgium, Italy, Japan, Sweden, and USA) whose main goal is to study demographic behaviors of past populations in a comparative perspective. For details, see Bengtsson, Campbell, Lee et al. (2004).

primarily in the main village, but a part of the population lived directly on farms scattered over the territory. The population was largely employed in agricultural labors (around 70 percent), but for the most part they were landless with different types of contracts and relative well-being (Giorgetti 1974).[3] Sharecroppers and tenants were best-off among the landless, while paid farm laborers and day laborers lived under worse economic conditions.[4] Poor artisans, shopkeepers, and a minority of bourgeois and nobles formed the nonagricultural sector of the population. Finally, some people were involved in textile proto-industrial activities such as embroidery and silk industries.

In the period studied, the population rose continuously (Figure 1.1). Once the last great mortality crisis of the nineteenth century—the typhus epidemic of 1817—was over, the number of inhabitants increased from 1,906 in 1819 to 2,697 in 1859, with a mean annual growth rate of 8.5 per thousand (Breschi, Derosas, and Manfredini 2004). The upward trend was interrupted in the period 1854–1855 by a serious cholera epidemic that hit the community (Manfredini 2003a) and a large part of Tuscany and Northern Italy. As far as households are concerned, the trend was similar. In 41 years, the number of households increased from 400 to 534, with a mean annual growth rate of 7.1 per thousand, a figure very close to that computed for the whole population.

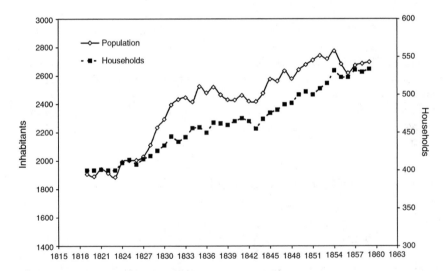

Figure 1.1 Population and households, Casalguidi, 1819–1859

---

[3] It is, however, not possible to exclude the possibility that some day laborers could own very small plots of land.

[4] We want to specify that the distinction among the various agricultural professions was not always clear in parish registers. The indication "farmer" was a generic category including sharecroppers, tenants, and other agricultural persons living on a farm. On the contrary, day laborers were clearly specified as such.

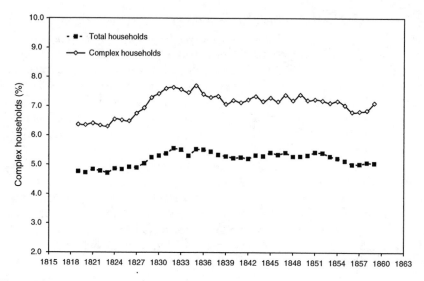

Figure 1.2   Mean household size, Casalguidi, 1819–1859

Household size did undergo a constant increase in the mean number of members, reaching a maximum in 1832 with 5.6 individuals per household on average (Figure 1.2). This level remained quite constant up to 1852–1853, when the spread of the epidemic and the consequent higher mortality both lowered the mean household size (about 5.0 individuals per household) and undermined the whole network of kin and relations. The trend for complex households was quite similar, with an average over the period of 7.1 members per household.

4   Sources Used and the Methodology Adopted

For this study, we reconstructed the life histories of the inhabitants of Casalguidi by linking two kinds of parish registers. These include the typical ecclesiastical vital registers—baptism, burial and marriage acts—along with *Status Animarum* (Register of Souls). The first books are well known and they have been the basis of almost every work in Italian historical demography, while the second type of register needs further comment. The *Status Animarum* was a sort of annual census the parish priest recorded on pastoral visits to families during Easter. For each household residing in the parish territory, the parson recorded name, surname, age, marital status, and relationship of each of the household's members to the household head. Information about the property of the household was present as well. Since the complete series of annual *Status Animarum* for the period studied is available, the nominative linkage of information between the two sources (census and vital registers) allowed us to reconstruct the life histories of individuals and families for the time they spent in Casalguidi (Manfredini 1996). By assigning a unique code number to each person and his/her parents and spouse(s), we were able to identify the individual kinship network by tracing relationships both horizontally and vertically in the genealogy line. Thanks to the information on coresidential patterns provided by *Status Animarum*, it is now possible to determine the kinship network of each person year after year, specifying the relatives living both outside and within the ego's household. According to this methodology, the reconstruction of non-coresidential kinship is inevitably limited to the local network of kin.

As for marriages, the parish registers provide information about the wedding date, name and surname of spouses and parents, marital status at the moment of marriage, current spouses' places of residence and domicile, and sometimes, age at marriage. Traditionally, couples married in the bride's parish so that parish marriage registers never contained acts of wife-exogamous unions, and Casalguidi is no exception (Manfredini 2003b). Since there is no trace of marriages between local men and foreign women, it has been necessary to turn to other sources to fill this gap. Due to the good continuity of *Stati Animarum* (only 1 year missing in the period studied), it has been possible to remedy this lack of information. This can be easily accomplished by checking all the men who changed their marital status from unmarried (or widowed) to married between two consecutive *Stati Animarum* (Manfredini 1996). This is a novelty for Italian studies on historical populations, which usually have been based solely on parish marriage registers. We stress that this selection bias in marriage registers can yield possible misinterpretations of the process of population evolution if not properly and carefully considered. In fact, we observed that wife-exogamous marriages celebrated elsewhere established their residence in Casalguidi, thereby contributing to its demographic and microevolutionary process. On the other hand, husband-exogamous unions, which were present in the marriage registers of the local church, went to live in the groom's parish after marriage and never played a role in the microevolution of the local population.

Along with parish books, another register was exploited, namely the Family Tax Register. It reported the sum each household had to pay annually according to its socioeconomic status (Breschi, Manfredini, and Pozzi 2004). For the purposes of this study, we collapsed the various classes of payment into just three groups, typifying three different levels of well-being: rich (high and medium tax), poor (low tax), and indigent (exempt from tax). A nominative linkage between parish books and the tax register enabled us to include and take into account this last piece of information in the reconstruction of individual and household life histories.

The reconstructed longitudinal data allowed the adoption of statistical tools normally used in contemporary population studies, such as event history analysis—one of the best and most powerful statistical tools in dealing with this kind of data (Trussell and Guinnane 1993). In this case, a discrete-time approach was used due to annual repeated observations.

5   Getting Married in Casalguidi

In the period 1820–1858, 1,028 marriages involving people of Casalguidi took place. The marriages were mainly celebrated in the local parish church, but 235 of them were held in churches outside the parish territory. This latter subset was made up exclusively of wife-exogamous unions—couples formed by a man from Casalguidi and a woman resident in the village where the ceremony was celebrated. As previously noted, this selection is the result of the custom of virilocality associated with the practice of performing the wedding ceremony in the bride's parish. This tradition was so common that the largest part of endogamous and wife-exogamous unions established their residence in Casalguidi, with proportions ranging from 87.1 percent for the former and 96.6 percent for the latter. Conversely, husband-exogamous unions were much less likely to remain in Casalguidi (24.8 percent); evidence of a differential gender pattern yielding out-migration of local married women from Casalguidi, a constant stream of just-married brides leaving their native families.

Accordingly, the computation of geographical endogamy provides different figures if based on the whole set of unions or on the sole fraction of resident marriages. In the former case; the endogamy rate is 49.6 percent, a level clearly identifying a nonisolated population, while in the second case it drops to 37.6 percent (Table 1.1)—further evidence of the propensity of local women involved in exogamous marriages to migrate. From an evolutionary point of view, it emerges that resident couples had more conservative marriage behaviors, and that the local biodemographic evolution was more dependent on endogamous marriages than what could be expected.

The utmost degree of endogamy is represented by consanguinity. The relationship between this peculiar practice and the kin network is much stronger as the mate choice is performed not simply within one's own community, but within one's own circle of relatives, with obvious genetic effects on future generations such as the reduction of genetic variability and higher risks of generating genetically ill children. The significant increase of consanguineous marriages that occurred in Italy in the second half of the nineteenth century was believed to have strong connections with variations in kinship size. In fact, many authors interpreted the rise of that practice—pursued in order to avoid land dispersal and excessive fractioning of the farm—as a response to the rapid population growth of that period (Cavalli-Sforza and Bodmer 1971; Pettener 1985). In Casalguidi, however, population growth was not associated with any increase in the practice of consanguinity,

Table 1.1 Endogamy and exogamy rates, total and resident marriages, Casalguidi, 1820–1858

	Endogamous	Exogamous	N
Total	50.3	49.7	1,028
Resident marriages	62.4	37.6	723

not even in the period where it caused a strong increase in the household size. Estimates of total consanguinity from isonymy, that is, spouses carrying the same surname, result in both a low overall inbreeding coefficient (Ft = 0.005420) and lack of noteworthy variation over time ($Ft_{1820-1844}$ = 0.005439, $Ft_{1845-1858}$ = 0.005392). These findings still address the issue of the open nature of the community of Casalguidi, and make clear how the presence of almost only landless peasants made the practice of consanguineous marriages definitely useless, regardless of the structure and size of the household. This is in line with other studies claiming a limited level of consanguineous marriages in the sharecropping societies of North and Central Italy (Arioti 1988; Grilli 2005; Solinas 1997).

If such a practice was not strategic in the economic context of the rural society of Casalguidi, what instead produced striking differences in the marriage pattern was the form of land tenure, or, in other words, the type of agricultural contract. Such contracts determined the tie with the land, the permanence and stability in the territory and the form of coresidence. The marriage pattern was only a further element of peasant life whose characteristics were shaped accordingly, and one of its most important aspects was the link between age at first marriage and household size. As displayed in Figure 1.3, the larger the household, the higher the age at first marriage of males, which increased by circa 1.5 years on average from small to very large households. On the contrary, no significant variations in the access to marriage emerged on the female side.

A dichotomy between sharecroppers and day laborers emerges, illustrating contrasts that highlight the complex interrelationship between many facets of the kin network and the marriage pattern. Very schematically, sharecroppers lived in large

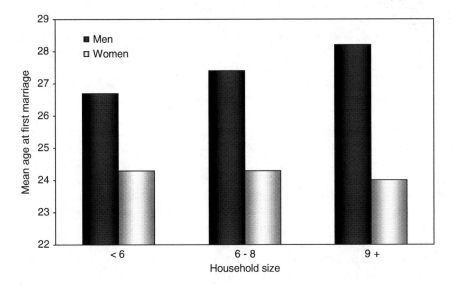

Figure 1.3 Mean age at first marriage by household size, Casalguidi, 1819–1859

Table 1.2 Some features of the socioeconomic groups of Casalguidi, 1820–1858

Head's occupation	Age at first marriage		Celibacy[a]		People in complex households (%)	Kindred households[b] (%)	Household turnover rate[c]
	Males	Females	Males	Females			
Sharecroppers and farmers	28.5	24.6	17.8	10.1	54.4	55.9	44.3
Day laborers	27.3	24.9	8.3	6.1	40.8	47.5	88.6
Artisans and shopkeepers	27.1	25.4	12.1	5.5	39.4	55.6	54.6
Middle-class and nobles	30.9	26.7	7.9	20.0	53.4	46.5	29.0
Total	28.2	24.6	14.5	10.0	49.0	53.4	67.6
N	807	853	4,971[d]	4,794[d]	92,432[d]	18,553[d]	18,553[d]

[a]Percentage values of never-married people 45–54 years.
[b]Proportion of households with at least one kin of whatever degree living in another household of Casalguidi.
[c](In-migrant + out-migrant households)/total resident households.
[d]Total figures (N) are expressed in either household- or person-years.

and complex households (5.9 persons per household, 55.4 percent of individuals living in complex households), and followed a patrilocal pattern of living arrangement after marriage; and both men and women married at relatively old age (Table 1.2). Conversely, day laborers lived in simple family groups (4.6 persons per household, 40.8 percent of individuals living in complex households), and established a new independent family after marriage; and men married at a younger age than sharecroppers did (Barbagli 1990; Kertzer and Hogan 1991).

Sharecroppers were landless people who lived on the farm and had to give half of the crop to the landowner. Usually, the whole household was employed as a single working unit, whose size was often contractually determined according to the specific necessities of the farm work. Under these conditions, the relative well-being of the household was closely associated to the delicate equilibrium between household size and the resources that the members could produce, i.e., its labor capacity (Doveri 2000; Poni 1982; Viazzo 2003).

Thus, household demography had to be carefully controlled in order to avoid losing the farm: a significant variation in the household size could compromise either its working capacity or welfare, leading the landowner to evict the sharecroppers or move them to another farm of different size. In this view, marriage and individual mobility, with their present and future implications on household size, were two demographic mechanisms the household head and, to a higher degree, the landowner himself personally controlled.

These behaviors had to act as preventive checks aimed at guaranteeing the permanence of the household on the farm and avoiding downward social mobility. Unlike rural societies characterized by the diffuse presence of smallholders, whose efforts were directed to preserving the possession of the land and avoiding its dispersal, sharecropping societies were much more interested in safeguarding a sort of immaterial good such as the household labor capacity. Each element of the marriage pattern was therefore intended to meet this fundamental need, putting the household perspective before the individual will. While patrilocality was the key to maximize the male labor force within the household, delay in the access to marriage and permanent celibacy of males could represent common strategies to avoid unbalance between consumers and producers (Cocchi et al. 1996; Della Pina 1990; Rettaroli 1993). The figures in Table 1.2 confirm this theoretical scheme: sharecroppers present the highest age at first marriage (28.5 years) and the highest celibacy rate (17.8 percent) among farm workers.

In Casalguidi, these sociodemographic behaviors did combine to lead to the formation of multiple households constituted by two conjugal units (about 86 percent of multiple family groups). Households including three couples accounted for about 13 percent, whilst only a very few included four units. The majority of households composed by two couples were actually stem families (78 percent), with one parental nucleus along with another one involving a married son. This family system can be seen as the result of many factors, such as the small size of farms, the use of backward techniques of cultivation unable to guarantee enough resources to sustain larger households, the rigidity of many contracts that specified a fixed and invariant household size according to a given landholding size, and many others. Notwithstanding its resemblance, this pattern has little to do with Le Play's stem family system, which described peasant societies concerned with avoiding fractioning of their own land, not households of landless farmers contractually tied as single working units to landowners. At the same time, it is evident how a complex-household system in this case was associated with late marriage and high celibacy rates rather than early and quasi-universal marriage, as assumed by Laslett's Mediterranean pattern.

At the other extreme, day laborers lived in poorer economic conditions than sharecroppers. They had no stable tie to the land, were employed in temporary jobs in farms scattered over the territory, but lived in poor houses in the center of the village. The instability of such employments made the category of day laborers very mobile, as proved by the figure of the household turnover rate displayed in Table 1.2 (88.6 per thousand), which was twice that of sharecroppers and tenants (Manfredini 2003c).[5] The short permanence of day laborers in a community made them unable to create a network of kindred households in loco: only 47.5 percent of the households had at least one kinsman of whatever degree living in another family group of Casalguidi (Manfredini 2005). There was neither social authority imposing its rules of family formation, nor social or economic reasons for day laborers to live in large and complex households. Indeed, this light structure could make it easier and less burdensome to move. A weaker tie to the land and a different socioeconomic niche in the agricultural economy of Central Italy made the family

---

[5]The household turnover rate is calculated as the ratio between out-migrant plus in-migrant households and the total number of resident households. We decided to adopt this indicator since it provides a realistic picture of the propensity to move of the different socioeconomic groups.

formation system and the nuptiality pattern of day laborers antithetic to that of sharecroppers (Rettaroli 1990).

In conclusion, this community offers the opportunity to analyze the relationship between marriage and kin structure of day laborers and sharecroppers that, according to Reher's definition (1998), it is possible to characterize as weak and strong family systems respectively. The objective is to understand what role these striking contrasts in living arrangements, mobility, and kin networks might have had on the chances of the single household members to marry.

6   Kin Network and the Marriage: An Individual Approach

When discussing the multifaceted relationship between kinship, household structure, and SES (i.e., socioeconomic status) and marriage pattern, it is best to investigate such connections in a dynamic perspective. Descriptive analyses provide only partial snapshots of dynamic processes, such as the household life cycle, and are not useful in arranging and interpreting events in the context of individual and family life histories. Furthermore, the complexities of the explicative framework make descriptive statistics unfit to take exhaustive account of the multidisciplinary nature of such issues. The statistical technique of event history analysis has, for all these reasons, been adopted to deal with longitudinal data such as those employed in this research. Because of the discrete-time nature of the data available, a logistic regression has been used.

Three risk models have been estimated. The first one is a general model, while the other two concern sharecroppers and tenants on the one hand and day laborers on the other. Each model has been run for males and females separately. In order to appreciate properly the connections between marriage, kinship, and the family formation system, the population at risk is defined as never-married people between 18 and 44 years who did not live alone at the moment of marriage.

The covariates used to check the role of the kinship network on the risk of marriage, concern the kin structure both beyond and within the household where the ego lived. The focus is primarily on the presence (and influence) of both ever-married and unmarried siblings, analyzed also in terms of hierarchy by birth order. The underlying hypothesis is that the more complex the household, the lower the risk of marriage. This could obviously be the case with sharecroppers and tenants, whose household size and structure had to be calibrated on the landholding size, and whose living arrangement after marriage required that married men remained within the native households. For differences in the typology of living arrangement after marriage, the household composition effect is then expected to be less pronounced for women than for men, and less for day laborers than for sharecroppers. Nonetheless, this is not a foregone outcome. Alter and colleagues (2000) found a generalized significant impact of the presence of siblings on the likelihood to marry in a society—the Land of Herve, in Belgium—characterized by a large prevalence of simple families.

Another important coresidential factor is the presence of parents. This covariate aims at capturing possible effects associated with the necessity to substitute for a dead or absent parent. The purpose is therefore to test to what extent siblings could be encouraged to get married in order to bring into the family a person who would be able to take over the duties previously carried out by the absent parent.

A covariate accounting for the number of kindred households outside the household of the ego has been included in the models as well. Despite the limitations of this indicator, in our opinion, this kind of variable provides a more precise picture of the real extension of connections and relations within the parish territory than the simple number of relatives would do.[6] The rationale is that a larger local kin network might be helpful in finding local spouses, also with the purpose of widening and reinforcing the local network of family alliances.

Other factors have been included as control variables. Profession and tax class are used to describe the socioeconomic status at the household level. In this way, it is possible to control not only for the head's occupation but also for the relative well-being of the household in terms of family tax.

The grain price is intended to capture variations in the general macroeconomic picture. Its inclusion stems from the necessity to take into account the economic nature of marriage, given the burden that this event could put upon families and individuals. While men inherited land and properties or were obliged to guarantee or find agricultural contracts, women were provided with a dowry on marriage as a substitute for inheritance. The payment of a dowry to the groom's family was a common custom among Italian populations, a practice that in hard times could be difficult to sustain and guarantee. The mean annual grain price aims simply at capturing years of meagre harvest, when prices went up and farmers might have faced economic hardship. The price has been considered at both year t and $t - 1$ on account of the seasonality of marriages, characterized by marked peaks in February and November.

The last two variables concern the migratory experience of individuals and an indicator of the local marriage market. The former singles out the most mobile part of the population of Casalguidi, trying to understand whether recent in-migration (<3 years) might yield some effect on the risk of marriage. People recently moved into Casalguidi, without relations and with difficulties in finding a partner, might be isolated.

The marriage market index has been constructed as the ratio between unmarried men aged 25–35 years and unmarried women 22–28 years old.[7] The obvious hypothesis is that the higher the ratio, the lower the number of eligible spouses with respect to unmarried men, with a consequent decrease of the risk of marriage.

Looking at Table 1.3, there is no doubt about the differential role played by kinship and household composition on the risk of marriage among males and females.

---

[6] Each household where at least one ego's relative lived was regarded as related. Both close and distant relatives were likewise taken into account, and in particular parents, spouses, children, siblings, grandparents, grandchildren, cousins of whatever order, aunts, uncles, nephews and nieces. No differential weight was assigned to the various kin. However, our possibility to identify distant relatives outside the household depends on the length of his or her permanence in Casalguidi. The longer the time spent in Casalguidi, the wider the quantity of documentation and religious acts at our disposal to link the ego to his or her relatives.

[7] The age brackets chosen to construct this indicator are defined as the central 50 percent of the distributions of the observed ages at marriage for each gender.

Table 1.3 Odds of first marriage, 18–44 years. Total marriages, Casalguidi, 1820–1858[a]

Covariates	Males			Females		
	Mean	Odds	p-values	Mean	Odds	p-values
Age (ref. 18–34 years)	88.0	1.000		91.2	1.000	
35–44 years	12.0	0.638	0.013	8.8	0.415	0.000
Older brothers ever-married (ref. Absent)	81.0	1.000		83.3	1.000	
Present	19.0	0.722	0.026	16.7	1.254	0.056
Older brothers unmarried (ref. Absent)	71.6	1.000		72.6	1.000	
Present	28.4	0.542	0.000	27.4	0.880	0.219
Younger brothers ever-married (ref. Absent)	96.4	1.000		97.4	1.000	
Present	3.6	0.470	0.036	2.6	1.257	0.425
Younger brothers unmarried (ref. Absent)	52.1	1.000		54.7	1.000	
Present	47.9	0.758	0.018	45.3	1.033	0.749
Older sisters ever-married (ref. Absent)	99.7	1.000		98.6	1.000	
Present	0.3	0.721	0.653	1.4	1.168	0.655
Older sisters unmarried (ref. Absent)	81.4	1.000		82.1	1.000	
Present	18.6	0.517	0.000	17.9	0.605	0.000
Younger sisters ever-married (ref. Absent)	99.8	1.000		99.7	1.000	
Present	0.2	0.964	0.973	0.3	0.551	0.560
Younger sisters unmarried (ref. Absent)	54.6	1.000		57.9	1.000	
Present	45.4	0.947	0.653	42.1	1.175	0.103
Parents (ref. Both present)	44.6	1.000	0.011	46.2	1.000	0.604
Only father	12.4	1.662	0.000	11.5	1.076	0.601
Only mother	17.1	1.323	0.058	18.3	1.083	0.529
No parents	25.9	0.915	0.614	24.0	0.982	0.902
Number of kindred households	1.4	1.019	0.454	1.2	1.013	0.591
Head's occupation (ref. Day laborers)	17.7	1.000	0.055	20.9	1.000	0.079
Sharecroppers and farmers	65.7	0.855	0.222	57.7	1.090	0.461
Artisans and other non-agricultural activities	12.8	1.107	0.544	15.1	1.077	0.612
Bourgeois and nobles	2.3	0.434	0.078	4.0	0.741	0.320
Unknown	1.5	0.560	0.233	2.3	0.393	0.047
Tax class (ref. Untaxed)	23.3	1.000	0.016	30.7	1.000	0.648
High and medium tax class	27.3	1.036	0.821	20.4	0.851	0.270
Low tax class	49.4	1.366	0.018	48.9	1.009	0.930
Migrant in the previous 3 years (ref. No)	75.4	1.000	0.450	76.4	1.000	0.277
Migrant	19.3	1.142	0.294	17.9	1.020	0.873
Unknown	5.3	1.199	0.408	5.7	1.286	0.200
Marriage market at year t – 1[b]	1.1	0.751	0.055	1.1	0.982	0.900
Logged price of wheat at year t	3.1	0.558	0.132	3.1	1.035	0.922
Logged price of wheat at year t – 1	3.1	0.973	0.942	3.1	0.643	0.202
–2 Log likelihood		3658.55			4091.3	
Person-years		9,022			7,098	

[a]Values associated to reference categories are *p*-values of joint significance.
[b]Unmarried men 25–34 years/unmarried women 22–28 years.

In particular, the differential role was stronger and more remarkable among the males, while it was weaker and less noticeable among the females. For men, we found a significant depressive effect associated with the presence of coresident brothers of whatever age and marital status. In particular, the most striking variations in the odds of marriage are associated with the presence of older unmarried brothers (−46 percent) and younger ever-married brothers (−53 percent).

Considering that sharecroppers and tenants represent around 65 percent of male total person-years, and that the results in Table 1.3 closely mirror those of Table 1.4, relative to sharecroppers and tenants only, it was no surprise to find household

Table 1.4 Odds of first marriage, 18–44 years. Sharecroppers and tenants, Casalguidi, 1820–1858[a]

| Covariates | Males | | | Females | | |
	Mean	Odds	p-values	Mean	Odds	p-values
Age (ref. 18–34 years)	87.0	1.000		92.0	1.000	
35–44 years	13.0	0.541	0.008	8.0	0.498	0.018
Older brothers ever-married (ref. Absent)	78.9	1.000		80.7	1.000	
Present	21.1	0.678	0.031	19.3	1.282	0.080
Older brothers unmarried (ref. Absent)	68.3	1.000		66.5	1.000	
Present	31.7	0.538	0.000	33.5	0.843	0.173
Younger brothers ever-married (ref. Absent)	96.0	1.000		96.8	1.000	
Present	4.0	0.392	0.041	3.2	0.938	0.868
Younger brothers unmarried (ref. Absent)	49.8	1.000		47.6	1.000	
Present	50.2	0.734	0.035	52.4	1.099	0.475
Older sisters ever-married (ref. Absent)	99.8	1.000		98.4	1.000	
Present	0.2	0.995	0.996	1.6	1.011	0.980
Older sisters unmarried (ref. Absent)	80.5	1.000		80.7	1.000	
Present	19.5	0.413	0.000	19.3	0.541	0.000
Younger sisters ever-married (ref. Absent)	99.9	–		99.8	–	
Present	0.1	–	–	0.2	–	–
Younger sisters unmarried (ref. Absent)	52.3	1.000		54.0	1.000	
Present	47.7	0.944	0.715	46.0	1.064	0.620
Parents (ref. Both present)	46.4	1.000	0.031	52.2	1.000	0.489
Only father	13.7	1.731	0.002	12.6	0.977	0.899
Only mother	14.6	1.530	0.025	15.8	1.155	0.366
No parents	25.3	0.918	0.711	19.4	1.065	0.742
Number of kindred households	1.5	0.996	0.889	1.5	1.053	0.071
Tax class (ref. Untaxed)	21.4	1.000	0.236	27.6	1.000	0.845
High and medium tax class	24.4	0.789	0.248	16.8	0.953	0.793
Low tax class	54.2	1.041	0.804	55.6	1.047	0.733
Migrant in the previous 3 years (ref. No)	82.4	1.000	0.820	84.5	1.000	0.707
Migrant	14.2	0.916	0.634	11.8	1.140	0.451
Unknown	3.4	1.186	0.596	3.7	1.059	0.858
Marriage market at year t − 1[b]	1.2	0.907	0.681	1.2	1.220	0.376
Logged price of wheat at year t	3.1	0.872	0.785	3.1	1.343	0.525
Logged price of wheat at year t − 1	3.1	1.274	0.604	3.1	0.781	0.577
−2 Log likelihood		2239.0			2446.7	
Person-years		5,927			4,089	

[a]Values associated to reference categories are p-values of joint significance.
[b]Unmarried men 25–34 years/unmarried women 22–28 years.

composition variables to be so responsive in a context of strong predominance of patrilocal pattern of living arrangement after marriage. In the model concerning sharecroppers and tenants, the effects associated with the presence of brothers are even stronger. Living with an older unmarried brother reduced the likelihood of marriage by 47 percent, while living with a younger ever-married brother induced a 61 percent reduction of the odds. If the former variable points out the importance of hierarchy by birth order, the second provides further evidence of the very limited number of couples the sharecropping households living in Casalguidi could sustain. If hierarchy by age was not respected and a younger son got married, the chances for the older one of finding a spouse were strongly reduced. Behind this family strategy, there was a strong competition among brothers due to the necessity to preserve the delicate equilibrium between producers and consumers; a condition which the acquisition of a new household member by marriage (along with possible prospective children) might alter.

This interpretation finds further support in the models relative to day laborers. Since they usually left the native family on marriage, the presence of coresident brothers had less effective and influential results on the risk of marriage. Thus, younger ever-married brothers did not negatively affect the marriage chances of the other siblings. The only determinant factor governing access to marriage was birth order, as evidenced by a 52 percent reduction of the odds with the presence of older unmarried brothers in the household (Table 1.5).

Table 1.5 Odds of first marriage, 18–44 years. Day laborers, Casalguidi, 1820–1858[a]

Covariates	Males			Females		
	Mean	Odds	p-values	Mean	Odds	p-values
Age (ref. 18–34 years)	87.9	1.000		91.0	1.000	
35–44 years	12.1	0.861	0.700	9.0	0.182	0.023
Older brothers ever-married (ref. Absent)	84.3	1.000		85.7	1.000	
Present	15.7	0.779	0.505	14.3	1.328	0.319
Older brothers unmarried (ref. Absent)	77.0	1.000		80.1	1.000	
Present	23.0	0.498	0.036	19.9	0.979	0.935
Younger brothers ever-married (ref. Absent)	96.8	1.000		97.9	1.000	
Present	3.2	0.923	0.914	2.1	1.746	0.401
Younger brothers unmarried (ref. Absent)	56.8	1.000		61.5	1.000	
Present	43.2	0.964	0.901	38.5	0.989	0.960
Older sisters ever-married (ref. Absent)	99.7	1.000		99.1	1.000	
Present	0.3	1.690	0.642	0.9	3.508	0.075
Older sisters unmarried (ref. Absent)	83.9	1.000		82.8	1.000	
Present	16.1	0.577	0.133	17.2	0.822	0.462
Younger sisters ever-married (ref. Absent)	99.8	1.000		99.8	–	
Present	0.2	2.759	0.364	0.2	–	–
Younger sisters unmarried (ref. Absent)	59.5	1.000		61.4	1.000	
Present	40.5	1.032	0.914	38.6	1.321	0.234
Parents (ref. Both present)	45.7	1.000	0.094	49.4	1.000	0.453
Only father	11.1	1.564	0.186	13.3	0.900	0.722
Only mother	14.1	1.790	0.088	12.0	0.800	0.558

(continued)

Table 1.5 (continued)

Covariates	Males			Females		
	Mean	Odds	p-values	Mean	Odds	p-values
No parents	29.1	1.127	0.761	25.3	0.814	0.562
Number of kindred households	0.9	0.975	0.752	0.9	0.961	0.486
Tax class (ref. Untaxed)	36.0	1.000	0.041	38.2	1.000	0.489
High and medium tax class	15.3	0.830	0.588	14.8	1.012	0.973
Low tax class	48.7	1.653	0.095	47.0	1.294	0.364
Migrant in the previous 3 years (ref. No)	51.3	1.000	0.369	60.7	1.000	0.137
Migrant	36.1	1.216	0.400	29.5	0.839	0.456
Unknown	12.7	0.798	0.570	9.8	0.943	0.876
Marriage market at year t − 1[b]	1.1	0.719	0.162	1.1	0.852	0.564
Logged price of wheat at year t	3.0	0.184	0.045	3.1	0.591	0.493
Logged price of wheat at year t − 1	3.0	0.890	0.890	3.1	0.602	0.511
−2 Log likelihood		734.7			816.1	
Person-years		1,598			1,478	

[a]Values associated to reference categories are p-values of joint significance.
[b]Unmarried men 25–34 years/unmarried women 22–28 years.

Going back to the general model, the picture is complicated by the presence of other household members. In the presence of older unmarried sisters, the odds of marriage shows a marked reduction for both men (−48 percent) and women (−40 percent). In the latter case, the depressive effect reflects a strict hierarchy by birth order in the access to marriage, with the younger sisters awaiting their turn to marry and leave home. Still, the presence of an older unmarried sister could make the arrival of another woman into the household unnecessary and undue, thereby blocking the chances of marriage for her younger brothers, especially if they practiced a patrilocal living arrangement after marriage. Once again, it is among sharecroppers that this effect is much stronger, but even among day laborers there is evidence of a reduction of the risk of marriage, although not at a statistically significant level.

As far as the absence of one of the parents is concerned, we found clear-cut differences between males and females, on the one hand, and sharecroppers and day laborers, on the other hand. Unmarried men stand out as the only household members whose risk of marriage is positively affected by the absence of either father or mother. This finding supports the hypothesis of households as single working-units, where the subdivision of roles and duties among the members was carefully and clearly defined. Once a member disappeared, there was the necessity to fill his or her social and economic niche within the household. Since this argumentation entails a patrilocal residence after marriage, it was not unexpected to find sharecroppers more responsive than day laborers. Among the former, the odds of marriage increases significantly, by 73 percent and 53 percent, in case of a mother's or father's absence respectively (Table 1.4). Relative to day laborers, the model shows no significant effect for the absence of the mother. A 79 percent odds increase was observed in the case where the mother was solely present, at a 10 percent level of statistical significance.

The question of presence or absence of other coresident kin was less relevant to the risk of marriage of unmarried women, perhaps due to their almost universal departure from the household on marriage. What remains is a gender-oriented hierarchy regulating access to marriage by age and social status, evidenced by the almost generalized decrease of risk of marriage when older unmarried sisters are present in the house. Once again, it is among sharecroppers that the risk of marriage was more responsive to household compositional factors. In addition, daughters of sharecroppers were also sensitive to the kinship network size beyond the household. In a context where this factor did not affect the odds of marriage for sharecropping men and day laborers, the likelihood of marriage increased for women by 5 percent for each unitary increase in the number of related households living in the territory of Casalguidi. If we consider that this result concerned only endogamous unions and not exogamous ones (models here not shown), these marriages can be seen as strategic in reinforcing local family alliances. Not only could a large kinship network beyond the household increase local connections, relations and friendships, but it could also encourage endogamous marriage in order to reinforce and make more solid the position of the family in the local community.

As for the control variables of socioeconomic nature, people belonging to the upper class stand out as the least likely to marry, especially the men. This outcome substantiates their higher age at first marriage (Table 1.2) and could be related to the narrowness of their social marriage market, which could cause a delay in finding the right bride.

A last important remark about economic factors concerns the depressive impact of periods of high prices on the chances of marriage of day laborers. Landless and without the ability to live on farm produce, people of this social group had to buy food on the local market and were therefore much more sensitive than other groups to rises in prices. These difficulties could, in turn, affect their decision to marry, perhaps postponing weddings to more propitious times.

7 Conclusion

In this chapter, we investigated the role of kinship in marriage patterns existent in a peasant community of mid nineteenth century Italy. Going beyond the often simplistic categorizations of family formation systems, we probed the deepest mechanisms of the family life cycle to gain an insight into two almost antithetic marriage patterns—those of sharecroppers and day laborers respectively.

We clarified the homeostatic nature of the demographic regime of this rural society, where the diverse family formation systems played different roles according to the head's profession. They were functional not only to the niche the household occupied within the rural economic system, but also to the different roles people had within the household. Accordingly, the marriage pattern of sharecroppers differed from that of day laborers, and norms governing access to marriage varied between males and females of the same social category.

The stem family system of sharecroppers was the result of strategic behaviors that addressed two basic economic requirements: a maximization of the number of men within the household; and differentiation of well-defined roles among the household members. Thus, patrilocality guaranteed the permanence of men within the household but, at the same time, strongly favored competition among coresident brothers for marriage. According to the number of married sons a farm could sustain (usually only one in our case study), this competition could lead to either late marriage or permanent celibacy of the unmarried brothers. On the other hand, marriage could be strategically used to introduce a new member into the household in order to take over the role and duties of an important missing member, i.e., the father or mother.

Conversely, for those people whose presence within the household was not necessary or even disadvantageous, a neolocal family formation system contributed to relax the constraints imposed by the coresidential pattern. According to this scheme, women belonging to sharecropping households showed behaviors that were paradoxically much more similar to day laborers than to sharecropping males. In this latter scheme, hierarchy by birth order could represent the only factor determining timing of and access to marriage.

As for kinship outside the household, it was only effective in modifying the risk of marriage for women living in sharecropping households. Thus, large and deep-rooted networks of relations favored a woman's access to marriage, especially when a local man was involved, suggesting that marriage is sometimes used to establish and reinforce local family alliances.

Our work is limited by the genealogical depth enabled by a 40-year-period. In future work, efforts will be required to increase the genealogical depth, allowing a more precise reconstruction of genealogical trees and of the local kin network. Such an extended genealogy will permit us to check the consistency of the conclusions that have emerged here about the role of kinship, especially the fraction outside the household, in the decision to marry.

References

Alter, G., M. Neven, and M. Oris. 2000. Individuals, households and communities facing economic stresses: A comparison of two rural areas in 19th century Belgium, in M. Neven and C. Capron (eds.), *Family structures, demography and population: A comparison of societies in Asia and Europe*, Laboratoire de Démographie, Université de Liège, Liège, pp. 185–210.

Angeli, A. and A. Bellettini. 1979. Strutture familiari nella campagna bolognese a metà dell'Ottocento. *Genus* 35: 155–72.

Arioti, M. 1988. *Non desiderare la donna d'altri. Gruppi sociali parentela e matrimonio nella comunità mezzadrile di Prodo*. Angeli, Milan.

Barbagli, M. 1984. *Sotto lo stesso tetto. Mutamenti della famiglia in Italia dal XV al XX secolo*. Il Mulino, Bologna.

Barbagli, M. 1990. Sistemi di formazione della famiglia in Italia, in Società Italiana di Demografia Storica, *Popolazione, società e ambiente. Temi di demografia storica italiana (secc. XVII-XIX)*, Clueb, Bologna, pp. 3–43.

Bengtsson, T., C. Campbell, J.Z. Lee et al. (eds.). 2004. *Life Under Pressure: Mortality and Living Standards in Europe and Asia, 1700–1900*. MIT, Cambridge, MA.

Berkner, L.K. and F. Mendels. 1978. Inheritance systems, family structure, and demographic patterns in Western Europe, 1700–1900, in C. Tilly (ed.), *Historical studies of changing fertility*, Princeton University Press, Princeton, pp. 209–23.

Biagioli, G. 1986. La diffusione della mezzadria nell'Italia centrale: Un modello di sviluppo demografico ed economico. *Bollettino di Demografia Storica* 3: 59–66.

Breschi, M., R. Derosas, and M. Manfredini. 2004. Mortality and environment in three Emilian, Tuscan, and Venetian communities, 1800–1883, in T. Bengtsson, C. Campbell, J.Z. Lee (eds.), *Life under pressure: Mortality and living standards in Europe and Asia, 1700–1900*, MIT, Cambridge, pp. 209–52.

Breschi, M., M. Manfredini, and L. Pozzi. 2004. Mortality in the first years of life: Socio-economic determinants in an Italian nineteenth-century population, in M. Breschi and L. Pozzi (eds.), *The determinants of infant and childhood mortality in Europe during the last two centuries*, Forum, Udine, pp. 123–38.

Bourdieu, P. 1962. Celibat et condition paysanne. *Études Rurales* 5/6: 32–136.

Campbell, C. and J. Lee. 2003. Social mobility from a kinship perspective: Rural Liaoning, 1789–1909. *International Review of Social History* 48: 1–26.

Castro De Guerra, D., H. Arvelo, and J. Pinto-Cisternas. 1999. Population structure of two black Venezuelan populations studied through their mating structure and other related variables. *Annals of Human Biology* 26: 141–50.

Cavalli-Sforza, L.L. and W. Bodmer. 1971. *Human Population Genetics*. Freeman, San Francisco.

Cocchi, D., D. Crivellaro, G. Dalla Zuanna, and R. Rettaroli. 1996. Nuzialità, famiglia e sistema agricolo in Italia, negli anni '80 del XIX secolo. *Genus* 52(1/2): 125–59.

Corsini, C.A. 2000. Introduction, in M. Neven and C. Capron (eds.), *Family structures, demography and population: A comparison of societies in Asia and Europe*, Laboratoire de Démographie, Université de Liège, Liège, pp. 1–11.

Crow, J.F. and A.P. Mange. 1965. Measurement of inbreeding from the frequency of marriages between persons of the same surname. *Eugenics Quarterly* 12: 199–203.

Da Molin, G. 1990. Family forms and domestic service in Southern Italy from the seventeenth to the nineteenth centuries. *Journal of Family History* 15: 503–27.

Das Gupta, M. 1997. Kinship systems and demographic regimes, in D. Kertzer and T. Fricke (eds.), *Anthropological demography: Towards a new synthesis*, Chicago University Press, Chicago, pp. 36–52.

Delille, G. 1985. *Famille et proprieté dans le royaume de Naples (XVᵉ–XIXᵉ siècle)*. EHESS, Rome-Paris.

Della Pina, M. 1990. Famiglia mezzadrile e celibato: le campagne di Prato nei secoli XVII e XVIII, in Società Italiana di Demografia Storica, *Popolazione, società e ambiente. Temi di demografia storica (secc. XVII–XIX)*, Clueb, Bologna, pp. 125–40.

Derosas, R. 2002. Si sposi chi può, resti chi deve: Matrimonio e relazioni familiari nella Venezia di metà Ottocento. *Popolazione e Storia* 1: 35–68.

Doveri, A. 1982. Famiglia coniugale e famiglia multinucleare: Le basi dell'esperienza domestica in due parrocchie delle colline pisane lungo il secolo XVIII. *Genus* XXXVIII(1/2): 59–95.

Doveri, A. 1990. Sposi e famiglie nelle campagne pisane di fine '800. Un caso di matrimonio mediterraneo? in Società Italiana di Demografia Storica, *Popolazione, società e ambiente. Temi di demografia storica italiana (secc. XVII-XIX)*, Clueb, Bologna, pp. 141–60.

Doveri, A. 2000. Land, fertility and family: A selected review of the literature in historical demography. *Genus* LVI(3/4): 19–59.

Dribe, M. and C. Lundh. 2005. Finding the right partner: Rural homogamy in nineteenth-century Sweden. *International Review of Social History* 50: 149–77.

Ehmer, J. 2002. Marriage, in D.I. Kertzer and M. Barbagli (eds.), *Family life in the long nineteenth century*, Yale University Press, New Haven/London, pp. 282–321.

Giorgetti, G. 1974. *Contadini e proprietari nell'Italia moderna: Rapporti di produzione e contratti agrari dal secolo XVI ad oggi*. Einaudi, Turin.

Grilli, S. 2005. Reti d'alleanza. Lo spazio matrimoniale di una fattoria senese, in M. Breschi and A. Fornasin (eds.), *Il matrimonio in situazione estreme: Isole e isolati demografici*, Forum, Udine, pp. 63–92.

Hajnal, J. 1965. European marriage patterns in historical perspective, in D. Glass and D.E.C. Eversley (eds.), *Population in history*, Aldine, Chicago, pp. 101–43.

Herlihy, D. and C. Klapisch-Zuber. 1985. *The Tuscans and Their Families: A Study of the Florentine Catasto of 1427*. Yale University Press, New Haven.

Kertzer, D.I. 1991. Household history and sociological theory. *Annual Review of Sociology* 17: 155–79.

Kertzer, D.I. 2002. Living with kin, in D.I. Kertzer and M. Barbagli (eds.), *Family life in the long nineteenth century*, Yale University Press, New Haven/London, pp. 40–72.

Kertzer, D.I. and C. Brettell. 1987. Advances in Italian and Iberian family history. *Journal of Family History* 12(1/3): 87–121.

Kertzer, D.I. and D.P. Hogan. 1991. Reflections on the European marriage pattern: Sharecropping and proletarianization in Casalecchio, Italy, 1861–1921. *Journal of Family History* 16(1): 31–45.

Kertzer, D.I. and R.P. Saller. 1991. *The Family in Italy from Antiquity to the Present*. Yale University Press, New Haven/London.

Kertzer, D.I., D.P. Hogan, and N. Karweit. 1992. Kinship beyond the household in a nineteenth-century Italian town. *Continuity and Change* 7(1): 103–21.

Lasker, G.W., C.G.N. Mascie-Taylor, and D.A. Coleman. 1986. Repeating pairs of surnames in marriages in Reading (England) and their significance for population structure. *Human Biology* 58: 421–5.

Laslett, P. 1977. *Family Life and Illicit Love in Earlier Generations. Essays in Historical Sociology*. Cambridge University Press, Cambridge.

Laslett, P. 1983. Family and household as work group and kin group: Areas of traditional Europe compared, in R. Wall et al. (eds.), *Family forms in historic Europe*, Cambridge University Press, Cambridge, pp. 513–63.

Le Play, F. 1871. *L'organisation de la famille selon le vrai modèle signalé par l'histoire de toutes les races et de tous les temps*. Alfred Mame et fils, Tours.

Levi, G. 1990. Family and kin—A few thoughts. *Journal of Family History* 15(4): 567–78.

Madrigal, L. and B. Ware. 1999. Mating pattern and population structure in Escazù, Costa Rica: A study using marriage records. *Human Biology* 71: 963–75.

Manfredini, M. 1996. L'utilizzo degli Status Animarum nelle ricostruzioni nominative: Miglioramenti informativi qualitativi e quantitativi. Il caso di Madregolo (1629–1914). *Bollettino di Demografia Storica* 24/25: 113–29.

Manfredini, M. 2003a. La mobilità di un paese rurale durante l'epidemia di colera del 1854–55, in M. Breschi, R. Derosas, and P.P. Viazzo (eds.), *Piccolo è bello. Approcci microanalitici nella ricerca storico-demografica*, Forum, Udine, pp. 93–104.

Manfredini, M. 2003b. The use of parish marriage registers in biodemographic studies: Two case-studies from nineteenth century Italy. *Human Biology* 75(2): 255–64.

Manfredini, M. 2003c. Families in motion: The role and characteristics of household migration in a 19th-century rural Italian parish. *The History of the Family: An International Quarterly* 8(2): 317–43.

Manfredini, M. 2005. Coresident and non-coresident kin in a nineteenth-century Italian rural community. *Annales de Démographie Historique* 1: 157–72.

Mascie-Taylor, C.G.N., G.W. Lasker, and A.J. Boyce. 1987. Repetition of the same surnames in different marriages as an indication of the structure of the population of Sanday Island, Orkney Islands. *Human Biology* 59: 97–102.

Moring, B. 1996. Marriage and social change in south-western Finland, 1700–1870. *Continuity and Change* 11(1): 91–113.

Perrenoud, A. 1998. The coexistence of generations and the availability of kin in a rural community at the beginning of the nineteenth century. *The History of the Family* 3(1): 1–15.

Pettener, D. 1985. Consanguineous marriages in the upper Bologna Apennine (1565–1980)—microgeographic variations, pedigree structure and correlation of inbreeding secular trend with changes in population size. *Human Biology* 57: 267–88.

Poni, C. 1982. *Fossi e cavedagne benedicon le campagne*. Il Mulino, Bologna.

Reher, D.S. 1998. Family ties in Western Europe: Persistent contrasts. *Population and Development Review* 24(2): 203–34.

Relethford, R. 1992. Analysis of marital structure in Massachusetts using repeating pairs of surnames. *Human Biology* 64: 25–33.

Rettaroli, R. 1990. Età al matrimonio e celibato nell'Italia del XIX secolo: Un'analisi regionale, in Società Italiana di Demografia Storica, *Popolazione, società e ambiente. Temi di demografia storica italiana (secc. XVII–XIX)*, Clueb, Bologna, pp. 213–26.

Rettaroli, R. 1993. Maritu a chi troa, moglie a chi tocca. Nuzialità e famiglia nell'Italia mezzadrile del primo Ottocento, in Società Italiana di Demografia Storica, *La popolazione delle campagne italiane in età moderna*, Clueb, Bologna, pp. 505–26.

Rowland, R. 1983. Sistemes matrimoniales en la peninsula ibérica: Una perspectiva regional, in V. Perez and D.S. Reher (eds.), *La demografia historica de la peninsula ibérica*, Tecnos, Madrid, pp. 39–55.

Segalen, M. 1991. Mean age at marriage and kinship networks in a town under the influence of the metropolis: Nanterre, 1800–1850. *Journal of Family History* 16(1): 65–78.

Solinas, P.G. 1997. L'exogamie parfaite, l'espace généalogique dans une société complexe, in T. Barthélemy and M.C. Pingaud (eds.), *La généalogie entre science et passion*, Editions du Comité des travaux historiques et scientifiques, Paris, pp. 65–86.

Tittarelli, L. 1991. Choosing a spouse among nineteenth-century Central Italian sharecroppers, in D.I. Kertzer and R.P Saller (eds.), *The family in Italy from antiquity to present*, Yale University Press, New Haven/London, pp. 271–85.

Trussell, J. and T. Guinnane. 1993. Techniques of event-history analysis, in D. Reher and R. Schofield (eds.), *Old and new methods in historical demography*, Oxford University Press, Oxford, pp. 181–205.

van Leeuwen, M.H.D. and I. Maas. 2002. Partner choice and homogamy in the nineteenth century: Was there a sexual revolution in Europe? *Journal of Social History* 36: 101–23.

Viazzo, P.P. 2003. What's so special about the Mediterranean? Thirty years of research on household and family in Italy. *Continuity and Change* 1(18): 111–37.

Viazzo, P.P. and D. Albera. 1990. The peasant family in Northern Italy, 1750–1930: A reassessment. *Journal of Family History* 15: 461–82.

Chapter 2
Mortality in the Family of Origin and Its Effect on Marriage Partner Selection in a Flemish Village, 18th–20th Centuries

Bart Van de Putte[1], Koen Matthijs[2], and Robert Vlietinck[3]

Abstract This chapter addresses the role of health-related characteristics as a basis of marriage partner selection in a preindustrial population with a low level of social differentiation and a high level of mortality. We measured health characteristics by the level of infant and child mortality in the family of origin of the marriage partners. We observed a homogamous marriage pattern according to mortality in the family of origin. We argue that mortality in the family of origin was probably used to evaluate potential marriage partners. The level of infant and child mortality in a family can be seen as an indicator of health status, (future) social position, physical appearance, or reputation of the potential partner and his family.

Keywords marriage, homogamy, health selection, mortality, preindustrial

1 Introduction

Partner selection leads to a solid, sometimes lifelong, union between two individuals, their families and friends. It offers a tool to attract new people into the family network. Hence, it is a crucial decision and the choices made concerning partner selection, whether instrumental or expressive, always reveal important characteristics of society.

In this chapter we address the role of health-related characteristics as a criterion in marriage partner selection in a preindustrial population with high mortality. In mainstream historical-sociological research, the significance of health for partner selection is not that often discussed. There are, however, good reasons for addressing the topic. Health was a central issue in preindustrial society. Apart from the high level of mortality, which simply made health a daily concern, there are more indirect ways in which health issues mattered. Preindustrial (agricultural) labor required a substantial

[1] Department of Sociology, Faculty of Political and Social Sciences, Ghent University, Belgium, and Centre for Sociological Research, Catholic University of Leuven, Belgium

[2] Center for Sociological Research, Catholic University of Leuven, Belgium

[3] Center of Human Genetics, Catholic University of Leuven, Belgium

T. Bengtsson and G.P. Mineau (eds.), *Kinship and Demographic Behavior in the Past.*
© Springer Science+Business Media B.V. 2009

physical input (De Beule 1962) which evidently required good health. The importance of health and physical strength is, for example, reflected by the higher prices in the United States that were paid for taller slaves, presumably because tallness was associated with greater productivity (Margo and Steckel 1982). Also, in contemporary developing countries, there is a relationship between height and wages (Strauss and Thomas 1998). Furthermore, health evaluations played a role in many decisions, for example in the selection of wet-nurses (Hedenborg 2001).

Consequently, health is a crucial determinant of life chances and therefore presumably a central element in partner selection strategies. Shorter (1975, 145) confirms this by citing preindustrial sources: "You chose the richest person [...], aside from that, the morality and health of the parents were taken into account". There are some indications that this view is correct. Indirect evidence comes from research on the effect of marital status on mortality. One of the reasons why higher mortality rates are observed for the unmarried is, it seems, that the unhealthy have a lesser chance of marrying (Murray 2000; infra). There is also some direct evidence. For some preindustrial (and modern) populations it is shown that physical characteristics such as stature, strength, body weight or previous health experience and health behavior affect marriage partner selection (Baten and Murray 1998; Sköld 2003; Fu and Goldman 1996; Helmchen 2002).

All this shows that in a preindustrial high mortality environment, health was possibly a criterion in partner selection. However, partner selection research mainly focuses on socioeconomic (e.g., class, wealth) and cultural factors (e.g., religion) without much reference to possible physical characteristics. There is an enormous amount of literature on partner selection that is based on the idea that wealth (and not health) matters. In this chapter we try to integrate the ideas on the role of health in mainstream partner selection research.

We aim to respond to four specific questions. First, is the partner selection pattern homogamous according to health? Second, if so, is this a consequence of the intentional use of health as a criterion or is it simply the unintentional consequence of structural causes, such as the association between social position and health? Third, what is the relationship with other criteria? When does one use health instead of wealth? And finally, can we give more precise reasons why health is important?

In sections 2 and 3 we discuss theoretical and methodological issues concerning the relationship between health and partner selection. In section 4 we perform an empirical analysis of the importance of health-related characteristics (infant and child mortality in the family of origin) for marriage in a preindustrial Flemish village.

2 Theory

In order to evaluate the role of health and to integrate it into partner selection theory, we first take a closer look at the assumptions underlying the view that health matters for partner selection. In section 2.2 we turn to a more systematic approach that incorporates the discussion of these assumptions.

2.1   The Health Selectivity of Marriage: Basic View and Assumptions

The view that marriage is selective upon health characteristics is grounded on the idea that partner selection strategy, as a means of attracting new people into the family network, will be based on any criterion that enhances one's life chances. If health is a crucial determinant of life chances, then health-related characteristics are likely to be a target for partner selection strategies.

However, this view relies on several assumptions. A first assumption is that it is possible to choose partners based on health criteria. Before being entered into the partner evaluation process, health conditions need to be visible, and they must be evaluated as positive or negative for the future health of yourself or your family. To clarify this issue, it is important to distinguish between different aspects of health. Fu and Goldman (1996) provide a useful framework. These authors distinguish between three types of health characteristics: health conditions (physical and mental illnesses and limitations), physical attributes that may be associated with past or future health (obesity, short stature), and health-related behaviors (smoking, drinking, taking drugs, risk-taking behavior). In case health conditions are not directly visible, individuals use physical attributes and health-related behavior as signals to detect and evaluate the health conditions of the potential partner. Often, detection is very evident. The health conditions of the limp, deaf, blind, and disabled are very visible. But the detection of health conditions is often not an easy job. And sometimes this is practically impossible as some diseases even require high-tech screening. Nevertheless, even in a preindustrial society, or perhaps especially in such a society, evaluating health is not impossible. Diseases may affect one's physical appearance. Smallpox, for example, leaves scars on the face (Sköld 2003; Bruneel 1998). Villagers probably also knew very well about the number of infants and children that died in a given family, about the history of diseases in specific families, and so on (infra). These characteristics can be used to distinguish between "healthy" and "unhealthy" partners.

A complicating issue is that health attributes and behavior are not evaluated in a uniform way. These health characteristics may be interpreted as signals for other characteristics and may be used for other reasons. Drinking behavior, for example, may refer to a specific lifestyle, and this lifestyle can be evaluated regardless of its effects on health conditions. Similarly, some health attributes may not only reveal past or future health threats, they can also result in a lower sex appeal, depending on the societal norms in a given population (e.g., obesity, scars, height). All this implies that there is no direct relation between health and partner selection. Health characteristics are subjected to a complicated evaluation process and its impact on partner selection is dependent upon the outcome of this evaluation.

Even if humans are able to detect the health status of possible partners, there are no reasons why they automatically would use this information in partner selection. This leads us to the second assumption, which holds that (a) humans choose their partners instrumentally to enhance one's own and one's family's life chances; and

(b) health characteristics are used rather than wealth characteristics, consciously or unconsciously.[1] This assumption is not valid for every societal context. First, in some societies, partner selection strategies are to some extent not instrumental. Partners are sometimes chosen because of romantic reasons (e.g., Shorter 1975), or because of the existence of group bonds between the families of groom and bride (e.g., van de Putte 2003). Second, even if we assume that partner selection is based on purely instrumental grounds, it is not necessarily health that matters. Even if health indicates future economic well-being, it makes no sense to use health as a criterion if there are, in a given societal context, more direct and more visible characteristics, such as landholding, that offer more precise information about future economic well-being. Partner selection is not the same in every period or location, nor is it the same for every social group.

The third assumption is that partner selection is a matter of free individuals being able to make a free choice of marriage partner. Yet, partner selection is constrained by the "marriage market". The distribution of health characteristics in a population, the difference between the number of unhealthy males and females, the restriction of meeting opportunities between healthy and unhealthy individuals, and so on; all these factors influence the partner selection pattern according to health in a given society and therefore these have to be accounted for.

2.2 Health, Partner Selection, and Marriage Access

In this section we turn to a systematic overview of how health may affect both partner selection and marriage access. In section 2.3 we apply this approach to a specific health characteristic, namely the level of infant and child mortality in the family of origin.

2.2.1 Partner Selection

In most partner selection research the basic notions are homogamy (a marriage between a groom and a bride with similar characteristics) and heterogamy (a marriage between a groom and a bride with dissimilar characteristics). We give an overview of the reasons why there possibly is homogamy according to health characteristics. To organize the discussion, we use a simple framework of partner selection determinants. We distinguish between three main groups of determinants: structure, preferences, and social control (van Poppel et al. 2001; van Leeuwen and Maas 2002; Van de Putte 2005).

By structural determinants we refer to the (supply) effects of the marriage market on the partner selection pattern. The supply of potential partners has an effect

---

[1] The latter view is prominent in biological theory. See section 2.4.

on the partner selection pattern since the specific composition of the group of potential partners—the distribution of characteristics such as health and wealth in a population—strongly determines the level of homogamy (Van de Putte 2005). The chance to marry healthy or unhealthy partners depends on the precise number of potential partners that are healthy or unhealthy in a given society in a given period. As such this is not a very interesting factor, but to measure the preference for a specific type of partner, we have to control for this structural effect, although this depends on the specific methodological strategy (see methodology section).

The role of the marriage market is even more complex. The marriage market is composed of intermediate structures that mold the supply of potential partners. Often societal organization unites people with similar characteristics. For example, schools and neighborhoods often recruit people with a specific social background. If, for this reason, healthy people have a greater chance of meeting other healthy people, homogamy according to health will be observed, irrespective of the preference of healthy persons to marry a healthy partner. For example, if health is unevenly distributed over villages and parishes, and if people tend to meet and, for that reason, marry more frequently persons living in the same village or parish, then we will inevitably observe homogamy according to health characteristics. As both the association between health and location (Reid 1997) and homogamy according to place of residence have been frequently observed, this is likely to be a cause of homogamy according to health. This effect we call the meeting opportunities effect (Kalmijn and Flap 2001).

A special case of the meeting opportunities effect is the so-called by-product effect (Uunk 1996). If there is an association between two variables (e.g., health and social class) and if there is homogamy according to one of these variables (social class), homogamy according to the other variable (health) will be observed. This by-product effect is possibly present for class and health, but also for migration and health, since migrants often marry within their own group (Van de Putte 2003), and since their geographical background and common social situation may lead to specific health characteristics (Anderton, Beemer, and Hautaniemi 2005).

A second group of determinants of partner selection involves the preferences of marriage candidates. Marriage candidates have preferences which are expressed in the evaluation criteria they use. Health characteristics can be used as direct (to estimate health) or indirect (to estimate other characteristics) criteria. We distinguish between three types of evaluation criteria. Firstly, there are instrumental criteria. Visible health characteristics that are evaluated as important or even crucial to the survival chances of the household are a logical target for partner selection (supra). Apart from this direct use of health, there is possibly also an indirect instrumental use. Health may be used as a signal for past, present, and future social position. There is some empirical evidence for such an effect. Baten and Murray (1998, 124–35) explain the relation between stature and marriage chances by claiming that stature indicated physical strength and therefore economic position. This aspect of the relation between social position and health has to be distinguished from the by-product effect which does not assume a conscious evaluation of health characteristics.

Secondly, there are romantic-expressive criteria. In some cases partners are chosen because they are the only true, irreplaceable partner. It is difficult to connect this with health. Perhaps related to this is the role of physical attraction. Fu and Goldman (1996) on contemporary United States, Murray (2000) on nineteenth-century United States, and Sköld (2003) on preindustrial Sweden show that health may be important for marriage access and partner selection as it sometimes has severe consequences for one's physical appearance.

A third evaluation criterion is group membership. People often wish to marry a partner belonging to the same social group as their own. These groups may, for example, be based on lifestyle or on the occupational identity of the parents. Partner selection based on occupational groups, as is illustrated by traditionally high levels of homogamy among miners, farmers, and weapon makers, is not uncommon (Van de Putte, Matthijs, and Vlietinck 2005). As health is often related to values, tastes, and lifestyles (e.g., smoking behavior) and as these are often markers for reputation and group membership, homogamy according to health characteristics is probable (Fu and Goldman 1996). Also in this case, health is used as a signal for other characteristics (indirect effect).

A third determinant of partner selection is social control. Social control simply refers to the preferences of third parties, such as parents and colleagues. Even if marriage candidates do not intend to use health as a criterion, social control actors may force them to do so. The role of the parents in providing information on the health history of the families of potential partners is likely to be a (subtle) strategy that shapes their children's preferences. But as such, this factor does not introduce new arguments into the debate since the preferences of such social control actors likewise are shaped by the above-mentioned criteria.

Some additional factors require discussion. First, although wealth and health often are correlated, this is by no means a one-to-one relationship. Therefore, health is in competition with other characteristics. Second, the use of health characteristics in partner selection does not necessarily lead to homogamy. Another possible pattern is that health and wealth are exchanged. Third, health may also be related to the decision to marry, irrespective of the evaluation of marriage candidates.

2.2.2 Competition with Other Criteria

The possibility cannot be excluded that under some conditions the criteria of health and wealth may be combined. In that case, even if there is no priority given to health, we will observe homogamy according to health characteristics. The possibility to combine both criteria is probably strongest for large social groups. If farmers account for 50 percent of the total population in a society and if they do not differ strongly in terms of property, it is easy to find another farmer and other characteristics can be used as a partner selection criterion.

If it is difficult to combine both characteristics, marriage candidates have to choose. If there is a priority for wealth, then no homogamy according to health will be observed. A crucial question is, therefore, to which criterion people give priority. It is difficult to determine under what conditions people choose health as the main characteristic. Perhaps the role of health is most important in societies that have high levels of mortality and hard living and working conditions that put a lot of pressure on the physical condition of its population.

Also social position matters. We can consider health as a necessary condition that needs to be fulfilled in order to fully realize one's economic potential. Yet, this does not count for everybody to the same extent. Individuals who have secure access to property (e.g., farmers with very large property) or who are employed in physically less demanding occupations (e.g., civil servants, teachers), will probably be less dependent upon their health to ensure their life chances. At least they will be less dependent upon their health to attract a marriage partner. Also, for groups that have no secure access to land at all (ordinary workers, day laborers, etc.), we assume that there is more reason to select partners based on purely economic reasons (land or skill). This implies that health is particularly important for the partner selection of the middle groups, e.g., farmers with more or less secure access to land. In other words, health is used on the condition that some wealth characteristics are met.

It is even harder to determine under what conditions romantic criteria and group belonging are important. However, we expect that if these are important criteria, they are also most likely adopted by groups that to some extent have the economic freedom to use them, making both the highest and the lowest social categories less likely to adopt them.

2.2.3 Exchanging Wealth for Health?

So far we have assumed that health was important for both partners. This is not necessarily the case. First, it has been argued that, in the breadwinner task-distribution of the household, it is usually the men's task to bring in economic resources, while women are mainly evaluated by their social, domestic, and physical qualities (Fu and Goldman 1996, 73). This would imply that health characteristics are not equally important for males and females. However, in an agricultural society everybody in the household was exposed to hard living conditions. Hence, everybody benefited largely from good health and physical strength. In our view, there is no clear argument for expecting that there is, by definition, a greater need for good health for one of the sexes.

Second, partners may bring in different resources. Men or women with property can use this to "buy" health belonging to the other partner. If this is the case, we will not measure homogamy according to health: resourceful men or women may have a greater chance of attracting healthier partners. While leading to a different partner selection pattern, such a *differential exchange effect* also indicates the importance of health for partner selection.

2.2.4   Access to Marriage

So far, we have discussed health selectivity in terms of its consequences for partner selection. Health selectivity may, however, also be expressed via restrictions on marriage access. In the discussion of partner selection, we framed health selection in terms of the desirability of potential marriage partners. Desirability is also important for marriage access. One reason for a marriage candidate to remain unmarried is that he or she does not find a (suitable) partner. Yet, there are more reasons to remain unmarried, and these cannot be reduced to desirability (Fu and Goldman 1996). An individual may simply not want to marry (this individual is no marriage candidate); or other involved parties, such as parents, can decide that the marriage candidate should not marry (that person is not a *de facto* marriage candidate). This may occur irrespective of the evaluation by a potential partner, say, as a principled decision.

This decision not to marry is usually debated in terms of the Malthusian marriage pattern and is connected with the norm that one should be able to establish an economically independent household. Hence, if health conditions are so bad that it strongly affects the chance of running a household, it may lead to celibacy. There is an important argument in favor of this view. It has been shown that mortality rates are higher for unmarried people than for married people. This may be caused by the protection marriage offers. It could, however, also be caused by a selection effect. In view of this, the unhealthy simply have lesser chances of marrying (Ben-Shlomo et al. 1993; Hu and Goldman 1990, 233–50; van Poppel 1976). Also, physical attributes such as the height of both men (Whaples 1995) and women (Baten and Murray 1998) seem to be associated with marriage access.

The existence of a selection effect cannot be ignored. Yet, it is important to stress that for the large majority of people, bad health as such does not withhold them from developing a wish to marry. For the unhealthy, the question is rather to find a partner. Here the marriage market enters the debate. If we assume that the distribution of health characteristics is not different for men and women, there are always potential marriage partners with the same bad health characteristics. Consequently, mating opportunities for unhealthy people will exist. This *assortative mating effect* implies that there is no health selection that regulates marriage access. In this view, the relation between marriage and health is mainly a matter of the desirability of the marriage partner and not of a Malthusian limitation to marriage access.

The question is under what conditions these two principles, assortative mating versus Malthusian limitation, determine marriage access. First, for the extremely unhealthy, marriage access will be limited. Although they may of course develop a wish to marry, and we cannot exclude the possibility of assortative mating, social control actors may play an important role in preventing them from marrying. Furthermore, in practice, the fact that there will be only a few potential partners with the same extreme absence of health hinders their marriage chances. These individuals may have difficulties in meeting each other as, for example, in preindustrial society there were fewer "hospitals" in which to meet.

Second, for the others, those who are in poor, but not extremely poor health, there will always be potential marriage partners on the marriage market. Nevertheless, preindustrial societal conditions are often favorable for a strong selection effect. The role of the societal context is important here. The number of never-marrying persons might differ quite strongly between preindustrial populations. Stronger marriage selection, as revealed by the level of celibacy, probably implied a stronger effect of health characteristics on marriage access. According to a strict Malthusian marriage pattern, we can expect that entry into marriage is restricted to the extent that health-related characteristics are used along with direct economic requirements, such as the possibility of establishing an independent household.

Third, the assortative mating effect on marriage access will not be present if there is a difference in access to marriage between men and women. A quantitative disadvantage may result in stronger selection of the disadvantaged sex and this may result in a difference between males and females with regard to the possibility of entering the marriage market if unhealthy.

To sum up, if the possibility to marry is limited, selection is hard and this may lead to greater chances of marrying for the healthy. Furthermore, it is very possible that health selection is present for both marriage access and partner selection. As long as health selection on marriage access does not reduce all health variability in the group of those who marry, homogamy according to health characteristics is possible.

2.3 Partner Selection According to Infant and Child Mortality in the Family of Origin

In the next step, we apply this theoretical framework to a specific health characteristic. The first question is, Which health characteristics can be measured? The historical sources impose a serious limit on the possibility of analyzing the role of health. In standard historical demographic databases, there are not many variables that indicate the health characteristics of marriage partners. An interesting feature that can be measured is the level of infant and child mortality in the family of origin (the number of siblings of the spouses that died as infants or children). The level of infant and child mortality in the village under observation, as in many other places, was high (reaching a peak level of about 300 infants dying per thousand births in the last decade of the nineteenth century, infra). This made it a very visible characteristic.

Furthermore, the level of infant and child mortality differed between families (see section 3). It differed so strongly that this phenomenon has been described as the "clustering" of mortality in some families (Edvinsson et al. 2005; Das Gupta 1997; Guo 1993). For both contemporary and historical populations, it is observed that a limited number of families accounted for a large proportion of all infant mortality. For example, in some regions in Northern Sweden, about 10 percent of the women accounted for more than 50 percent of the total number of infant deaths (Edvinsson et al. 2005). This clustering suggests that there was no general culture of indifference towards infant mortality: quite the contrary. The indifference was probably strongest in populations with high and evenly spread infant mortality. In short, clustering of infant deaths made mortality in the family of origin a very marked characteristic that was not necessarily seen as something normal (see Edvinsson et al. 2005; Woods 2003).

As contemporaries were able to distinguish between low and high mortality in families, it is important to know which factors were linked to such differences. The level of infant and child mortality is a symptom of other underlying causes and consequences, and these can be interpreted in the partner selection scheme (see Table 2.1). Let us start by considering the causes. First, the biological constitution of the family is important. Genetic causes are thought of as being important for infant and child mortality (Johansson 2004, 117–8; Edvinsson et al. 2005, 328). Therefore, if health considerations determine partner selection, it may be worthwhile to evaluate infant and child mortality.

Second, poverty can lead to infant and child mortality (Johansson 2004, 113; Scott and Duncan 2000). Intermediate variables are bad housing conditions (e.g., crowding), malnutrition, and lack of decent medical care. If there is a strong effect of poverty on infant and child mortality, this implies that information on the level of infant and child mortality enables a better assessment of a family's social position and that it could be used as an indirect criterion in instrumental partner selection. Yet, research does not systematically confirm the relation between infant

Table 2.1 Overview of the possible role of infant and child mortality in the family of origin for partner selection

Determinants of partner selection	Infant and child mortality related to:
Structural	
– Distribution of health characteristics among marriage candidates	
– Meeting opportunities	Parish
– By product effect	Class, migration
Preferences	
1. Instrumental	
– Direct	Health (e.g., physical/genetic constitution, health in later life)
– Indirect	Negative economic qualities (e.g., poverty, expected social mobility)
	Positive economic qualities (e.g., no competing siblings)
2. Expressive-romantic	
– Beauty	Appearance (e.g., scars, stature)
3. Group belonging	
– Indirect	Reputation (e.g., breast-feeding, hygiene, child care)
Social control	
Preferences of third parties	

mortality in particular and class (Bengtsson 1999, 121). The main reason for this is the strong effect of breast-feeding practices.

Third, infant and child mortality may reflect values and lifestyles and therefore possibly be connected to group membership. There are several reasons why values are at play. Hygiene and childcare practices (such as the time spent in food preparation, housecleaning, care of the sick, and prevention of accidents, see van Poppel 2000), breast-feeding practices[2] (Bengtsson 1999, 121), parents' ideas about the time and effort to invest in their children (Johansson 2004, 116), and patriarchal values about internal family food distribution[3] may all affect mortality. Breast-feeding may be of crucial importance here. It is known that breast-feeding was not a generally applied habit in Catholic regions. Breast-feeding was a target for all kinds of prejudices; the yellow/orange color of the colostrum was "devilish", sexual intercourse "could have bad consequence for the quality of the mother milk", etc. (Jachowicz 2002). In short, infant (and child) mortality is related to hygiene, childcare, and breast-feeding practices and these were probably central elements of the reputation of families. If so, these families were seen as nonchalant, or even worthless. Reputation is typically a solid basis for group membership, and therefore homogamy according to health characteristics can be expected.

The consequences of infant and child mortality in the family of origin might also be a target of partner selection strategies. First, poor living conditions and high disease load may have consequences for the rest of one's life. Fogel (1994), Barker (1998), Bengtsson and Lindström (2003), and Fridlizius (1989) confirm that early-life conditions affect health in later life. Research on the effect of early-life conditions also shows how social mobility is affected (Svensson, Bröström, and Oris 2004). Poor living conditions and high disease load can be made visible for contemporaries by high levels of infant and child mortality, but also height can be a crucial intermediate variable. If this effect on later life is strong and if this mechanism is visible for contemporaries, then infant and child mortality will be used in a direct (future health) or indirect (future social position) instrumental way. Second, not only one's physical strength but also one's physical appearance may be affected by disease experience during childhood (supra).

So, infant and child mortality may act as a signal of reputation, physical appearance, and past, present, and future health and wealth. Yet, while the number of infants and children that died is probably visible in a given village, it may be less clear, even for contemporaries, what the underlying causes are. Perhaps it is the combination of these factors that is seen as the underlying cause. It seems plausible that in a society in which mortality is high and in which social stratification is not

---

[2] Religious groups have for instance different breastfeeding practices (van Poppel 2005; Kintner 1987). Also farmers, because of the availability of substitutes (milk), might possibly breastfeed their children less (Bengtsson 1999, 121).

[3] The position of females and their level of education is an important cause of decreasing infant and child mortality in contemporary societies. A better position of women seems to be associated with a more democratic distribution of medical care and allocation of food (Caldwell and McDonald 1982).

extremely sharp (all individuals are exposed to poor living conditions), infant and child mortality is one of the best indications of whether a family has problems coping with their poor living conditions, and is, therefore, possibly a good indicator of the general quality of a family. It may, in the absence of other features, be good practice not to ignore this aspect.

A complicated question is whether there is a difference between infant and child mortality. There are some reasons why it might be useful to separate the effect of infant mortality from that of child mortality. First, different causes are important during the first month of life (endogenous causes), the period of breast-feeding, and the period after breast-feeding (here the effect of poverty may be stronger). Second, the divergent visibility between infant and child mortality may be important. Infant mortality was typically higher, which created more variation amongst families in terms of the number of deaths. The majority of families did not experience child mortality (defined as dying between ages 1 and 5) and the large majority would only experience the death of a child once, at the most (section 3). So, in principle it might be useful to analyze infant and child mortality separately. However, it is very hard to assume that contemporaries were able to distinguish between the levels of infant and child mortality or between their different underlying causes. It is, in our view, the combined level of infant and child mortality which was evaluated and which led to a distinction between high and low mortality families, with infant mortality being its strongest component. Furthermore, there are some technical reasons that make it more convenient to analyze the effect of the level of infant and child mortality combined (section 3.4).

A final issue concerns the possible positive effects of the level of infant and child mortality. So far, we have treated infant and child mortality as a signal of negative characteristics of the family of origin. But as infant and child mortality may limit the number of surviving children in a family, this may increase the chances of the surviving children to receive larger proportions of the resources present in the family. It can therefore not be excluded that the level of infant and child mortality in the family of origin has a positive effect. In particular in families in which there is no egalitarian inheritance system, this might make a huge difference.

In this section we have focused on the way the level of infant and child mortality can be intentionally used to shape preferences for a specific type of marriage partner. The relationship of mortality with structural determinants and with marriage access is very dependent on the specific societal context. This will be discussed in more detail below in the section that presents context information on the village under research (section 3.2).

2.4 The Biology of Partner Selection

We conclude this theoretical section with a short discussion on biological views on partner selection. In biological theories of partner selection, health-related characteristics play a crucial role as a basis for mate selection. The biological discussion of partner selection starts with Charles Darwin (2002/1871). Darwin worried about the effects of increasing civilization on the process of natural selection since improved health care increased the survival chances of the "weak and inferior".[4] This implied that their characteristics would be passed on to the next generation. There is one major threshold: the "weak and the inferior" do not "marry as freely as the healthy people do". Contemporary biological approaches have reframed this discussion in terms of genetics (Jaffe 2002).

The central concepts are sexual selection and mate selection. The former refers to competition between individuals of the same sex and selection of the best of these individuals by the other sex (Darwin 2002/1871, 262). This competition is based on the selection of good genes (Jaffe 2002). It is assumed that populations have a partner selection system in which individuals with good genes have greater chances of being selected as a marriage partner. The concept of mate selection is somewhat more general and refers to the process by which individuals select a partner for reproduction. This leaves the possibility open that not all individuals of one sex desire the same individual of the opposite sex, which reduces the level of competition (Jaffe 2002). Also, a marriage pattern in which individuals with similar genes marry each other (e.g., assortative mating) has evolutionary advantages as, for example, it accelerates the extinction of suboptimal genetic combinations (Jaffe 2002).

The question is then how humans detect good genes, or good health. Psychological theory offers some possible mechanisms that may explain this. Evolutionary psychologists claim that, for example, facial symmetry, body size, and odors make it possible to unintentionally select the healthiest partner, or the one with the best genes. Downes (2005) reviews three dominant views. First, it has been proposed that men prefer women with a waist/hip ratio near to 0.7. The waist/hip ratio seems to be correlated with a woman's reproductive endocrinological status and long-term health risk. According to Singh (1993), humans have perceptual and cognitive mechanisms for utilizing the waist/hip ratio to infer attributes of women's health, youthfulness, attractiveness, and reproductive capacity. Second, there is the "fluctuating asymmetry approach". The central idea is that if an individual is able to undergo identical development on both sides of a bilaterally symmetrical trait, this development can be susceptible to environmental and genetic stresses. Asymmetry therefore is a signal of these underlying causes. Third, the "chemical signaling approach" is based on the idea that animals rely on chemical signaling to mediate successful mating. Some animals are able to use a male's odor to obtain disease-resistance genes, as it increases the chance to mate with males carrying dissimilar Myosin Heavy Chain genes.[5]

The vision underlying this biological mate-selection theory is basically that in the course of history, humans acquired an increased ability to detect resourceful

---

[4] Darwin referred to a broader category than what we nowadays would call "unhealthy", as he, for instance, also referred to intelligence.

[5] A Myosin Heavy Chain gene encodes a Myosin Heavy Chain isoform. Each fibre type in mammalian skeletal muscles contains a different Myosin Heavy Chain isoform.

partners that are willing to invest in childrearing. In our view this is not problematic. Yet, translating this to the preindustrial population under research in this chapter is far from evident. We agree here with Downes (2005, 184) that: "Human behavior is unusual in that almost none of our behavior is inevitable. Given a particular cue, generally speaking, a certain behavior will result, but this need not be the case. We have many internal proximate causes that could produce the same behaviour …". We think that these proximate causes are not only internal. The ones that are listed in the framework provided above play a role as well. Partner selection is a complex process in which wealth, health, the marriage market, visibility, interpretation and evaluation of characteristics, and trade-offs between health and wealth is important. We do not want to reduce the level of infant and child mortality in the family of origin in the partner selection process to a target unconsciously used by humans to detect good genes. This would lead to nonrecognition of all these factors. Furthermore, it is difficult to see how the level of infant and child mortality can be linked to the characteristics that are the targets for biological mate selection, such as an odor and the waist/hip ratio. All this clearly does not mean that we exclude the possibility that there is an ultimate motivation of human behavior that may be interpreted in biological terms. But it is difficult to envisage the consequences for the empirical analysis that will be presented in the next sections.

2.5 Hypotheses

On the basis of this overview we derived the following hypotheses:

1. Under conditions other than extremely poor health, with weak Malthusian pressure on marriage and no different significance of health for one of the sexes, marriage access is not strongly determined by one's health as there is the possibility of assortative mating according to health. Yet, these conditions require almost modern living conditions. In preindustrial society, health was probably related to marriage access.
2. Health is important for the partner selection pattern. There are many potential reasons for why there is homogamy according to health characteristics. Structural reasons (distribution of health in a population, meeting opportunities, by-products), but also preferences for partners with specific health characteristics are possibly important, in direct instrumental ways (health) or as a signal for other characteristics (wealth, reputation, physical appearance).
3. We expect that health is most important for the partner selection of the (large) middle groups, that is, those with some secure access to land.

3   Data, Context, and Methodology

In this section we give a description of the data, present some information on the socioeconomic and mortality characteristics of the village under observation, and discuss the methodology.

3.1   Data

The database includes information from parochial and civil registers (Matthijs, Van de Putte, and Vlietinck 2002; Van de Putte, Matthijs, and Vlietinck 2004). It contains information on individuals who were born, married, or died in Moerzeke. In the analysis, we have information on the marital behavior and the mortality in the family of origin of individuals born between 1727 and 1908. The number of observations is about 1,800 for the analysis of marriage access and about 1,400 for the analysis of partner selection.

The family reconstitution database represents the so-called stable population. This restricts the analysis in two ways. First, as we need information on infant and child mortality in the family of origin, the research will be limited to spouses whose parents lived in the village. There is almost no information available on the mortality experience or the marital behavior of migrants' parents. This implies that we might, for example, miss the effect of mortality in the family of origin on marriages outside the village. This effect might be stronger than for marriages within the village, if we assume that those born in higher mortality families have lesser chances of marrying and therefore have to migrate and find a spouse elsewhere. Nevertheless, this does not mean that the expected effect should not be visible for the stable population. It simply means that we might not measure all effects of mortality in the family of origin.[6]

Second, the figures on infant and child mortality shown below are probably somewhat biased. We do not have information on the precise age at death of out-migrants, nor do we have information on the precise migration date. Children who out-migrated and who died before their fifth birthday are not included in the number of dead children of a given family. We assume that out-migrants survived their fifth birthday. Hence, if we refer to the level of infant and child mortality of a given family, we refer to the observed and therefore minimal level of mortality.

However, this bias will not be very strong. The bias is only present if someone who married in Moerzeke (and with parents living in Moerzeke) had siblings that out-migrated and died before their fifth birthday. Out-migration before the age of 5 years was likely to be a family event. This implies that the marrying individual probably also out-migrated (with his family of origin); and in particular, given the low level of in-migration (infra), there was not much chance of this individual returning to the village to marry. But the possibility cannot be excluded that the family out-migrated with very young children and later came back with at least one child (the marrying child), though not with the other children (for whom we do not have information on age at death).

3.2   Context

Moerzeke is a small village in the center of Flanders (Belgium), in the province of Eastern Flanders. The population of Moerzeke rose from approximately 2,000 in 1761 to 4,706 in 1950 (De Beule 1962). It is geographically isolated as it is almost

---

[6] As will be shown in note 16, there is a somewhat greater chance of out-migrating if one is born in a high or medium infant-mortality family.

completely surrounded by the river Scheldt. Moerzeke was a rather closed society in terms of geographical mobility. In-migration, in particular, was very limited (De Beule 1962).

We first briefly discuss the economy and the social structure. The agricultural sector was dominant until well into the twentieth century. During the second half of the nineteenth century, the rural textile industry gradually became more important, although about 60 percent of the employed males were still involved in farming in 1960 (De Beule 1962). To classify the occupations present in the database, we followed De Beule (1962), who distinguished between three important groups in Moerzeke. The largest group consisted of farmers. The large majority of them had access only to a small piece of land. The average size of the landholding in 1846 was about 3.4 ha. About 61 percent of the farms were smaller than 2 ha. In the course of the nineteenth century, the plots of land became even smaller. The average landholding size was 1.96 ha in 1895, with 76 percent of farms being smaller than 2 ha (Vanhaute and Wiedemann s.d.). Moreover, the large majority of farmers were tenants. The other occupations can be divided into a lower status group of occupations such as workers, day laborers, and domestic servants ("lower class"), and a higher status group of occupations such as bakers, doctors, owners, and civil servants ("elite"). This social differentiation was echoed in the level of homogamy according to social origin. The odds for sons of farmers to marry daughters of farmers were 1.6 times higher than the odds for sons of lower status fathers ($p = 0.001$).[7] The odds for sons of elite fathers to marry daughters of elite fathers were 2.8 times higher than the odds for sons of lower status fathers ($p < 0.001$).

Marriage access was rather restricted. First, men and women married late. For those born in the period 1727–1908, the mean age at first marriage was about 31.4 for men and about 28.7 for women. Second, the level of celibacy was rather high. For those who were born in the period 1721–1908, and who died in Moerzeke after their 50th anniversary, about 20.3 percent of the meh were unmarried, while about 28.3 percent of the women were unmarried. Especially elite and farmers' sons had lesser chances of marrying, as will be shown in section 4.1. All this implies that societal conditions favored a hard selection on marriage access.

Next we provide some general information on mortality in Moerzeke. The level of infant and child mortality was high (De Ridder 1986). Table 2.2 shows the percentages of children born in Moerzeke that died at a given age. Of males born in Moerzeke, 9.7 percent died within 1 month, 14.5 percent after their first month and before their first anniversary, and some 10 percent between ages 1 and 5 years. This means that about 35 percent died as infants or children. The pattern for females was not very different, but with only 7.2 percent of deaths within the first month.

Table 2.3 shows the number of dead children by age for couples born in Moerzeke. For neonatal mortality, we observe that about 65 percent of the couples that had at least one child did not experience a single death of any of their children during their

---

[7] Data not shown. Measured using multinomial logistic regression with social origin of bride as dependent variable and controlled for group sizes and year of birth of the groom.

Table 2.2 Percentages of individuals dying at a given age, Moerzeke, 1727–1908

Age at death	N	Percentage
Males		
Died within first month	643	9.7
Died after first month and before first year	961	14.5
Died between 1 and 5 years	687	10.3
Died after fifth year	2,829	42.6
Missing/emigrant	1,518	22.9
Total	6,638	100.0
Females		
Died within first month	450	7.2
Died after first month and before first year	917	14.6
Died between 1 and 5 years	667	10.6
Died after fifth year	2,808	44.8
Missing/emigrant	1,422	22.7
Total	6,264	100.0

Table 2.3 Percentage of families experiencing a specific number of neonatal, infant, child, and infant and child deaths, Moerzeke, 1727–1908

Number of deaths	Neonatal	Infant	Child	Infant and child
0	65.54	28.95	61.33	18.85
1	25.19	30.44	25.19	27.40
2	6.22	17.36	9.07	19.11
3	1.49	9.78	3.43	12.37
4	1.04	6.74	0.71	9.26
5	0.19	3.04	0.26	5.96
6	0.26	1.62		3.04
7	0.06	0.78		1.49
8		0.97		1.42
9		0.32		0.52
10				0.45
11				0.13
N	1,544	1,544	1,544	1,544

first month of life. For 25 percent of the couples, there was one death. These figures suggest that differentiation according to neonatal mortality was not very visible. This was different for infant mortality. Two extreme groups emerge. About 29 percent of the couples had no children dying during their first year, while 23 percent of the couples had at least three infants who died. This made differentiation in infant mortality a rather visible phenomenon. For child mortality, differentiation was not very visible, as about 86 percent of the couples did not have more than one dead child.

Let us next consider the causes of mortality. We do not have direct information on the causes of death so we have to limit the discussion to indirect information. In the eighteenth century, major mortality crises (mainly dysentery) occurred, but these became weaker as the century advanced (De Ridder 1986). The village under study was possibly strongly affected by malaria, as the ecological conditions there were favorable for the development of this disease (Devos 2001). Malaria patients had less resistance against, for example, dysentery, smallpox, and typhus. Both typhus and dysentery were related to hygiene and contaminated food and water. Smallpox was a "democratic" disease, affecting almost everyone regardless of social class (Bruneel 1998).

Malaria declined in Flanders during the nineteenth century (Devos 2001). From the late eighteenth century onwards, smallpox became less common due to the implementation of vaccination programs, although this was a rather slow process with quite strong regional variation (Bruneel 1998). Yet, in Moerzeke, infant mortality did not drop until the first decades of the twentieth century. On the contrary, the number of infants that died increased in the second half of the nineteenth century. While infant mortality was about 200 per thousand in the eighteenth century and in the first half of the nineteenth century, it gradually increased to more than 300 per thousand in the final decade of the nineteenth century.

Reduced breast-feeding is a plausible explanation for this effect. Breast-feeding gives advantages in terms of nutrition, immunity, and sterility (Kintner 1987). Infectious diseases therefore have a weaker impact on breastfed babies. In general, Catholics breastfed their children less often than others did (Wolleswinkel-van den Bosch et al. 2000). In Flanders, this habit became even less common in the late nineteenth century, although there was strong regional variation. According to Buysse (1997), breast-feeding practices became less common in the late nineteenth century in the neighboring village of Hamme. Furthermore, in an analysis restricted to children that died before their first birthday, we did not observe a relationship between the number of days a child lived and the length of the birth interval to the subsequent birth (data not shown). As the death of a child coincides with the end of the breast-feeding period, the number of days the child lived should be related to the birth interval to the next child if breast-feeding practices were strong.[8]

All this may indicate that diarrhoeal diseases such as typhus and dysentery could have had a strong impact (Wolleswinkel-van den Bosch et al. 2000). The seasonal pattern of infant mortality suggests the same development. In an analysis of some English villages, Huck (1997) claims that the observed, increased summer mortality was related to reduced breast-feeding practices. This reduction was associated with diarrhoeal diseases (dysentery) that typically led to peak mortality in July, August, and September. Respiratory diseases, on the contrary, were more dangerous in winter (Huck 1997, 378). Smallpox had a peak in spring (April, May, June) while it was at its lowest level in September, at least in Sweden (Sköld 1996, 149). In Moerzeke, the seasonal pattern of infant mortality also showed a clear peak in

---

[8] The relationship between infant death, breastfeeding, and birth interval is far more complicated. One of the factors that complicates this relation is the practice of "replacing" the dead child with a new one. The relationship may also be reversed: a long birth interval may increase survival chances of the previous child.

the late summer months of August and September. This peak was visible for males and females, and became stronger for infants born between 1851 and 1900 (more than 16 percent, compared to 10 percent per month for males and 8 percent per month for females during the period 1700–1800).

What does this mean for our analysis? First, recall that apart from a lack of breast-feeding, there were many other causes of diarrhoeal diseases. Analyses of developing countries show, for instance, that weaning procedures, including the type of food that is given to the child, are important (Scrimshaw, Taylor, and Gordon 1968, 230–40). Furthermore, diarrhoeal diseases lead to death mainly because of dehydration and overrestriction of the diet. Know-how concerning rehydration and the restriction of the diet is essential (Scrimshaw et al. 1968, 257). In short, this suggests that in preindustrial periods the quality of the childcare offered by families was crucial.

Second, what are the consequences of diarrhoeal diseases? The deterioration in nutritional status after an episode of diarrhoea frequently results in patient malnutrition (Scrimshaw et al. 1968, 216). The body's ability to generate a surplus for growth is dependent upon allocation of nutrients to other tasks, such as the claims of work and recovery from infections (Fogel 1986, 29). This has important implications. In less-developed countries where diarrhoeal diseases are highly prevalent and a major cause of death, it is recognized that synergism between diarrhoea and malnutrition seriously affects the general health of young children. Malnutrition commonly impairs resistance to other infections (Scrimshaw et al. 1968, 216) and, at the same time, exerts a lasting effect on growth (Scrimshaw et al. 1968, 55–216; Gopalan 1992, 25). Stunting is indeed an indicator of past malnutrition (Gopalan 1992, 44–5; Floud 1992). In addition to physical strength, mental development of children can be expected to be retarded because of the adaptation of children to energy deficiency by reducing play and other physical activities (Gopalan 1992, 26).

How is this related to the clustering of mortality in some families? Even if diarrhoeal diseases were widespread in the whole village, that is, present for every family, there might have been different health consequences for different families. High mortality families might have been the ones that combined diarrhoea with a higher susceptibility for other diseases, for instance, because of the families' genetic constitution, breast-feeding habits, childcare, and physical environment. Mortality, therefore, clearly revealed the characteristics of the family of origin. But as the children of these families might have been more exposed to diseases that depleted nutrition, the level of infant mortality in the family of origin might also have been associated with the level of physical strength.

Finally, we compare the levels of infant and child mortality in different groups. First, the by-product effect was probably not very large. The difference between farmers, the elite, and the lower class as regards the levels of infant and child mortality was not very strong, although mortality was somewhat lower for the elite in almost every category, except child mortality (Table 2.4).[9] For contemporaries, infant

---

[9] These figures might be misleading in the sense that family size was not taken into account. But it is difficult to control for this as mortality might also influence family size.

Table 2.4 Mean number of children dying at a specific age in a family; comparison by social position of the family, Moerzeke, 1727–1908

	Farmers	Elite	Lower class
Neonatal	0.43	0.44	0.51
Infant	1.52	1.33	1.54
Child	0.71	0.75	0.72
Infant and child	2.23	2.08	2.26
N	701	323	930

Table 2.5 Mean number of children dying at a specific age in a family; comparison by place of residence, Moerzeke, 1727–1908

	Centrum	Mixed	Kastel	Unknown
Neonatal	0.47	0.61	0.52	0.48
Infant	1.62	1.77	2.00	1.56
Child	0.50	0.61	0.69	0.58
Infant and child	2.12	2.37	2.69	2.14
N	303	145	132	1,013

and child mortality was probably not strongly associated with wealth. Second, as Moerzeke was composed of two parishes (Centrum and Kastel), there might have been a meeting opportunities effect according to parish. We can only make an indirect classification of the population by parish (see further). There were some limited mortality differences between the parishes, with Kastel consequently showing the highest figures (Table 2.5).

3.3 General Methodological Issues

Before we give details on the models and the variables, we address some general methodological issues. As we examine the partner selection of all individuals in the village, the analyses include brothers and sisters. This problem of nonindependent observations makes it necessary to adopt a multilevel strategy. We add a family identification variable to the model. We estimate a random intercept but do not estimate random slopes in every family cluster. The latter is not necessary since we do not intend to evaluate the different effects that the variables have in each family. Clearly, this does not make much sense in a case like this in which the level 2 units (families) have few or only one observation. In practice, the nonindependency of observations turned out to be unproblematic. As there are many persons that do not have brothers or sisters in the analysis, in particular in the partner selection analysis, adding this family identification variable did not lead to very different results than we would have obtained in an analysis without the multilevel design.

We look at information on the partner selection of first marriages. Although the partner selection of remarrying persons is not without significance, at this stage we aim to keep the analysis simple and avoid the issue of remarriage, which differs in many ways from first marriage (Matthijs 2003).

In order to estimate the number of dead infants and children in the family of origin, we look at the children of the biological parents of the individual for whom marriage access or partner selection is examined. This is the most direct estimation of the mortality of the family of origin. This implies, however, that information about children born to one of the biological parents with a new or previous partner is not counted. Thus, for some individuals, we will underestimate the level of mortality within their close environment. Yet, simply adding the number of dead infants and children of the subsequent or previous family of one of the biological parents is probably also misleading. Does one interpret the level of mortality of the "biological" family and the new or old family with stepfather/mother in the same way? Not using this information may lead to "noise", as the total amount of mortality is not counted, but that may be preferred to information that is mixed and difficult to interpret. Note, however, that about 87 percent of the spouses included in the analysis had a family of origin composed of both biological parents.

3.4   Models and Variables

3.4.1   Marriage Access Model

We will perform two sets of multilevel logistic regression analyses. First, we address the role of infant and child mortality for marriage access.[10] The analysis is straight-forward. We select individuals (men and women separately) having reached at least the age of 50 (ensuring that every individual undoubtedly had the opportunity to marry) and examine whether men and women born in families with high infant and child mortality had lesser chances of marrying than others. We start by using a basic model containing mortality and year of birth as independent variables (model A). In the next step, we add control variables to see whether the assumed effect of mortality can be explained by one of these (model B). In model C, we add interaction variables (social position and social origin) to evaluate whether the effect of mortality in the family of origin was different according to social position or origin.

Independent variables:

– Infant and child mortality in family of origin[11]

---

[10] We perform different analyses for marriage access and partner selection as they have different underlying selection mechanisms (see for example the principle decision of whether to marry or not, supra) and we do not want to mix up these differences.

[11] Another possibility is to use the "failure rate" (percentage of children in a given family that died as infants or children) instead of the absolute number of deaths. In our view, the absolute number is more revealing as for instance four infant deaths in nine children is probably more informative

1 (low) = number of infants and children that died is lower or equal to 1
2 (medium) = number of infants and children is equal to 2
3 (high) = number of infants and children that died is higher than 2
(reference category)

Control variables:

We add these variables as they may be related to both mortality and marriage access.

- Year of birth
- Birth rank
- Number of male siblings surviving until the age of 20
- Number of female siblings surviving until the age of 20
- Social origin (social position of father)

  1 = farmer
  2 = elite
  3 = lower class (reference category)

- Social position

Same categories as social origin; for women we added the category "no information".

- Parish of residence

The village under observation includes several parishes. Unfortunately, we do not have information on the place of residence. Some information, however, gives a hint. De Beule lists surnames that are typical for the village center (Centrum) and for Kastel. We constructed a variable that measures parish by using this information.

  1 = Centrum
  2 = Mixed (surnames not typical for either Centrum or Kastel, but strongly present in both)
  3 = Kastel
  4 = Unknown (reference category)

- Migration

  1 = birth and death in Moerzeke, the stable population
  2 = others (reference category)

---

for the contemporaries than a failure rate of 50 percent in a family with two children. Yet, the choice between these two types of categorizations is not problematic as the percentage and the number of deaths is strongly correlated. The high failure percentage families do also have a larger absolute number of deaths compared to low failure families. Furthermore, using a failure rate in the analyses did not lead to very different results (not shown).

3.4.2 Partner Selection Model

Second, we address partner selection. We analyze grooms and brides in separate analyses. We choose to use the characteristics of one of the spouses as the
dependent variable, rather than using characteristics of the marriage (homogamous or heterogamous according to mortality) as the dependent variable. The
models estimate the chance of grooms marrying a specific type of bride, and
vice versa. Homogamy was present in case high mortality grooms had greater
chances of marrying a high mortality bride. The strategy of using the characteristics of one of the partners as the dependent variable permits an interpretation
of each control variable within an exchange framework. If we observe that persons who belonged to a specific social category had greater chances of marrying a high mortality bride, a differential exchange effect was present. The
differential exchange effect would not be measured if we used homogamy as
the dependent variable. The models use a combined variable for infant and
child mortality for both the independent and the dependent variable (infra).

Dependent variable in the analysis of partner selection of grooms (brides):

– level of infant and child mortality in the family of origin of partner

   0 (low) = number of infants and children that died is lower or equal to 1
   1 (medium or high) = number of infants and children that died is higher than 1

Independent variables:

– level of infant and child mortality in family of origin groom (bride):

See description variables for marriage access models.

3.4.3 Structural Causes

Controlling for the basic structural effect of the distribution of the level of mortality
does not require a group size variable if the dependent variable is marrying a partner belonging to a specific mortality category. If 60 percent of the families of origin
of the brides had a low level of mortality, then every groom, irrespective of his
social background, had a 60 percent chance of marrying a bride belonging to this
category (in case of random partner selection). Controlling for group size is important when modeling frequencies of homogamy (as in loglinear analysis) or when
modeling chances of marrying homogamously.

   The by-product and the meeting-opportunities effect do require control variables. The general strategy is to add the variable for which such an effect is expected.
For example, if mortality was associated with social origin and if there was homogamy according to social origin, then some social groups had a greater chance of
marrying a partner with the same mortality level in the family of origin. By adding
the social origin variable, this by-product effect is controlled.

- Social origin of groom/bride (see marriage-access models for categories)[12]
- Migration (see marriage-access models for categories)
- Parish of residence (see marriage-access models for categories)
- Period, operationalized as the year of birth of the spouse[13]

3.4.4 Preferences

If there is an effect of the level of mortality of the family of origin, then this simply indicates homogamy. It is not possible to determine whether mortality was used as a signal for health, beauty, group bonds, or economic characteristics by simply introducing variables to the model.

3.4.5 Other Control Variables

- Social position of groom/bride
  With this variable we examine whether social position was used in exchange for health characteristics.
- Number of females and males surviving until their 20th anniversary
  Variable introduced to control for the positive effect of the mortality of siblings.
- Birth rank
  Although there is an egalitarian inheritance system, we cannot exclude an effect of birth rank on partner selection.
- Family of origin: identification number of the family
  Variable introduced to control for the multilevel effect.

We only use models with a combined variable of infant and child mortality. In a preliminary analysis (Van de Putte et al. 2005), we used supplementary models that included separate variables for infant mortality and for child mortality. This strategy has, in theory, the advantage that it enables you to observe whether infant rather than child mortality was used as a criterion. But there are good reasons for using a combined variable. First, although it is likely that infant mortality had the strongest effect (being the most visible of the two types of mortality), it seems reasonable that child mortality was not evaluated very differently, as if it were a different or irrelevant

---

[12]To control for the by-product it would, in theory, be more convenient also to add social origin of the partner to the model. Yet, differences in mortality according to social origin are not very strong (supra). More importantly, adding this variable to the model might lead to violation of the nonrecursivity assumption, as the dependent variable (mortality in the family of origin of partner) can also be a cause of an independent variable (social origin of the family of origin of the partner). The social origin of the partner might be the consequence of the selection of the partner according to mortality (if social origin and mortality are related). We tested supplementary models by introducing social origin of the partner as a variable. This did not change the results; parameter estimates and p-values were very similar.

[13]Technically, period also determines meeting opportunities. If subperiods have different mortality levels, and of course they usually do, then, inevitably, high levels of homogamy will be measured.

characteristic of the family of origin. Indeed, the impact of unlikely breast-feeding in this Catholic village probably made the difference between infant and child mortality less strong. Second, using separate variables also obscures the results. If the effect was caused by infant as well as child mortality, the latter strategy does not necessarily lead to any significant result as these variables are used in the same model and control for each other. This does not make sense if the villagers did not distinguish between both types of mortality. If we exclude one of the variables from the model, we risk losing information that was used by contemporaries—the remaining variable might not take enough of the effect into account to produce significant results.

For the village under consideration, both variables were indeed correlated. In a simple logistic regression analysis with child mortality as the dependent variable (no dead children versus at least one dead child) and year of birth as a control variable, the b-parameter for being born in a low infant mortality family versus being born in a high infant mortality family is 0.67 (p = <0.001; N = 6,071). Substantially, this means that it was not that important for the villagers to separate infant mortality from child mortality. Technically, this means that controlling for one of these variables makes it more difficult to find significant results for the other variable. Therefore, and for reasons of space limitations, we choose to report only the analysis with the variable that measures both infant and child mortality at the same time.

4   Results

4.1   Access to Marriage

Table 2.6 shows the results of the logistic regression analysis of the chance, for men, of getting married versus remaining unmarried.[14] The level of infant and child mortality in the family of origin is not as such related to marriage access (model A). The estimates for "infant and child mortality" increase after adding control variables (model B) but remain insignificant (for the category "low", $p = 0.12$). The estimates for social origin show that sons of farmers and of the elite had lesser chances of marrying. This could be compensated for by one's own social position. The farmers and the elite had greater chances of marrying. The positive effect of birth rank (the higher the birth rank, the greater the chance of marrying) and the negative effect of the number of female siblings that survive until their 20th anniversary were striking. The first can be seen as the consequence of the policy of parents to keep their oldest son at home to assist them in coping with the household's economic needs (De Beule 1962). The latter effect is puzzling. That the number of adult siblings had a negative impact on marriage access is plausible. Yet, why in particular the number of female siblings had such an effect is unclear.

The picture of the role of mortality in the family of origin on marriage access becomes clearer when we look at the results of model C, which includes interaction

---

[14] In the table, we show b-parameters, not exponents. We did not print the multilevel estimates of the intercept. Tolerance statistics for all analyses showed that there were no problems of multicollinearity.

Table 2.6 Logistic regression of the chance of marrying versus remaining unmarried; men (b-parameters), Moerzeke, 1727–1908

	Model A	Model B	Model C
Constant	6.30*	18.25***	17.89**
Infant and child mortality	(0.21)	(1.26)	(0.02)
Low (0 or 1)	0.125	0.38	0.38
Medium (2)	0.091	0.14	0.22
High (more than 2) (ref.)			
Year of birth	−0.002	−0.008**	−0.008**
Social origin		(8.14***)	(7.29***)
Farmer		−0.65**	−0.69*
Elite		−1.17***	−0.94
Lower class (ref.)			
Social position		(67.2***)	(63.9***)
Farmer		1.47***	1.28***
Elite		2.48***	3.34***
Lower class (ref.)			
Parish		(0.98)	(1.03)
Centrum		0.14	0.012
Mixed		−0.30	−0.36
Kastel		0.56	0.55
Unknown (ref.)			
Migration			
Born and died in the village		−0.21	−0.21
Migrant (ref.)			
Birth rank		0.11***	0.11***
Number of male siblings above 20		−0.08	−0.09
Number of female siblings above 20		−0.38***	−0.40***
INTERACTION EFFECTS			
Social origin × infant and child mortality			(0.29)
Farmers × low infant and child mortality			0.26
Farmers × medium infant and child mortality			−0.36
Elite × low infant and child mortality			−0.12
Elite × medium infant and child mortality			−0.50
Social position × infant and child mortality			(2.26*)
Farmers × low infant and child mortality			0.21
Farmers × medium infant and child mortality			0.43
Elite × low infant and child mortality			−1.61**
Elite × medium infant and child mortality			−0.43
N	1,834	1,565	1,565

For each categorical variable; F-values (and significance level) generated by F-tests are indicated between brackets.
*$p < 0.10$; **$p < 0.05$; ***$p < 0.001$.

terms. The main effects show the estimates for the reference groups included in the interaction terms. For this reference group (lower class), the estimate for low infant and child mortality is not significant (b = 0.38); yet, if we use farmers as the reference group, the effect of infant and child mortality is significant (t = 2.02; p = 0.04; not shown in table). Model C also shows that for sons who themselves belonged to the elite, infant and child mortality had a significantly weaker effect on marriage access.

It appears that the negative effect of high mortality was compensated for by upward social mobility.

The analysis shows somewhat different results for women (Table 2.7). Low mortality women had a greater chance of marrying (model A). The control variables

Table 2.7 Logistic regression of the chance of marrying versus remaining unmarried; women (b-parameters), Moerzeke, 1727–1908

	Model A	Model B	Model C
Constant	−3.25	−8.07	−7.98
Infant and child mortality	(2.59*)	(2.72*)	(3.01*)
Low (0 or 1)	0.38**	0.50**	0.40
Medium (2)	0.25	0.33	0.16
High (more than 2) (ref.)			
Year of birth	0.002	0.005**	0.005**
Social origin		(0.45)	(0.40)
Farmer		0.06	−0.18
Elite		−0.20	−0.71
Lower class (ref.)			
Social position		(85.4***)	(79.5***)
No occupation		−2.71***	−2.38***
Farmer		0.43	0.53*
Elite		−0.85	−0.87
Lower class (ref.)			
Parish		(0.46)	(0.41)
Centrum		0.17	0.17
Mixed		−0.14	−0.10
Kastel		0.31	0.30
Unknown (ref.)			
Migration			
Born and died in the village		−0.46	−0.47
Migrant (ref.)			
Birth rank		0.004	0.003
Number of male siblings above 20		−0.12*	−0.11*
Number of female siblings above 20		−0.07	−0.08
INTERACTION EFFECTS			
Social origin × infant and child mortality			(0.92)
Farmers × low infant and child mortality			0.16
Farmers × medium infant and child mortality			0.80
Elite × low infant and child mortality			0.68
Elite × medium infant and child mortality			1.15
Social position × infant and child mortality			(0.61)
No occupation × low infant and child mortality			−0.43
No occupation × medium infant and child mortality			−0.72
Farmers × low infant and child mortality			−0.05
Farmers × medium infant and child mortality			−0.50
Elite × low infant and child mortality			0.35
Elite × medium infant and child mortality			−0.72
N	1,616	1,372	1,372

For each categorical variable; F-values (and significance level) generated by F-tests are indicated between brackets.
*p < 0.10; **p < 0.05; ***p < 0.001.

do not explain this effect (model B). The effect of social origin and position on marriage access was less strong for women.[15] There were no interaction effects (model C). These results might signify that selection into marriage was generally somewhat stronger for women.[16] Or it might signify that it was somewhat easier for men to compensate for bad health characteristics by economic resources.

These results show, in general, that the level of infant and child mortality in the family of origin affected the chances of marrying. Given the absence of good agricultural ground and farms, it was not easy to establish an independent household in Moerzeke (De Beule 1962). And under such conditions, selection into marriage was strong. In this respect, it is important that for men, the strongest effect was observed for farmers' sons. In short, in this village, the selection effect, rather than the assortative mating effect, determined access into marriage.

4.2 Partner Selection According to Infant and Child Mortality in the Family of Origin

Before we turn to the logistic regression analysis, we first present a marital mobility table comparing the level of infant and child mortality of the family of origin of groom and bride (Table 2.8). These crude observations, not controlled for any variable, indicate that the percentage of men that married a low mortality bride was about 9 percent higher for men born in a low mortality family than for men born in a high mortality family. This confirms the presence of homogamy; yet, it is also clear from these results that this characteristic does not create an extremely sharp social boundary.

Table 2.9 shows the results, for men, of the logistic regression analysis of the chance of marrying a partner born in a high or medium level infant and child mortality family versus marrying a partner born in a low level mortality family. The conclusion is rather straightforward: there is homogamy according to the level of infant and child mortality in the family of origin (Table 2.9, model A). The estimate of −0.31 (b-parameter) signifies that the odds for men born in a low mortality family of origin to marry a bride born in a medium or high mortality family was 1.36 (exponent of the b-parameter) times lower than for men born in a high mortality family of origin.

[15] The effect of "no occupation" is probably misleading since for women who did not marry there was less of a chance of an occupation being recorded, as the main source of information on occupations was the marriage certificate.

[16] This difference between men and women might be related to some specific characteristics of the marriage market of the village. Out-migration was somewhat stronger for men (the percentage of out-migrating men was 2 percent higher) and in-migration stronger for women (the percentage of in-migrating women was 2 percent higher), creating a marriage market that was to some extent less favorable to women. Furthermore, for those women who reached the age of 20, the percentage of low infant mortality families was about 7 percent higher for natives than for out-migrants, suggesting that there was some stronger pressure for the unhealthy to move. For men, this was about 3 percent. For child mortality, no analogous differences were found.

Table 2.8 Marital mobility table by level of infant and child mortality in family of origin, Moerzeke, 1727–1908

Groom		Bride			
		Low infant and child mortality	Medium infant and child mortality	High infant and child mortality	N
Low infant and child mortality	Frequency	337	140	178	655
	Row %	51.5	21.4	27.2	
	Column %	52.2	47.8	43.4	
Medium infant and child mortality	Frequency	147	62	101	310
	Row %	47.4	20.0	32.6	
	Column %	22.8	21.2	24.6	
High infant and child mortality	Frequency	162	91	131	384
	Row %	42.2	23.7	34.1	
	Column %	25.1	31.1	32.0	
N		646	293	410	1,349

Model B shows that this effect is not explained by the control variables (social origin, parish, and migration status). Model B also shows that sons who belonged to the elite were less likely to marry a high mortality bride. This was not because they were also sons of elite fathers (the model controls for social origin), but suggests instead the existence of an exchange effect. These elite sons were possibly exchanging their socioeconomic position for the low mortality of the family of the bride. The estimates for farmers, though close to significant, were not significant ($p = 0.065$).

Model C adds interaction terms. The estimates show that the effect of infant and child mortality of the family of origin of the groom was strongest for sons of farmers. The effect does not differ between the elite and the lower class. This confirms that homogamy according to infant and child mortality was strongest in the "middle group" of the village's social structure. Among the lower class sons and daughters, the competition for scarce marriage candidates with land was probably extremely important, and therefore it was difficult for them to combine it with a rigorous application of health criteria. An illustrative example of this is the higher level of homogamy according to social position (of the couple) for sons and daughters of lower class fathers. Among this group, farmers' homogamy was much stronger than among sons and daughters of farmers.[17]

---

[17] For marriages composed of sons and daughters of the lower class (a category with a low level of homogamy according to health), homogamy of farmers is 1.5 times stronger than is the case for marriages composed of sons and daughters of farmers (a category with high homogamy according

Table 2.9 Logistic regression of the chance of marrying a medium or high infant and child mortality bride (b-parameters), Moerzeke, 1727–1908

	Model A	Model B	Model C
Constant	−7.09**	−14.15***	−14.3***
Infant and child mortality	(2.92*)	(3.52**)	(2.60*)
Low (0 or 1)	−0.31**	−0.39**	−0.31
Medium (2)	−0.17	−0.30	−0.53*
High (more than 2) (ref.)			
Year of birth	0.004**	0.008***	0.008***
Social origin		(0.36)	(0.93)
Farmer		0.11	0.52
Elite		−0.008	0.07*
Lower class (ref.)			
Social position		(3.72**)	(2.51*)
Farmer		−0.27*	−0.55**
Elite		−0.50**	−0.84**
Lower class (ref.)			
Parish		(0.33)	(0.21)
Centrum		−0.12	−0.10
Mixed		−0.16	−0.13
Kastel		−0.04	−0.04
Unknown (ref.)			
Migration			
Born and died in the village		0.11	0.10
Migrant (ref.)			
Birth rank		−0.02	−0.02
Number of male siblings above 20		−0.03	−0.03
Number of female siblings above 20		−0.01	−0.01
INTERACTION EFFECTS			
Social origin × infant and child mortality			(1.61)
Farmers × low infant and child mortality			−0.70**
Farmers × medium infant and child mortality			−0.39
Elite × low infant and child mortality			0.001
Elite × medium infant and child mortality			−0.55
Social position × infant and child mortality			(1.23)
Farmers × low infant and child mortality			0.25
Farmers × medium infant and child mortality			0.57
Elite × low infant and child mortality			0.22
Elite × medium infant and child mortality			1.07**
N	1,348	1,208	1,208

For each categorical variable; F-values (and significance level) generated by F-tests are indicated between brackets.

$*p < 0.10$; $**p < 0.05$; $***p < 0.001$.

to health). This is not to say that sons and daughters of farmers chose their partners irrespective of their social background. Yet, for farmers' children marrying farmers' children, health characteristics were more important than for children of lower class workers who still had to compete for the scarce potential spouses that had some land at their disposal.

Table 2.10 Logistic regression of the chance of marrying a medium or high infant and child mortality groom (b-parameters), Moerzeke, 1727–1908

	Model A	Model B	Model C
Constant	−7.39**	−6.87*	−7.38*
Infant and child mortality	(3.39**)	(3.74**)	(3.10**)
Low (0 or 1)	−0.34**	−0.41**	−0.33
Medium (2)	−0.11	−0.16	−0.14
High (more than 2) (ref.)			
Year of birth	0.004**	0.003**	0.004**
Social origin		(1.47)	(1.58)
Farmer		0.20	−0.09
Elite		−0.12	0.25
Lower class (ref.)			
Social position		(0.70)	(0.63)
No occupation		0.12	0.37
Farmer		−0.14	0.06
Elite		0.19	0.83
Lower class (ref.)			
Parish		(0.32)	(0.29)
Center		−0.15	−0.15
Mixed		−0.05	−0.04
Kastel		−0.13	−0.09
Unknown (ref.)			
Migration			
Born and died in the village		0.001	−0.01
Migrant (ref.)			
Birth rank		0.012	0.01
Number of male siblings above 20		−0.01	−0.07
Number of female siblings above 20		−0.06	−0.06
INTERACTION EFFECTS			
Social origin × infant and child mortality			(1.77)
Farmers × low infant and child mortality			0.20
Farmers × medium infant and child mortality			0.84**
Elite × low infant and child mortality			−0.60
Elite × medium infant and child mortality			−0.29
Social position × infant and child mortality			(1.07)
No occupation × low infant and child mortality			0.04
No occupation × medium infant and child mortality			−1.28*
Farmers × low infant and child mortality			−0.16
Farmers × medium infant and child mortality			−0.55
Elite × low infant and child mortality			−0.52
Elite × medium infant and child mortality			−1.38
N	1,230	1,068	1,068

For each categorical variable; F-values (and significance level) generated by F-tests are indicated between brackets.

$*p < 0.10; **p < 0.05; ***p < 0.001$.

Women born in a family with low infant and child mortality had greater chances of avoiding a medium and high mortality groom than high mortality women had (Table 2.10). For women, we did not observe interaction effects of social origin or position that were comparable to the ones found for men. Furthermore, there were no direct effects of social origin or position. These characteristics were not exchanged for health benefits, showing that one's social position was more crucial for men than for women.

5 Conclusion and Discussion

The starting point of this research was the idea that in a preindustrial high mortality environment, health characteristics were plausible criteria used in the selection of marriage partners. We measured health characteristics by the level of infant and child mortality in the family of origin of the marriage candidates.

A first important result is the observation of homogamy according to mortality in the family of origin. Spouses born in high mortality families had greater chances of marrying partners that were also born in high mortality families. Apart from this pattern of homogamy according to mortality in the family of origin, there was a differential exchange effect. Wealth was exchanged for health on the marriage market, as revealed by the greater chance of elite sons to marry a low mortality partner. Second, the effect was present after controlling for possible structural causes. Homogamy according to mortality was not simply the by-product of homogamy according to social origin or parish. This suggests that the level of infant and child mortality in the family of origin, or its causes and its consequences, was probably intentionally used in the partner selection process. A third conclusion is that homogamy according to mortality was to some extent related to social position. Sons of farmers had a higher level of homogamy according to mortality in the family of origin compared to elite sons—a smaller group that gave strong priority to social position as a criterion—and compared to sons of lower class fathers. The strong competition for access to land was one reason why the latter group gave priority to social position. Also the analysis of marriage access fits this picture. Children of low mortality families had greater chances of marrying. This supports the idea that in premodern conditions there was, probably, a health selection underlying the access to marriage, even though the selection might have been based on the causes or the consequences of the level of infant and child mortality.

The question as to why mortality characteristics were used is less easy to answer. The level of mortality in the family of origin may refer to four characteristics: health, wealth, physical appearance, and reputation. High exposure to disease in early life may have had effects on one's *physical appearance*. Yet, the mortality pattern in the village under study suggests that diarrhoeal diseases, such as dysentery, were probably more important than smallpox. We can only speculate whether, in this village, the surviving children of high mortality families had a different physical appearance, such as low stature, that was seen as less attractive or beautiful.

Physical characteristics should not be reduced to matters of beauty. The possible weaker *health* of children born in high mortality families may have been evaluated as a serious handicap in later life in general. Moreover, individuals born in high mortality families might have lacked physical qualities (such as physical strength) that were highly valued in farmers' communities because of their instrumental value. Therefore, health may have been evaluated as a good indicator of (future) *wealth*.

It is perhaps less likely that mortality was used as a more refined indicator of the economic position of the family of origin of the spouses—that is, without an intermediate variable of present physical characteristics. As it was mainly infant mortality that contributed to the distinction between low and high mortality families, and as the role of social position was usually most strongly expressed with regard to child mortality, we suggest that other factors were more important. But as breast-feeding practices were probably not very strong in this village, the present research is perhaps not a strong test of this effect.

The level of mortality might also have been used as an indicator of the lifestyle and the *reputation* of a given family. If mortality was related to the decision to breastfeed children (an option that was probably not automatically chosen by the inhabitants), hygiene, the care given to children, etc., then the level of mortality was very visible proof of this form of lifestyle. The bad reputation of the high mortality family might have been a subtle, but strong, handicap on the marriage market.

These explanations do not contradict each other. Perhaps the analytical distinction made here was not used by contemporaries. Mortality was maybe an indicator of the past, present, and future general quality of a family, both in terms of instrumental and symbolic value.

However, these conclusions do not close the debate. The analysis is based on the research of only one village. The village had a high level of infant mortality, was mainly populated by farm workers and farmers with limited access to landholding, presented hard physical conditions for agricultural work, was rather closed in terms of geographical mobility, and was characterized by a quite strong Malthusian pressure on marriage access. The possibility cannot be excluded that these conditions were very beneficial to selection based on health. On the other hand, these conditions were far from exceptional and, consequently, this pattern might not necessarily be observed exclusively in this village. The advantage of our research strategy is that replication does not require exceptionally well-documented databases with individual level information on such criteria as stature or cause of death. Comparative analysis of the impact of infant and child mortality on partner selection might lead to better insights as to the precise reasons underlying it.

Acknowledgments The authors wish to thank the Fund for Scientific Research Flanders (Belgium) for funding the project. The authors wish to thank Sam Clark, Christer Lundh, Jan Van Bavel, Kent Johansson, Kirk Scott, Martin Dribe, Michel Oris, Patrick Svensson, and Tommy Bengtsson for their attempts to fight the authors' ignorance in the field of mortality and agricultural history. The authors wish to thank R. Bijl, genealogist of VVF-Dendermonde, for permitting them to use his demographic database.

References

Anderton, D., J. Beemer, and S. Hautaniemi. 2005. Family Wealth and Mortality: An Analysis of Alternative 19th Century Data Sources. Presented at the Conference on Kinship and Demography, IUSSP, Salt Lake City, Utah.

Barker, D. 1998. *Mothers, Babies and Health in Later Life.* Churchill Livingstone, Edinburgh.

Baten, J. and J. Murray. 1998. Women's stature and marriage markets in pre-industrial Bavaria. *Journal of Family History* 2: 124–35.

Ben-Shlomo, Y., G. Davey-Smith, M. Shipley, and M.G. Marmot. 1993. Magnitude and causes of mortality differences between married and unmarried men. *Journal of Epidemiology and Community Health* 47: 200–5.

Bengtsson, T. 1999. The vulnerable child. Economic insecurity and child mortality in pre-industrial Sweden: A case study of Västanfors, 1757–1850. *European Journal of Population* 2: 117–51.

Bengtsson, T. and M. Lindström. 2003. Airborne diseases during infancy and mortality in later life in Southern Sweden, 1766–1894. *International Journal of Epidemiology* 2: 286–94.

Bruneel, C. 1998. Ziekte en sociale geneeskunde: De erfenis van de Verlichting, in J. De Maeyer, L. Dhaene, G. Hertecant and K. Velle (eds.), *Er is leven na de dood. Tweehonderd jaar gezondheidszorg in Vlaanderen*, Uitgeverij Pelckmans, Kapellen, pp. 17–32.

Buysse, S. 1997. Macrostudie over de touwindustrie te Hamme met nadruk op de 19de en 20ste eeuw, gevolgd door een casestudie over het touwslagersgeslacht Vermeire van de 16de eeuw tot de 20ste eeuw. Unpublished Licentiate's Thesis. University of Gent, Gent.

Caldwell, J. and P. McDonald. 1982. Influence of maternal education on infant and child mortality: Levels and causes. *Health Policy and Education* 3–4: 185–205.

Darwin, C. 2002/1871. *De afstamming van de mens en selectie in relatie tot sekse.* Uitgeverij Nieuwezijds, Amsterdam.

Das Gupta, M. 1997. Socio-economic status and clustering of child deaths in rural Punjab. *Population Studies* 3: 191–202.

De Beule, O. 1962. *Moerzeke. Religieus-sociale monografie van een plattelandsgemeente.* Katholieke Universiteit Leuven, Leuven.

De Ridder, J. 1986. *Moerzeke. 1710–1796. Een historisch-demografische analyse van een plattelandsparochie in Oost-Vlaanderen.* Belgisch Centrum voor Landelijke Geschiedenis, Leuven.

Devos, I. 2001. Malaria in Vlaanderen tijdens de 18de en 19de eeuw, in J. Parmentier and S. Spanoghe (eds.), *Orbis in Orbem. Liber Amicorum John Everaert*, Academia, Gent, pp. 197–233.

Downes, S. 2005. Integrating the multiple biological causes of human behaviour. *Biology and Philosophy* 20: 177–90.

Edvinsson, S., A. Brändström, J. Rogers, and G. Broström. 2005. High-risk families: The unequal distribution of infant mortality in nineteenth-century Sweden. *Population Studies* 3: 321–37.

Floud, R. 1992. Anthropometric measures of nutritional status in industrialized societies: Europe and North America since 1750, in S. Osmani (ed.), *Nutrition and poverty*, Oxford University Press, Oxford/New York, pp. 219–42.

Fogel, R. 1986. Nutrition and the decline in mortality since 1700. Some additional preliminary findings, NBER Working Paper No. 1802 (January 1986), National Bureau of Economic Research, Cambridge, MA.

Fogel, R. 1994. The relevance of Malthus for the study of mortality today: Long-run influences on health, mortality, labour force participation and population growth, in K. Lindahl-Kiessling and H. Landberg (eds.), *Population, economic development, and the environment. The making of our common future*, Oxford University Press, Oxford/New York, pp. 231–84.

Fridlizius, G. 1989. The deformation of cohorts: Nineteenth century mortality decline in a generational perspective. *Scandinavian Economic History Review* 3: 3–17.

Fu, H. and N. Goldman 1996. Incorporating health into models of marriage choice: Demographic and sociological perspectives. *Journal of Marriage and the Family* 58: 740–58.

Gopalan, C. 1992. Undernutrition: Measurement and implications, in S. Osmani (ed.), *Nutrition and poverty*, Oxford University Press, Oxford/New York, pp. 217–48.

Guo, G. 1993. Use of sibling data to estimate family mortality effects in Guatemala. *Demography* 1: 15–32.

Hedenborg, S. 2001. To breastfeed another woman's child: Wet-nursing in Stockholm, 1777–1937. *Continuity and Change* 3: 399–422.

Helmchen, L. 2002. *Marriage Market Incentives to Invest in Health*. University of Chicago, Chicago (http://home.uchicago.edu/~lahelmch/job_market_paper.pdf).

Hu, Y. and N. Goldman. 1990. Mortality differentials by marital status: An international comparison. *Demography* 2: 235–50.

Huck, P. 1997. Shifts in the seasonality of infant deaths in nine English towns during the 19th century: A case for reduced breast feeding? *Explorations in Economic History* 3: 368–86.

Jachowicz, A. 2002. Met de moedermelk ingegeven. Een onderzoek naar de houding tegenover borstvoeding in België tijdens de eerste helft van de twintigste eeuw. Unpublished Licentiate Thesis. University of Gent, Gent.

Jaffe, K. 2002. On sex, mate selection and evolution: An exploration. *Comments on Theoretical Biology* 2: 91–107.

Johansson, K. 2004. *Child mortality during the demographic transition. A longitudinal analysis of a rural population in Southern Sweden, 1766–1894*. Lund Studies in Economic History 30. Almqwist & Wiksell International, Lund.

Kalmijn, M. and H. Flap. 2001. Assortative meeting and mating: Unintended consequences of organized settings for partner choices. *Social Forces* 4: 1289–312.

Kintner, H. 1987. The impact of breastfeeding patterns on regional differences in infant mortality in Germany, 1910. *European Journal of Population* 3: 233–61.

Margo, R. and R. Steckel. 1982. Heights of American slaves: New evidence on slave nutrition and health. *Social Science History* 6: 516–38.

Matthijs, K. 2003. Frequency, timing and intensity of remarriage in 19th-century Flanders. *The History of the Family* 1: 135–62.

Matthijs, K., B. Van de Putte, and R. Vlietinck. 2002. The Inheritance of longevity in a Flemish village (18–20th century). *European Journal of Population* 1: 59–81.

Murray, J. 2000. Marital protection and marital selection: Evidence from a historical-prospective sample of American men. *Demography* 4: 511–21.

Reid, A. 1997. Locality or class? Spatial and social differentials in infant and child mortality in England and Wales, 1895–1911, in C. Corsini and P. Viazzo (eds.), *The decline of infant and child mortality: The European experience, 1750–1990*, UNICEF/Sides/Martinus Nijhoff, Leiden/Boston, pp. 129–54.

Scott, S. and C. Duncan. 2000. Interacting effects of nutrition and social class differentials on fertility and infant mortality in a pre-industrial population. *Population Studies* 1: 71–87.

Scrimshaw, N., C. Taylor, and J. Gordon. 1968. *Interactions of Nutrition and Infection*. World Health Organisation, Geneva.

Shorter, E. 1975. *The Making of the Modern Family*. Basic Books, New York.

Singh, D. 1993. Body shape and women's attractiveness: The critical role of waist-to-hip ratio. *Human Nature* 3: 297–321.

Sköld, P. 1996. *The two faces of smallpox. A disease and its prevention in eighteenth- and nineteenth-century Sweden*. Umeå University/Demographic data base, Umeå.

Sköld, P. 2003. The beauty and the beast—Smallpox and marriage in eighteenth and nineteenth-century Sweden. *Historical Social Research* 3: 141–61.

Strauss, J. and D. Thomas. 1998. Health, nutrition, and economic development. *Journal of Economic Literature* 36: 766–817.

Svensson, P., G. Broström, and M. Oris. 2004. Early-life conditions and social mobility in nineteenth century Belgium and Sweden. Paper presented at the 2004 Annual Meeting, SSHA: Chicago.

Uunk, W. 1996. *Who Marries Whom? The Role of Social Origin, Education and High Culture in Mate Selection of Industrial Societies during the Twentieth Century.* Katholieke Universiteit Nijmegen, Nijmegen.

Van de Putte, B. 2003. Homogamy by geographical origin. Segregation in 19th century Flemish cities (Leuven, Aalst and Ghent). *Journal of Family History* 3: 364–90.

Van de Putte, B. 2005. *Partnerkeuze in de 19de eeuw. Klasse, geografische afkomst, romantiek en de vorming van sociale groepen op de huwelijksmarkt.* Leuven University Press, Leuven.

Van de Putte, B., K. Matthijs, and R. Vlietinck. 2004. A social component in the negative effect of sons on maternal longevity in preindustrial humans. *Journal of Biosocial Science* 3: 289–97.

Van de Putte, B., K. Matthijs, and R. Vlietinck. 2005. Mortality in the family of origin and its effect on marriage partner selection in a Flemish village (18th–20th century). Presented at the Conference on Kinship and Demography, IUSSP, Salt Lake City, Utah.

Vanhaute, E. and T. Wiedemann, T. (s.d.) *Belgian Historical GIS,* Gent, Department of Modern History (website: http://www.flwi.ugent.be/hisgis).

van Leeuwen, M. and I. Maas. 2002. Partner choice and homogamy in Sweden in the nineteenth century: Was there a sexual revolution in Europe? *Journal of Social History* 1: 101–23.

van Poppel, F. 1976. Burgerlijke staat en doodsoorzaak: Een overzicht van de situatie in de 19e en het begin der 20e eeuw. *Bevolking en Gezin* 1: 41–66.

van Poppel, F. 2000. Children in one-parent families: Survival as an indicator of the role of parents. *Journal of Family History* 3: 269–90.

van Poppel, F. 2005. Differential infant and child mortality in three Dutch regions, 1812–1909. *Economic History Review* 2: 272–309.

van Poppel, F., A. Liefbroer, J. Vermunt, and W. Smeenk. 2001. Love, necessity and opportunity: Changing patterns of marital age homogamy in the Netherlands, 1850–1993. *Population Studies* 1: 1–13.

Whaples, R. 1995. The standard of living among Polish- and Slovak-Americans: Evidence from fraternal insurance records 1880–1970, in J. Komlos (ed.), *The biological standard of living on three continents,* Westview, Boulder, pp. 151–71.

Wolleswinkel-van den Bosch, J., F. van Poppel, C. Looman, and J. Mackenbach. 2000. Determinants of infant and early childhood mortality levels and their decline in the Netherlands in the late nineteenth century. *International Journal of Epidemiology* 29: 1031–40.

Woods, R. 2003. Did Montaigne love his children? Demography and the hypothesis of parental indifference. *Journal of Interdisciplinary History* 3: 421–42.

Chapter 3
Villages, Descent Groups, Households, and Individual Outcomes in Rural Liaoning, 1789–1909

Cameron Campbell[1] and James Lee[2]

Abstract We make use of a uniquely detailed and voluminous longitudinal, individual and household-level dataset from rural Liaoning in northeast China during the eighteenth and nineteenth centuries to compare the role of communities, kin networks, and households in determining individual social and demographic outcomes in late imperial China. We assess the importance of each level of social organization by examining how individual chances of attainment, fertility, marriage, and mortality were correlated with rates at the level of the household, the household group, the descent group, and the village. We then examine relations across outcomes by measuring how individual chances for each outcome were associated with rates for other outcomes at each of the four levels of social organization. Results indicate that each level of organization was important in the sense that clustering was apparent, though the precise pattern of associations varied by outcome. Finally, motivated by recent results for contemporary China that suggest that villages dominated by single kin groups or small numbers of kin groups have better provision of public goods (Tsai 2004), we carry out a preliminary assessment of the importance of "collective efficacy" in late imperial Liaoning villages by examining whether residents of villages that were more homogeneous in terms of their descent group composition had better provision of public goods, as reflected in more favorable demographic outcomes.

Keywords China, Liaoning, historical, community, household, fertility, mortality, marriage, descent group, kinship, kin networks, demographic behavior

1 Introduction

We examine the roles of kin and community in determining the individual social and demographic outcomes of a quarter-million Chinese peasants living in 500 villages in northeast China between 1774 and 1909. This exercise is part of our long-term effort

---

[1] University of California, Los Angeles, USA

[2] University of Michigan, USA

T. Bengtsson and G.P. Mineau (eds.), *Kinship and Demographic Behavior in the Past.*
© Springer Science+Business Media B.V. 2009

to apply techniques from demography and quantitative sociology to longitudinal, individual-level data to reconstruct the organization and behavior of social and kin networks in historical and contemporary China. While our previous work has focused on kin within the household, with this and other recent analyses we now consider the role of kin and other social networks outside the household as well.

Our primary goal is to examine how individual chances of attainment, mortality, fertility, and marriage correlated within households, administrative household groups, paternal descent groups, and villages. Analyzing these correlations identifies the loci of interactions, perceptions, and decisions that affected demographic and social outcomes and provides insight into the relative importance of each of these levels of social and economic organization. At the same time, such analyses reveal the interrelationships of attainment, mortality, fertility, and marriage within the demographic microregimes formed by social and kin networks at these different organizational scales.

Our related secondary goal is to examine how village and descent group organization interacted to shape individual outcomes. Inspired by Frankenberg's (2004) translation of the concept of "collective efficacy" (Sampson and Raudenbush 1999; Sampson, Raudenbush, and Earls 1997) from urban neighborhoods in developed countries to rural villages in developing countries, we hypothesize that villages dominated by single descent groups or a very small number of descent groups will have higher levels of "collective efficacy" and that this will be reflected in more favorable social and demographic outcomes for residents. In villages where residents are related to each other, mutual trust should be higher and collective provision of public goods should be easier (Tsai 2004). We expect the resulting higher levels of "collective efficacy" to be reflected in more favorable demographic rates, including earlier marriage, higher marital fertility, and later death.

We divide our chapter into four parts. First, we outline existing claims about the role of kin networks in late imperial Chinese society, and show how this analysis relates to the literature. In this context, we lay out our expectations about how village and descent group organization interact to affect "collective efficacy" and specify hypotheses about the influence of descent group diversity on demographic outcomes. We then introduce the data we use for this analysis and summarize the methods we use to calculate associations among demographic and social outcomes. Finally, we present our results and conclude with some brief remarks about the implications of these findings.

2   Background

There is a general consensus that the link between kinship and demographic and social behavior is virtually universal to all human societies. Most scholars distinguish between two ideal model family systems: a relatively simple conjugal family system characteristic of Western, particularly Northwestern, Europe, and a comparatively more extended family system characteristic of a much wider geographic area stretching from East Asia and South Asia to Eastern and Southern Europe. Many European demographic historians have focused on describing the West, especially the Northwest European conjugal family system, and the preventive population check that characterized its demographic behavior. Their general conclusion is that while the family organization of such societies was relatively simple, their demography, and particularly their nuptiality, were sensitive to economic circumstances (Goldstone 1986; Levine 1987; Schofield 1985; Weir 1984; Wrigley and Schofield 1981).

At least in theory, kinship should have been an important determinant of individual outcomes in China. Chinese kin groups are well known not only to influence demographic decisions, but in many cases actually to make such decisions (Lee and Wang 1999). Thus marriage, reproduction, education, employment, and even survivorship are often determined not by individuals but by kin, sometimes within and sometimes without the household. Many Chinese kin groups used to follow formal rules to define the jurisdiction of kin authority by residence, family relationships, and gender (Ebrey 1984, 1991; Liu 1959), as well as to transmit and manage power and resources, not just belonging to the kin group, but to individual members (Bian 1997).

International comparisons have confirmed the validity of some claims about European and Asian families, but have challenged our understanding of the links between kinship networks and demographic behavior. They have, for example, discovered little historical support for the long-held assertion that larger, more complex households better insulated members from economic pressure. Moreover, they have not been able to substantiate many of the behaviors claimed above. Mortality rates from a comparison of eighteenth- and nineteenth-century rural communities were equally sensitive to short-term economic stress in southern Sweden, eastern Belgium, and northern Italy, where households were relatively simple, as in northeastern China and northeastern Japan, where households were both larger and more complex. Such work on the importance of kinship in East Asian, particularly specific Chinese and Japanese populations, have documented how such social organization shielded individual behavior from short-term economic fluctuations but rendered them vulnerable to social circumstances (Bengtsson, Campbell, Lee et al. 2004; Lee and Campbell 1997).

A more complete understanding of the role of kinship networks in shaping demographic and social outcomes requires moving beyond the household to consider kin living elsewhere. The need for such analyses has long been recognized, but data limitations have hitherto precluded such research (Plakans 1984). Kin who lived apart interacted with each other in a variety of ways, sharing information as well as social, political, and economic resources. The genealogies that have been used in previous studies of kinship networks document kin ties, but do not provide information on residence; thus, it is impossible to compare effects of kin according to whether or not they lived in the same household or village. Household registers document residence, but usually do not have adequate generational depth to reconstruct pedigrees and identify kin who lived outside the household.

This analysis is accordingly a substantial advance over efforts by others to study associations between kinship and social and demographic behavior. By longitudinally linking individuals for whom we have historical household registers over as many as seven generations, we can trace a subset of our population from the middle of the eighteenth century to the beginning of the twentieth, and reconstruct their kin networks. From 1789 onwards, the registers organize individuals by household; thus, we can distinguish kin according to the closeness of their relationship, and whether they lived in the same household or village. We can compute measures of the aggregate characteristics of different units of kin organization, including the household, household group, and the descent group, and compare their effects, controlling for village of residence. In the future, with the additional collection of corollary auxiliary information on local economic, institutional, and social conditions, we expect to relate behavior not just to kinship, but also to environmental circumstances, including economic circumstances and occupational history.

This analysis is also a substantial advance over our own previous efforts to examine the associations between kinship and social and demographic outcomes. Most of our previous analyses have focused on effects of characteristics of kin in the same household, in particular, how the number, relationship, and positions held by close kin affected mortality outcomes (Campbell and Lee 1996, 2000; Lee and Campbell 1997). More recently, we explored the role that distant kin played in attainment processes, and showed that while having distant kin who held position increased an individual's own chances of attainment, descent lines were not able to monopolize official positions (Campbell and Lee 2003a). This analysis is distinguished from such previous analyses by its emphasis on the role of aggregate characteristics of kin networks at different scales, and the interaction among demographic and social processes.

Our data allow us to account for the communities in which kin networks were embedded. The community has long been recognized as a primary unit of social organization and a potentially important determinant of individual outcomes, demographic and otherwise. Ethnographies of urban neighborhoods and rural villages have been a staple of the fields of anthropology and sociology since their inceptions. Whether in an urban neighborhood or a rural village, the community is a physical, economic, and social context that individuals experience every day. It is accordingly a key locus for social interactions that circulate information and shape aspirations, expectations, preferences, and norms. In rural areas, the community may be the primary source of economic opportunity and access to education, health care, and other services.

In the United States, quantitative research on community effects focuses on the hypothesis that neighborhood context affects demographic, health, and socioeconomic attainment above and beyond what can be accounted for by individual and family characteristics (Wilson 1987). Empirical results have been mixed, reflecting the enormous complexity of the appropriate definitions, data, and methods (Jencks and Mayer 1990). Several specific mechanisms have been proposed to account for reported effects, including socialization through peer groups, physiological effects of stress from living in a poor neighborhood, social capital, and "collective efficacy" (Sampson, Morenoff, and Gannon-Rowley 2002). Recent studies assess the importance of hypothesized mechanisms, especially "collective efficacy," through innovative approaches to data collection and analysis (Sampson and Raudenbush 1999; Sampson et al. 1997).

Recent quantitative studies in developing countries focus on implications of community context for reproductive behavior and health. The potential importance of community context was recognized some time ago (Freedman 1974) and major data collections such as the World Fertility Survey and the Demographic and Health Survey included modules for community contextual variables. Early analyses based on these data examined how community characteristics, especially the presence of family planning programs or the availability of contraception, affected fertility-related behavior (Tsui et al. 1981; Entwisle, Casterline, and Sayed 1989; Entwisle et al. 1984, 1996). Other studies examine the importance of measured and unmeasured community characteristics on mortality, especially among infants and children (Sastry 1996). A number of mechanisms have been suggested to explain observed effects, including direct effects of availability of programs and services, social learning and influence via personal networks (Watkins, Behrman, and Kohler 2002; Rosero-Bixby and Casterline 1993; Entwisle et al. 1996), and better provision of public goods in villages with more social capital and higher levels of "collective efficacy" (Frankenberg 2004; Tsai 2004).

We take advantage of our data not only to assess the relative importance of kin group and community in determining individual outcomes, but to investigate how they interact. Following Frankenberg (2004), we assess whether villages with higher levels of "collective efficacy" had higher levels of well-being, as reflected in demographic outcomes. We capture the "collective efficacy" of a village with an entropy measure of descent group diversity. We assume that villages in which residents were more likely to be related to each other had higher levels of mutual trust and social cohesion that facilitated the provision of public goods such as security, irrigation, mutual assistance in fieldwork, and so forth. Tsai (2004) has already reported that in contemporary China, villages dominated by single descent groups appear to be more effective at provision of public goods.

3 Data

The data we use are a subset of one of the larger and longer individual-level longitudinal panel data sets assembled for microlevel historical studies. To construct this larger dataset, we have linked as many as 17 generations from the seventeenth century to the present with 275,000 individual histories, their households, their descent groups, and their demographic and social outcomes. For this analysis, we make use of household register data from 1749 to 1909 that come from triennial registers for almost 500 villages from Liaoning province. We have linked the register populations to other historical populations recorded in family genealogies and grave inscriptions from these same villages, and to other contemporary populations of their descendants recorded in current censal and household registers as well as retrospective surveys. We have also located and linked a variety of contextual information about the region and specific communities.

The household register data have four distinct features that make them uniquely suited to address a variety of substantive questions in historical demography and family sociology. First, they are longitudinal and individual level and include not only demographic information, but social, economic, and political information as well. Second, they locate individuals within their households and kin groups, distinguishing kin by relationship and coresidence. Third, they follow the population from the middle of the seventeenth century to the beginning of the twentieth. Fourth, the regions and villages covered by the data are numerous and varied enough to test many of the assertions about the relationships between kinship and demography over space and time. Thus, while the population covered by the data may not be representative of China or even Liaoning in a formal statistical sense, the great diversity of contexts suggests that these results transcend the specific populations under analysis.

We have been able to produce such historical data because of the internal consistency of the core household register data, their availability through the Genealogical Society of Utah and the Liaoning Provincial Archives, and the sustained efforts of teams of colleagues and data entry operators in the People's Republic of China. We have described the data and data entry operation elsewhere (Ding et al. 2004; Lee and Campbell 1997; Lee and Wang 1999). In addition, since 1998 an on-going collaborative project with the Liaoning Provincial Local History Office allows us to visit these villages to collect historical and contemporary population sources, survey specific lineages, and record analogous contemporary information to the historical records. All together, we have spent over 500 person-days in fieldwork visiting almost 50 of the largest villages to collect over 30 bound genealogies and over 50 genealogical charts and lists. We have also collected and transcribed dozens of long historical grave inscriptions, half a dozen other inscriptions, and half a dozen contemporary village census or household registers. Most importantly, we have completed retrospective and contemporary surveys in over a dozen villages recording each individual born in the village since 1949, their birth, marriage, death dates, education, occupation, and migration history and have linked these contemporary and historical populations.

Table 3.1 summarizes the currently linked data: 1.3 million observations of 250,000 individuals who lived between 1750 and 1909 of which 1,066,004 observations for 187,389 individuals have been checked and cleaned; 80 largely patrilineal genealogies with some 25,000 largely male descendents and their spouses who lived between 1650 and 2000; 30 inscriptions from 1770 to 1940 with as many as 1,000 linked relatives; and 11 retrospective surveys and 3 contemporary household registers with over 15,000 individuals born between 1880 and 2002. By supplementing the household registers with genealogies and other historical sources, we can trace 20,000 individuals from the arrival of their descent group founders in Liaoning in the late seventeenth century forward to the present. In addition, by surveying contemporary descendants from these historical populations and linking them to the registers, we can trace 50,000 people from the present back to the mid-eighteenth century.

For this analysis, we make use of the triennial historical household registers that provide detailed information on social outcomes, demographic behavior, and kinship

Table 3.1 Demographic sources for Liaoning (as of January 2006)

Location	Period	Registers	Observations	Coding	Genealogies	Inscriptions, etc.	Survey
Aerjishan	1813–1909	18	13,622	Done	7	5	5
Bakeshu	1759–1909	32	48,709	Done	10	14	4
Changzhaizi	1768–1909	25	46,810	Done			
Chengnei	1798–1909	24	55,671	Done			
Dadianzi	1756–1909	27	76,984	Done	2	1	
Dami	1759–1909	32	31,544	Done	2		
Daoyitun	1774–1909	35	118,633	Done	20	7	6
Daxintun	1749–1909	29	86,956	Done	10		1
Diaopitun	1768–1909	26	70,153	Done			
Feicheng	1756–1909	39	70,175	Done	8	5	
Gaizhou Manhan	1753–1909	20	50,110	Done			
Gaizhou Mianding	1789–1909	25	56,051	Done			
Gaizhou	1762–1909	27	42,834	Done	4		
Guosantun	1774–1909	34	35,073	Done	4	2	1
Haizhou	1759–1909	26	119,207	Done	14	5	2
Kaidang	1810–1852	7	4,476	Done			
Kaidang Toucong Baoyang	1792–1888	12	13,310	Done			
Langjiabao	1756–1909	25	47,340	Done	1	3	2
Nianmadahaizhai	1749–1909	29	53,882	Done	4	9	1
Niuzhuang Liuerbao	1780–1906	23	50,253	Done	16	20	5
Subai	1864–1910	9	3,787	Done			
Wangduoluoshu Rending	1792–1909	16	18,404	Done			
Wangduoluoshu Shengding	1864–1910	8	9,043	Done			
Wangzhihuitun	1765–1909	28	60,339	Done		5	
Waziyu	1777–1906	21	55,522	Done			
Wuhu	1789–1906	23	39,373	Done			
Zhaohuatun	1774–1909	26	50,865	Done	1	1	

organization for a population of hereditary royal peasants between 1749 and 1909. As summarized in Table 3.1, we have completed data entry and data cleaning of the household registers for 28 administrative populations. While we do not make use of the linked genealogies and other data in this analysis, we have begun to examine it in another publication (Campbell and Lee 2002).

The institutional contexts of these populations varied dramatically. While most of these populations produced grain, several of them produced more specialized goods. The Dami population gathered honey, the Gaizhou Mianding population raised cotton, and the Diaopitun population produced animal furs. While most of these populations consisted of royal peasants, some, such as Aerjishan, were royal serfs. Others, such as Gaizhou Mianding, were in-between. As a result of such institutional variation, the opportunities for economic, educational, political, and social advancement varied across populations. Members of some populations were eligible to take state examinations, serve in state offices, and to earn state titles; others were not.

The registers record these populations more completely than almost any other historic rural population in China because they were affiliated with the imperial household as royal peasants or royal serfs, and because they were organized under the Han Martial Banners and therefore liable for military service. The Imperial Household Agency surveyed and registered the population triennially beginning in 1749 with the establishment of the General Office of the Three Banner Commandry, and designed a system of internal cross-checks to ensure data consistency and accuracy. First, they assigned every person in the banner population to a residential household called a *linghu* and registered them on a household certificate. Then they organized households into local household groups called *zu*, and compiled annually updated local household registers. Finally, every 3 years, they compared these local registers and household certificates with the previous larger population and household register to compile a new register. They deleted and added people who had exited or entered in the last 3 years and updated the ages, relationships, and official positions, as well as any changes in their given names, of those people who remained. Each register, in other words, completely superseded its predecessor.

The registers list each individual one-to-a-column in order of their relationship to the household head, with his children and grandchildren listed first, followed by coresident siblings and their descendants, and uncles, aunts, and cousins. Wives are always listed immediately after their husbands, unless a coresident widowed mother-in-law supersedes them. For each person in the target population, the registers report the following information: relationship to their household head; name(s) and name changes; adult banner status; age; animal birth year; lunar birth month, birth day, and birth hour; marriage, death, or emigration, if any during the intercensal period; physical disabilities, if any; and if the person is an adult male; name of their household group head; banner affiliation; and village of residence. For adult males, the registers also record official titles and occupations that allow us to measure individual income or wealth. Of males, 4 percent held such titles at some point in their life; they and their families comprise the rural local elite. For working-age males, the registers also record whether or not they were considered disabled

(Campbell and Lee 2003b). Additional information, such as reproductive histories, is available through record linkage and comparison. Since individuals are listed in the same order in successive registers, longitudinal linkage of entries is straightforward.

As Figure 3.1 shows, the more than 500 Liaoning villages are arranged in four distinct regions over an area of $40,000\,km^2$, approximately the size of the Netherlands: a southern coastal region near Gaizhou on the Liaodong peninsula; a commercialized agricultural plain centered on Niuzhuang and Haicheng; an administrative center located on the Liaodong Plain around what is now Shenyang, the provincial capital; and a remote agricultural area in the hills and mountain ranges directly north and northeast of what is now Shenyang, near Tieling and Kaiyuan. These pronounced regional differences enable us to test a variety of hypotheses about socioeconomic conditions and demographic behavior, and measure regional characteristics as well as shared processes and relationships. The common immigration origins and institutional background of our communities allow us to control for such particular circumstances. While our results only illuminate the behavior of specific Chinese populations, we can draw from them implications for the demography not of China as a whole, but of specific social, economic, and political systems. This strategy, comparing local rather than national contexts, avoids the problem of representativeness normally inherent in community studies.

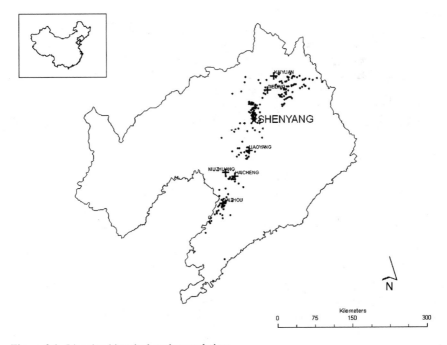

Figure 3.1 Liaoning historical study populations

These registers have a number of features that distinguish them as a source for historical demography. In contrast with historical Chinese demographic sources such as genealogies that only record adult males, the historical registers record most boys and some girls from childhood as well as all women from the time of their marriage. Unlike genealogies, they also provide detail on village and household residence. In contrast with parish registers, an important source for European historical demography, they allow for precise measurement of the population at risk of experiencing most demographic events and social outcomes. We have already used the registers to investigate the determinants of individual survivorship (Campbell and Lee 1996, 2000, 2002, 2004), marriage (Lee and Campbell 1998a, b), migration (Campbell and Lee 2001), ethnic identity (Campbell, Lee, and Elliott 2002), and social mobility (Campbell and Lee 2003a). We have also examined trends in demographic outcomes (Lee and Campbell 2005). These publications also detail the strengths and limitations of the register data relevant to the analysis of each outcome.

One of the most important features of the register data is that they follow families for as many as seven generations, from the middle of the eighteenth century to the beginning of the twentieth. The population is closed, in the sense that the registers followed families that moved from one village to another within the region. Entries into and exits from the region were rare, and when they did occur, their timing was recorded (Lee and Campbell 1997, 223–37; Lee and Wang 1999, 149–53). Through linkage within the registers, therefore, we can identify the paternal kin of individuals, even if they live in other households or even villages. Table 3.2 summarizes the results of the linkage we have already carried out within the household registers. We can locate a great-great-grandfather within the registers for 50.2 percent of men overall, and 83.0 percent of men who first appear after 1900. Figure 3.2 presents this information in graphical form, summarizing the proportion of children in each register for whom specified patrilineal ancestors can be located.

Through such linkage, we have grouped the individuals in the registers into descent groups defined by descent from a common male ancestor who may have lived before the earlier register in 1749. By assuming that households with the same surname who

Table 3.2 Males by number of generations of ancestry in registers (March 2004)

Paternal Ancestor	Percentage of males for whom specified ancestor can be located	
	All males	Appearing after 1900
Father	89.6	92.8
Grandfather	78.6	89.2
Great-grandfather	65.2	87.1
Great-great-grandfather	50.2	83.0
Great-great-great-grandfather	34.3	73.2
Great-great-great-great-grandfather	19.4	51.3
Great-great-great-great-great-grandfather	8.7	25.0
Great-great-great-great-great-great-grandfather	3.3	9.8
N	103,402	23,112

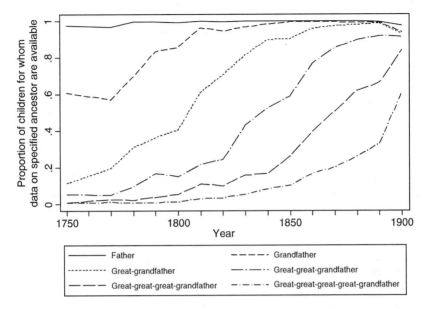

Figure 3.2 Proportions of children in each triennial register for whom specified paternal ancestors can be located via linkage within the database, 1750–1900

are listed consecutively in a register are related, these descent lines can be further aggregated into 2,136 descent groups defined by descent from a male founder who preceded the registers. The 743 largest groups account for 95 percent of the population. The small descent groups with only a few identified members consist mostly of members of households that were first recorded in the registers in the late nineteenth century or beginning of the twentieth and could not be linked to a larger group.

The registers also identify an analytically interesting unit of family organization between the residential household and the descent group: the household group. Household groups were administrative units that consisted of one or more closely related residential households, all in the same village and in close proximity to each other, and all part of the same descent group. Headship of the household group was an unsalaried official position and the lowest rung in the administrative hierarchy. Household group heads had a variety of powers and responsibilities.

Our data allow for an analysis that distinguishes the roles of each of four levels of social and family organization in accounting for individual social and demographic outcomes: village, descent group, household group, and household. Table 3.3 provides the mean numbers of lower levels of organization within each level. Thus, it provides the average numbers of observations, and distinct individuals, households, household groups, and descent groups per village, and so on. The data are clearly adequate to distinguish correlations across and within levels of organization. There are an average of 5.12 descent groups per village, 3.60 household groups per descent group, 2.91 households per household group, and 9.11 individuals per household.

Table 3.3 Average numbers of lower level units within each unit

	Villages	Descent groups	Household groups	Households	Individuals	Observations
Average numbers of Observations	1173.76	227.11	63.10	21.71	2.38	
Distinct individuals	492.54	95.30	26.48	9.11		
Distinct households	54.06	10.46	2.91			
Distinct household groups	18.60	3.60				
Distinct descent groups	5.17					
N	541	2,796[a]	10,064	29,247	266,463	635,005

[a] There are 2,136 distinct descent groups in the registers. 2,796 is a count of distinct descent groups within villages, in which descent groups spread across multiple villages are counted once for each village their members appear in.

4 Methods

We first assess the relative importance of the household, household group, descent group, and village as units of social organization through discrete-time event history analyses of four outcomes: male attainment of official position, male first marriage, male marital fertility, and mortality by sex. For the three binary outcomes, i.e., attainment of position, first marriage, and mortality, we estimate logistic regressions. The dependent variable in each case is the probability of experiencing the outcome of interest in the period between the current register and the next. For female marital fertility, the dependent variable is the number of male births between the current register and the next that survive to be registered. Since this is a count, we estimate a Poisson regression. For all four event history analyses, analysis is restricted to the registers where the one immediately succeeding or the one after that is available; thus, the outcomes of interest occur in either the next 3 or 4 years.

We model the individual probabilities of attainment, male marriage, male fertility, and mortality as functions of the incidence or prevalence of these outcomes in the village, descent group, household group, and household, along with a set of control variables. For mortality and fertility, we calculate the relevant rates per 1,000 at risk at each level. For male marriage, we use prevalence, in the form of the number of males per 1,000 aged 16–55 *sui* currently married. For attainment, we also use prevalence, in the form of the number of males per 1,000 aged 16–55 *sui* who currently hold a position. When we generate incidence or prevalence indices for these outcomes at each level, to use as right-hand side variables, we exclude the experience of the index individual's unit from the calculation for the unit above. Thus, measures for the village exclude the individual's descent group; measures for the descent group exclude the individual's household group; measures for the household group exclude the individual's household; and measures for the household exclude the individual. Since this measure is undefined in situations when the unit at the level above contains only one unit from the level below, for example, when a household group includes only one household, observations from such clusters are excluded from the analysis.

Equations 1 and 2 summarize the basic forms of the models we estimate. The first model, summarized by equation 1, examines associations within outcomes. The transformed probability of an outcome y for an individual at time t is a linear function of a constant term, a set of control variables, the village average for that outcome x_v, the descent group average x_{vd}, the household group average x_{vdg}, and the household average x_{vdgh}. As noted above, each average excludes information from the level below that contains the individual. Coefficients reflect the association between the individual's chances of experiencing the outcome and the rates at the different levels. The second model, summarized by equation 2, examines associations across outcomes. $\mathbf{X}_v$ is a vector of averages at the village level for the four outcomes; $\mathbf{X}_{vd}$ is a vector of averages at the descent group level, and so forth. Table 3.4 summarizes the means and standard deviations of the right-hand side measures X at each level. Controls not listed in Table 4 include fixed effects of register year and region. With these fixed effects, the coefficients for the characteristics of the four units of social organization reflect comparisons within the same geographic region at the same point in time. We also include controls for the age of the index individual.

Table 3.4 Means of the right-hand side variables used in analyses of associations across and within outcomes

	Mean	S.D.
Male deaths in next 3 years (per 1,000)		
Village, excluding descent group	51.39	31.54
Descent group, excluding household group	49.91	41.72
Household group, excluding household	54.51	64.11
Household, excluding self	52.70	81.72
Female deaths in next 3 years (per 1,000)		
Village, excluding descent group	64.16	28.28
Descent group, excluding household group	63.49	41.58
Household group, excluding household	69.01	77.05
Household, excluding self	67.03	106.07
Adult males 16–55 *sui* currently married (per 1,000)		
Village, excluding descent group	644.74	116.76
Descent group, excluding household group	659.19	128.65
Household group, excluding household	656.14	184.39
Household, excluding self	696.59	240.43
Adult males 16–55 *sui* with official position (per 1,000)		
Village, excluding descent group	61.62	177.87
Descent group, excluding household group	61.30	196.09
Household group, excluding household	56.95	192.67
Household, excluding self	59.68	200.94
Male births in next 3 years (per 1,000 married adult females 16–45 *sui*)		
Village, excluding descent group	167.09	57.41
Descent group, excluding household group	171.63	80.33
Household group, excluding household	171.04	120.92
Household, excluding self	175.95	172.99

$$f(p(y_{vdghit})) = a_0 + \mathbf{B_0 X} + b_1 x_v + b_2 x_{vd} + b_3 x_{vdg} + b_4 x_{vdgh} \tag{1}$$

$$f(p(y_{vdghit})) = a_0 + \mathbf{B_0 X} + \mathbf{B_1 X_v} + \mathbf{B_2 X_{vd}} + \mathbf{B_3 X_{vdg}} + \mathbf{B_4 X_{vdgh}} \tag{2}$$

By including the prevalence or incidence of the outcome at each level in each event history analysis, we identify the units of kinship or community organization that were the most important loci for determining the chances of the outcomes of interest. To the extent that one of the four levels that we consider was meaningful for determining a particular outcome, an individual's chances of experiencing that outcome should be correlated with the incidence or prevalence of the outcome at that level. If a particular level is unimportant for determining an outcome, correlations between individual risks and the incidence or prevalence at that level should be zero. Effects of common membership in higher or lower levels are accounted for by the incidence or prevalence measures at those levels.

Through this approach, we identify the units of organization that were meaningful in the sense of forming the world that on a day-to-day basis dominated the interactions, decisions, perceptions, and resource flows that governed demographic and social outcomes. To the extent that the individuals who composed one unit had relevant interactions with each other but not with members of the larger unit one level up, estimations should reveal associations with prevalence or incidence within the lower level unit but not within the higher level one. If the interactions that an individual had with other members of one level were entirely accounted for by their common membership of a higher level, only a correlation with the higher level should be apparent.

Thus, for example, if the primary units of organization in late imperial Chinese society were the household and village, event history analysis should reveal that individual risks of each of the four outcomes were most tightly correlated with rates in the household and village and uncorrelated with rates in the household group and descent group. If the interactions between kin who lived in separate households had more concrete implications, whether because they shared tangible resources like land or labor or intangible resources like prestige, then analysis should reveal that individual outcomes were also correlated with rates for the same outcome in the household group or descent group.

To address such questions, of course, our preferred approach would have been variance decomposition through estimations of multilevel models that allowed for correlations within each of the levels. At the time we were carrying out the analysis, however, that was not practical. The combination of binary outcome measures with the large number of levels, clusters at each level, and observations, precluded estimation of an appropriate model with any of the software available to us. We have begun to experiment with multilevel linear-probability models and more capable computing equipment, and hope to report results from those efforts in the near future. In the meantime, we believe that the results we report here are broadly indicative of underlying patterns and associations.

We examine associations in attainment and male marriage indices to measure the flow of economic, social, and political resources, tangible and intangible, within each unit of organization. Thus, we include the prevalence of official positions among males to measure directly how the social, economic, and political status of a unit affected the outcomes of members. Official positions measured with the attainment indices carried with them considerable prestige, substantial salaries and perquisites, and in many cases administrative power. The prevalence of male marriage is intended as a more indirect measure of how the social, economic, and political standing of a unit affected outcomes for its members. In late imperial China, male marriage was highly competitive because of an overall shortage of marriageable females; thus, units of organization with higher than expected proportions married shared something tangible, like economic resources, or intangible, like prestige, that advantaged their men in the competition for brides.

Male marriage chances in late imperial Chinese society depended not only on individual characteristics, but also on family economic, political, and social status. Identifying the unit of organization within which marriage chances were correlated locates the boundaries of kin groups within which economic resources as well as less tangible social and political resources like power and prestige circulated. For example, to the extent that male marriage chances were determined largely by local marriage market characteristics and the characteristics of their own household, not the household group or descent group, marriage chances should be correlated within households, but not within household groups or descent groups. Since we consider the proportion married indicative of economic, social, or political status, we are of course interested in how it affects attainment, fertility, and mortality chances.

Our inclusion of the mortality and fertility rates is more exploratory and motivated by a desire to understand how interrelationships between demographic processes affected each other, the marriage market, and attainment chances. We are especially interested in seeing how fertility and mortality affected the chances of other outcomes. We expect mortality to have increased male marriage chances, and for two reasons. First, kin networks may have responded to the loss of the labor of a member through death by bringing in a bride for a never-married male. To the extent that males in a kin group competed for brides, in effect forming a queue and marrying in order of seniority, higher death rates may have improved marriage chances by advancing the queue more quickly.

In a separate set of models, we examine the interaction between village and kin group organization. Following Tsai (2004) and Frankenberg (2004), we hypothesize that the villages that are more homogeneous with respect to descent groups will generate higher levels of "collective efficacy", and have better provision of public goods that require coordination and cooperation such as security, irrigation, mutual assistance, and land improvement. We expect that, in a rural setting, higher levels of "collective efficacy" will generate favorable social and demographic outcomes, including earlier marriage, higher marital fertility, later death, and higher social attainment.

We summarize the variables in this analysis in Table 3.5. To measure descent group diversity within a village, we calculate an entropy-based index. We use an entropy measure of descent group diversity, summarized by equation 3. In the equation,

Table 3.5 Means of the right-hand side variables used in the assessment of effects of descent group diversity

	Mean	S.D.	Minimum	Maximum
Population				
Village	211.0		1	2361
Descent group	92.4		1	1119
Household group	26.0		1	344
Household	9.4		1	117
Population (log base 1.1)				
Village	56.15	12.87	0.00	81.49
Descent group	47.49	12.07	0.00	73.66
Household group	34.19	10.00	0.00	61.28
Household	23.46	8.81	0.00	49.97
Entropy measures of diversity				
Descent groups within village	1.35	0.90	0.00	3.14
Descent group among villages	0.48	0.52	0.00	2.38
Proportion of village same descent group	0.44	0.35	0.00	1.00

N is the total population of the village, and n_i is the number of individuals in the village who are members of descent group i. Thus, the measure is the products of the proportion of village population in each descent group and the log of that proportion. For a village in which there is only one descent group, the measure will be zero. Higher values correspond to increasing diversity. A village evenly divided between two descent groups will have a value of 0.69, and a village evenly divided between 10 descent groups will have a measure of 2.3.

$$E = - \Sigma \, (n_i/N) \, \text{In} \, (n_i/N) \qquad (3)$$

We also assess the importance of the share of village population accounted for by the individual's descent group. We expect that larger descent groups within the village should have enjoyed returns to scale. They should have been able to offer more assistance to their members, whether by backing them in local disputes or carrying out collective projects. We expect that the numerically dominant descent groups within a village were also better poised to capture the benefits from public goods generated within the village. The measure ranges from just above zero for individuals who had no kin living in the same village, to one for individuals living in villages made up of a single descent group.

We also examine how the geographic spread of a descent group affected the outcomes of its members. We hypothesize that descent groups whose members were distributed among more than one village will have more favorable outcomes. One of the roles frequently claimed for descent groups in China was that of safety net. Individuals who had kin living in other villages should have been less affected by local shocks specific to the village in which they lived because of the availability of help elsewhere. Kin in other villages should also have been a source of information about opportunities, economic and otherwise. We measure the geographic spread of a descent group with another entropy measure, constructed as in equation 3, where n_i is the number of descent group members living in village i, and N is the total number of members of the descent group.

5 Results

We organize our discussion of results of the assessment of the importance of village, descent group, household group, and household by outcome. We begin with male first marriage, followed by attainment of official position, female marital fertility based on male births, and mortality. For each of the four outcomes, we begin by considering how individual chances correlated with rates for the same outcome within the village, descent group, household group, and household. To gain insight into the interrelationships across outcomes, we then examine how individual chances for each outcome correlated with the rates of the other three outcomes at each of the four levels of organization. We present the relevant results in Tables 3.6 through 3.9. As mentioned earlier, this identifies the loci within which the interactions that shaped outcomes occurred. Later, after completing the discussion of relationships within and across outcomes at different levels, we discuss the results on village descent group diversity.

5.1 Marriages

Every level of social organization, from the household up to the village, played a role in influencing male marriage prospects. Male marriage chances were correlated with rates at every level even when rates observed at other levels were accounted for. The results for male first marriage in column A of Table 3.6 reveal that men who lived in villages where higher proportions of men were already married were themselves more likely to marry. This likely reflects geographic variation in marriage market conditions. Within the village, marriage chances for men varied further according to which descent group they were in. The men in the descent groups in which higher proportions of males were already married were themselves more likely to marry. Within the descent group, men in household groups where higher proportions of males were married were themselves more likely to marry. Finally, within a household group, the men in the households in which higher proportions of males were married were themselves more likely to marry.

When it came to male marriage prospects, the benefits of the economic, social, and political resources associated with being related to someone with an official position were limited to members of the residential household. Table 3.7 presents associations across outcomes for the different levels of organization. According to the results for male marriage in column A, men who lived in households in which higher proportions of men held official positions were themselves more likely to

Table 3.6 Event history analyses of associations within outcomes

	Male first marriage (A)		Male attainment (B)		Female marital fertility (based on male births) (C)		Male mortality (ages 1–75 *sui*) (D)		Female mortality (ages 1–75 *sui*) (E)	
	Coeff.	p	Coeff.	p	Coeff.	p	Coeff.	p	Coeff.	p
Village, excluding descent group	0.0006	0.00	0.0003	0.47	0.0009	0.00	0.0022	0.00	0.0016	0.00
Descent group, excluding household group	0.0007	0.00	0.0020	0.00	0.0004	0.00	0.0001	0.64	−0.0001	0.86
Household group, excluding household	0.0008	0.00	0.0030	0.00	0.0006	0.00	0.0013	0.00	0.0013	0.00
Household, excluding self	0.0009	0.00	0.0036	0.00	0.0006	0.00	0.0015	0.00	0.0015	0.00
Observations	34,505		146,333		93,018		261,965		162,939	
Log likelihood	−19075.8		−3326.3		−45106.4		−46216.8		−35862.6	
Pseudo R squared	0.032		0.0937		0.0232		0.0891		0.06	

Table 3.7 Event history analyses of associations within and across outcomes

	Male first marriage (A)		Male attainment (B)		Female marital fertility (based on male births) (C)		Male mortality (ages 1–75 *sui*) (D)		Female mortality (ages 1–75 *sui*) (E)	
	Coeff.	p	Coeff.	p	Coeff.	p	Coeff.	p	Coeff.	p
Male deaths in next 3 years (per 1,000)										
Village, excluding descent group	0.0006	0.47	0.0002	0.96	−0.0003	0.50	0.0011	0.05	0.0016	0.01
Descent group, excluding household group	0.0000	0.94	−0.0006	0.66	−0.0001	0.66	0.0000	0.90	0.0001	0.87
Household group, excluding household	−0.0005	0.12	0.0005	0.66	−0.0001	0.77	0.0009	0.00	0.0006	0.01
Household, excluding self	−0.0002	0.17	0.0001	0.92	−0.0002	0.26	0.0012	0.00	0.0024	0.00
Female deaths in next 3 years (per 1,000)										
Village, excluding descent group	−0.0005	0.39	0.0017	0.43	0.0001	0.77	0.0011	0.01	0.0010	0.04
Descent group, excluding household group	0.0009	0.02	−0.0027	0.09	0.0002	0.39	0.0003	0.32	−0.0001	0.67
Household group, excluding household	0.0006	0.00	−0.0008	0.31	0.0003	0.03	0.0007	0.00	0.0011	0.00
Household, excluding self	0.0001	0.65	−0.0012	0.06	−0.0001	0.53	0.0015	0.00	0.0011	0.00
Adult males currently married (per 1,000)										
Village, excluding descent group	0.0006	0.00	−0.0003	0.62	−0.0002	0.11	0.0000	0.94	0.0002	0.10
Descent group, excluding household group	0.0007	0.00	0.0008	0.08	0.0001	0.15	0.0000	0.84	0.0000	0.75
Household group, excluding household	0.0008	0.00	0.0000	0.95	0.0000	0.81	0.0001	0.10	0.0001	0.08
Household, excluding self	0.0009	0.00	0.0013	0.00	0.0001	0.06	0.0001	0.00	−0.0005	0.00
Adult males with position (per 1,000)										
Village, excluding descent group	−0.0001	0.63	0.0004	0.33	0.0001	0.22	0.0000	0.72	−0.0001	0.39
Descent group, excluding household group	−0.0002	0.30	0.0022	0.00	−0.0004	0.00	−0.0002	0.24	0.0003	0.06
Household group, excluding household	−0.0004	0.04	0.0032	0.00	−0.0002	0.07	−0.0001	0.54	−0.0002	0.15
Household, excluding self	0.0006	0.00	0.0032	0.00	0.0003	0.00	0.0003	0.00	0.0000	0.95
Male births in next 3 years (per 1,000 married adult females)										
Village, excluding descent group	−0.0002	0.36	0.0004	0.65	0.0009	0.00	0.0004	0.02	0.0000	0.93
Descent group, excluding household group	0.0004	0.03	−0.0004	0.52	0.0004	0.00	0.0002	0.14	0.0002	0.24
Household group, excluding household	0.0004	0.00	0.0005	0.20	0.0006	0.00	0.0003	0.00	0.0003	0.00
Household, excluding self	0.0006	0.00	0.0008	0.00	0.0006	0.00	0.0001	0.03	0.0001	0.24
Observations	34,505		146,333		93,018		261,965		162,939	
Log likelihood	−19015.4		−3291.01		−45082.4		−46027.7		−35692.2	
Pseudo R squared	0.035		0.1033		0.0237		0.0928		0.0645	

marry. Households within the same group appeared to have competed in the marriage market: there was actually an adverse effect of having higher proportions of males in the household group who held official position.

Males were also more likely to marry if their kin had higher rates of marital fertility. According to the results for effects of female marital fertility at the bottom of Table 3.7, unmarried men in descent groups that had higher marital fertility were more likely to marry. There was further correlation within household groups that were part of the same descent group, and within households that were part of the same descent group. This was not the result of local variations in marital fertility determining marriage markets: there was no general effect of marital fertility at the village level. Neither was this due to some general effect on marriage and marital fertility of the prosperity of kin. As noted earlier, possession of position by kin benefited males only if the kin who held position lived in the same household.

5.2   Attainment

Kin networks played a key role in stratification in rural society. Variation in attainment of official position among descent groups within the same village was more important than variation between villages. Results in column B of Table 3.6 reveal that living in a village in which higher proportions of males held official position did not increase the chances that a male would himself attain an official position. Within the village, however, membership in a descent group in which higher proportions of men held an official position raised the chances of obtaining one. There was further differentiation among household groups in the same descent group, and among households in the same household.

As noted earlier, interrelationships between attainment and demographic behavior again appear to have been confined to members of the same household. Results in column B of Table 3.7 indicate that men in households in which higher proportions of men were married were more likely to attain an official position. Results in the same column indicate that men living in households that had higher levels of marital fertility were also more likely to attain an official position. In light of the results for determinants of male marriage in column A, the implication is that within households, attainment, male marriage chances, and marital fertility were interrelated. Households that were especially successful at one outcome were more successful at the others.

5.3   Fertility

For female marital fertility, correlations with rates at every level of organization were apparent. According to column C of Table 3.6, married women had higher chances of bearing children in the next 3 years if they lived in villages in which other women had higher marital fertility, or were members of descent groups, household groups, or households in which the other women had higher marital fertility. Given that the measures of fertility rely on births that survived to registration, this may either reflect correlations in actual fertility, or correlations in mortality in infancy and early childhood. Either way, it is clear that there was substantial variation in the success with which the residents of villages and the members of kin networks reproduced themselves.

As was the case with male marriage, relationship to someone who held an official position was only beneficial if they lived in the same household. Women who lived in households in which higher proportions of males held official position had higher birth rates. Kin with official positions who resided in other households or other household groups actually depressed the chances that a woman would have a child, just as they depressed the chances that an unmarried man would marry in the next 3 years. This is further evidence that marriage, reproduction, and attainment covaried at the level of the household, so that households successful at one were successful at the others.

5.4 Mortality

The village was a much more important source of variation in mortality than the descent group. According to columns D and E of Table 3.6, living in a village in which death rates were high raised the chances of dying. Among residents of the same village, being a member of a descent group that had higher death rates had no effect on the chances of dying. Variation in death rates between descent groups in the same village, in other words, was random. At lower levels of organization within the descent group, there were associations. Being a member of a household group or a household in which death rates were high raised the chances of dying. This likely reflects common exposure to the same sources of infection. Household groups generally consisted of adjacent households. Their members had more contact with each other than they did with other members of the same descent group. They were also more likely to experience the same local environment.

Mortality was intertwined with other demographic outcomes, but the relationships are less consistent than the ones among marriage, attainment, and fertility, reflecting the complexity of the determinants of mortality. Male mortality was higher in households in which higher proportions of males were married; but female mortality in such households was actually lower. Male mortality was higher in households in which higher proportions of men held position, consistent with the price of privilege that we have observed in previous analyses, according to which higher status males in Liaoning actually experienced higher mortality risks (Lee and Campbell 1997). Finally, males experienced higher mortality in villages, household groups, and households in which female marital fertility was higher.

To illuminate the mechanisms underlying these mortality patterns, we consider mortality by age group and sex in Tables 3.8 and 3.9. The results indicate that for mortality,

Table 3.8 Event history analyses of associations within mortality outcomes for each age group and sex

	Male mortality						Female mortality					
	1–15 *sui*		16–55 *sui*		56–75 *sui*		1–15 *sui* (Central Region)		16–55 *sui*		56–75 *sui*	
	Coeff.	p	Coeff.	p	Coeff.	p	Coeff.	p	Coeff.	p	Coeff.	p
Village, excluding descent group	0.0028	0.00	0.0018	0.00	0.0000	0.91	0.0052	0.10	0.0027	0.00	0.0007	0.00
Descent group, excluding household group	0.0013	0.00	0.0002	0.54	-0.0001	0.52	0.0001	0.94	-0.0001	0.84	0.0005	0.05
Household group, excluding household	0.0011	0.00	0.0014	0.00	0.0004	0.00	-0.0009	0.31	0.0007	0.00	0.0007	0.00
Household, excluding self	0.0009	0.00	0.0010	0.00	0.0003	0.00	0.0015	0.00	0.0012	0.00	0.0005	0.00
Observations	71,553		155,640		17,335		3,493		122,497		18,203	
Log likelihood	-10660.67		-22529.52		-7375.44		-737.44		-22301.84		-6974.61	
Pseudo R squared	0.04		0.04		0.03		0.06		0.02		0.04	

Table 3.9 Event history analyses of associations between outcomes and mortality for each age group and sex

	Male mortality								Female mortality			
	1–15 sui		16–55 sui		56–75 sui		1–15 sui (Central Region)		16–55 sui		56–75 sui	
	Coeff.	p	Coeff.	p	Coeff.	p	Coeff.	p	Coeff.	p	Coeff.	p
Male deaths (per 1,000)												
Village, excluding descent group	0.0002	0.85	0.0014	0.09	0.0014	0.17	0.0112	0.04	0.0016	0.06	0.0016	0.12
Descent group, excluding household group	0.0005	0.39	-0.0004	0.37	0.0003	0.54	-0.0038	0.29	0.0002	0.53	-0.0002	0.72
Household group, excluding household	0.0008	0.06	0.0009	0.00	0.0009	0.02	0.0010	0.53	0.0004	0.25	0.0008	0.04
Household, excluding self	0.0009	0.00	0.0012	0.00	0.0014	0.00	0.0024	0.01	0.0027	0.00	0.0021	0.00
Female deaths (per 1,000)												
Village, excluding descent group	0.0001	0.90	0.0024	0.00	0.0001	0.86	-0.0040	0.22	0.0012	0.07	0.0013	0.08
Descent group, excluding household group	0.0002	0.76	0.0004	0.35	0.0002	0.67	0.0003	0.91	-0.0007	0.12	0.0003	0.54
Household group, excluding household	0.0002	0.43	0.0006	0.00	0.0012	0.00	-0.0002	0.85	0.0010	0.00	0.0015	0.00
Household, excluding self	0.0014	0.00	0.0016	0.00	0.0014	0.00	0.0021	0.00	0.0011	0.00	0.0012	0.00
Adult males currently married (per 1,000)												
Village, excluding descent group	-0.0001	0.59	0.0002	0.31	-0.0001	0.60	0.0012	0.32	0.0003	0.12	0.0002	0.39
Descent group, excluding household group	-0.0004	0.05	0.0002	0.17	0.0001	0.51	-0.0007	0.28	0.0000	0.87	0.0001	0.55
Household group, excluding household	-0.0001	0.34	0.0001	0.23	0.0003	0.02	-0.0006	0.10	0.0001	0.19	0.0002	0.12
Household, excluding self	0.0003	0.00	0.0001	0.28	0.0001	0.08	0.0005	0.15	-0.0010	0.00	-0.0001	0.39
Adult males with position (per 1,000)												
Village, excluding descent group	-0.0001	0.42	0.0001	0.69	0.0000	0.92	0.0003	0.48	-0.0001	0.35	-0.0001	0.64
Descent group, excluding household group	-0.0003	0.28	0.0001	0.73	-0.0002	0.33	0.0001	0.85	0.0002	0.30	0.0005	0.07
Household group, excluding household	-0.0001	0.74	-0.0002	0.30	0.0003	0.23	-0.0010	0.10	-0.0001	0.71	-0.0002	0.42
Household, excluding self	0.0007	0.00	0.0002	0.21	-0.0002	0.43	0.0004	0.28	0.0000	0.96	-0.0002	0.41
Male births (per 1,000 married adult females)												
Village, excluding descent group	0.0011	0.00	0.0001	0.82	0.0004	0.20	-0.0010	0.58	0.0005	0.05	-0.0007	0.04
Descent group, excluding household group	0.0009	0.00	0.0000	0.83	0.0000	0.98	0.0017	0.14	0.0001	0.80	0.0002	0.50
Household group, excluding household	0.0003	0.07	0.0003	0.00	0.0002	0.10	-0.0005	0.37	0.0003	0.01	0.0004	0.00
Household, excluding self	0.0008	0.00	-0.0003	0.00	0.0001	0.19	0.0002	0.59	0.0001	0.33	0.0000	0.78
Observations	79,273		155,640		27,052		5,855		122,497		29,241	
Log likelihood	-11723		-22395.6		-11627.3		-1204.8291		-22098.4		-11210.5	
Pseudo R squared	0.0473		0.0434		0.0353		0.0573		0.0258		0.0436	

the relevant units of organization varied slightly according to age and sex; male child mortality was correlated with rates at each of the four levels; adult male mortality was correlated within villages, household groups, and households; and elderly mortality was correlated only within household groups and households. Female child mortality was correlated only within households, though this result is subject to the caveat that it was based only on data from a region around what is now Shenyang that had less incomplete registration of daughters. Adult female mortality, like adult male mortality, varied within villages, household groups, and households. Elderly female mortality varied with each level.

Relationships between mortality by age and sex and the other demographic outcomes were complex. The most consistent relationship was that male child mortality was actually higher in villages, descent groups, household groups, and households that had higher levels of marital fertility. Whether this was cause or effect, of course, remains unclear. Couples experiencing higher child mortality may have had higher birth rates, or couples with higher birth rates may have experienced higher levels of male mortality.

5.5   Village and Descent Group Interactions

Contrary to our expectations, descent group diversity within a village was generally associated with beneficial demographic outcomes, not adverse ones. According to Table 3.10, the effects of descent group diversity were strong for all of the demographic outcomes, though not attainment. Villages that were diverse in terms of their descent group composition had earlier male first marriage, lower male death rates, and lower female death rates. Early male first marriage, of course, is likely to reflect conditions in the local marriage market. Custom dictated against marrying someone with the same surname, especially if they were members of the same patrilineal descent group. Families in single descent group villages had to search for brides in neighboring villages. In more diverse villages, families had the opportunity to find brides locally, without searching neighboring villages. The apparent beneficial effects of descent group diversity on mortality may similarly reflect the implications of such diversity for patterns of exposure to disease. Villagers were most likely to interact with kin. Among villages of the same size, residents of a single surname village may have been liable to interact with anyone, because village residents were all kin. In another, more diverse village of the same size, a resident had smaller circle of kin with whom they interacted, reducing the chances that they would be exposed to disease. Table 3.11, which distinguishes effects on mortality by age and sex, offers some confirmation. Effects of descent group diversity were much stronger for male child mortality and male elderly mortality than for male adult mortality. Children and the elderly were much more vulnerable to the infectious diseases that spread through casual contact.

The higher marital fertility of residents of less diverse villages, meanwhile, suggests that residents of such villages actually did enjoy some important advantages.

Table 3.10 Event history analyses of associations of outcomes with population size and diversity

	Male first marriage		Male attainment		Female marital fertility (based on male births)		Male mortality (ages 1–75 *sui*)		Female mortality (ages 1–75 *sui*)	
	Coeff.	p	Coeff.	p	Coeff.	p	Coeff.	p	Coeff.	p
Population (log base 1.1)										
Village	0.0004	0.84	0.0169	0.02	0.0082	0.00	0.0096	0.00	0.0069	0.00
Descent group	-0.0009	0.61	-0.0121	0.10	0.0016	0.16	-0.0021	0.09	-0.0013	0.37
Household group	0.0029	0.06	0.0329	0.00	0.0024	0.02	0.0064	0.00	0.0088	0.00
Household	0.0187	0.00	0.0480	0.00	0.0048	0.00	-0.0014	0.17	-0.0078	0.00
Entropy measures of diversity										
Descent groups within village	0.0662	0.01	-0.0434	0.67	-0.0902	0.00	-0.0738	0.00	-0.0703	0.00
Descent group among villages	0.0189	0.50	0.0815	0.44	-0.0556	0.00	-0.0060	0.77	-0.0156	0.50
Proportion of village same descent group	0.0719	0.31	0.4287	0.15	-0.0252	0.58	0.0324	0.53	-0.0773	0.19
Observations	53,917		220,843		140,738		388,910		245,987	
Log likelihood	-28960		-4663.42		-66498.9		-69552.8		-54305.8	
Pseudo R squared	0.02		0.06		0.02		0.09		0.05	

Table 3.11 Event history analyses of associations of mortality by age group and sex with population size and diversity

	Male mortality						Female mortality					
	1–15 *sui*		16–55 *sui*		56–75 *sui*		1–15 *sui*		16–55 *sui*		56–75 *sui*	
	Coeff.	p	Coeff.	p	Coeff.	p	Coeff.	p	Coeff.	p	Coeff.	p
Population (log base 1.1)												
Village	0.009	0.00	0.006	0.00	0.013	0.00	0.021	0.04	0.008	0.00	0.006	0.01
Descent group	0.002	0.44	−0.004	0.06	−0.002	0.29	−0.007	0.45	−0.002	0.38	0.000	0.84
Household group	0.008	0.00	0.004	0.02	0.009	0.00	0.000	1.00	0.009	0.00	0.010	0.00
Household	0.010	0.00	−0.006	0.00	−0.001	0.44	−0.015	0.09	−0.010	0.00	−0.005	0.00
Entropy measures of diversity												
Descent groups within village	−0.127	0.00	−0.018	0.53	−0.112	0.00	−0.190	0.20	−0.063	0.03	−0.085	0.02
Descent group among villages	−0.058	0.21	0.012	0.70	−0.008	0.81	−0.185	0.19	0.002	0.94	−0.047	0.20
Proportion of village same descent group	−0.122	0.32	0.118	0.12	−0.010	0.91	−0.027	0.94	−0.053	0.50	−0.119	0.20
Observations	109,976		234,292		44,642		7,325		185,688		45,883	
Log likelihood	−15925		−34385		−18927		−1507		−33764		−17523	
Pseudo R squared	0.04		0.04		0.03		0.04		0.01		0.03	

It is hard to attribute the fertility effect of descent group diversity to patterns of contacts implied by different levels of diversity. Indeed, if the same network-based mechanisms we offered to account for marriage and mortality effects were relevant for fertility, we would expect diversity to be associated with higher fertility. Our fertility measures are based on children who survived infancy and early childhood and were registered by their parents. To the extent that infant and early childhood mortality was correlated with mortality in later childhood, more diverse villages should have seen more children surviving to be registered by their parents. This is not the case. We suggest that the higher marital fertility of less diverse villages is partial evidence that such villages had higher levels of "collective efficacy" and that these were reflected in improved demographic outcomes.

5.6 *Implications*

Villages and kin groups were all important determinants of demographic and social outcomes. For each demographic and social outcome, there were strong correlations within different levels of organization. Patterns of associations varied, implying that the loci of interactions that were relevant for determining each outcome varied. For marriage, village and concentric layers of kin were all important. For attainment, village was unimportant, but the various layers of kin were. For mortality, village was important, as were household and household group, but descent group was not.

There were associations across outcomes as well. The clearest was the interrelationship of attainment, marriage, and reproduction at the household level. Households that were especially successful at one of these outcomes appear to have been successful at the other two as well. Beyond the household, interrelationships among outcomes were more complex. Kin who held official position but lived in other households appear, if anything, to have been competitors in the marriage market, and even seemed to suppress marital fertility.

Our tests of the effects of descent group diversity, meanwhile, yielded mixed results. By some measures, in particular marriage and mortality, descent group diversity within the village appeared to have beneficial effects. We explained such effects in terms of the implications of descent group diversity for local marriage markets and patterns of exposure to disease. By another measure, i.e., fertility, descent group homogeneity within the village appeared beneficial. More homogeneous villages had higher marital fertility. We are unable to explain that as an artifact, as we did the effects on marriage and mortality, and suggest that Tsai (2004) is correct in that Chinese villages that were more homogenous with respect to descent group are better at the provision of public goods, and that this is reflected in demographic outcomes.

Acknowledgments Versions of this chapter were presented at the Population Association of America session "Historical Transitions and Demographic Responses," Philadelphia, April 2005, the UCLA California Center for Population Research colloquium in March 2005, the University of Wisconsin Center for Demography and Ecology in May 2005, and the IUSSP International

Conference on Kinship and Demographic Behavior, Salt Lake City, Utah, October 2005. We are grateful to the discussants and audiences at each venue for their comments and suggestions. The research on which this work was based was supported in part by NICHD 1R01HD045695-A2, "Demographic Responses to Community and Family Context." The authors were also supported by fellowships from the John Simon Guggenheim Memorial Foundation.

References

Bengtsson, T., C. Campbell, J.Z. Lee et al. 2004. *Life Under Pressure: Mortality and Living Standards in Europe and Asia, 1700–1900.* MIT, Cambridge, MA.

Bian, Y.J. 1997. Bringing strong ties back in: Indirect ties, network bridges, and job searches in China. *American Sociological Review* 62(3): 366–85.

Campbell, C. and J.Z. Lee. 1996. A death in the family: Household structure and mortality in rural Liaoning, life-event and time-series analysis, 1792–1867. *The History of the Family: An International Quarterly* 1(3): 297–328.

Campbell, C. and J.Z. Lee. 2000. Price fluctuations, family structure, and mortality in two rural Chinese populations: Household responses to economic stress in eighteenth and nineteenth century Liaoning, in T. Bengtsson and O. Saito (eds.), *Population and the economy: From hunger to modern economic growth*, Oxford University Press, Oxford, pp. 371–420.

Campbell, C. and J.Z. Lee. 2001. Free and unfree labor in Qing China: Emigration and escape among the bannermen of Northeast China, 1789–1909. *History of the Family: An International Quarterly* 6(4): 455–76.

Campbell, C. and J.Z. Lee. 2002. When husbands and parents die: Widowhood and orphanhood in late imperial Liaoning, 1789–1909, in R. Derosas and M. Oris (eds.) *When Dad died: Individuals and families coping with family stress in past societies*, Peter Lang, Bern, pp. 301–22.

Campbell, C. and J.Z. Lee. 2003a. Social mobility from a kinship perspective: Rural Liaoning, 1789–1909. *International Review of Social History* 47: 1–26.

Campbell, C. and J.Z. Lee. 2003b. Disability, disease, and mortality in Northeast China, 1749–1909. California Center for Population Research (www.ccpr.ucla.edu), Working Paper CCPR-038-03.

Campbell, C. and J.Z. Lee. 2004. Mortality and household in seven Liaodong populations, 1749–1909, in T. Bengtsson, C. Campbell, J.Z. Lee et al. (eds.), *Life under pressure: Mortality and living standards in Europe and Asia, 1700–1900*, MIT, Cambridge, MA, pp. 293–324.

Campbell, C. and J.Z. Lee. 2002. State views and local views of population: Linking and comparing genealogies and household registers in Liaoning, 1749–1909. *History and Computing* 14(1+2): 9–29.

Campbell, C., J.Z. Lee, and M. Elliott. 2002. Identity construction and reconstruction: Naming and Manchu ethnicity in northeast China, 1749–1909. *Historical Methods* 35(3) Summer: 101–16.

Ding Y., S. Guo, J.Z. Lee, and C. Campbell. 2004. *Liaodong baqi yimin shehui* (Liaodong banner immigration and rural society). Shanghai shehui kexue chubanshe, Shanghai.

Ebrey, P. 1984. *Family and Property in Sung China: Yuan Ts'ai's Precepts for Social Life.* Princeton University Press, Princeton, NJ.

Ebrey, P. 1991. *Confucianism and Family Rituals in Imperial China: A Social History of Writing About Rites.* Princeton University Press, Princeton, NJ.

Entwisle, B., J.B. Casterline, and H.A.-A. Sayed. 1989. Villages as contexts for contraceptive behavior in rural Egypt. *American Sociological Review* 54: 1019–34.

Entwisle, B., A.I. Hermalin, P. Kamnuansilpa, and A. Chamratrithirong. 1984. A multilevel model of family planning availability and contraceptive use in rural Thailand. *Demography* 21(4): 559–74.

Entwisle, B., R.R. Rindfuss, D.K. Guilkey, A. Chamratrithriong, S.R. Curran, and Y. Sawangdee. 1996. Community and contraceptive choice in rural Thailand: Case study of Nang Rong. *Demography* 33: 1–11.

Frankenberg, E. 2004. Sometimes it takes a village: Collective efficacy and children's use of preventive health care. California Center for Population Research (**www.ccpr.ucla.edu**), Working Paper CCPR-028-04.

Freedman, R.C. 1974. Community-level data in fertility surveys. WFS Occasional Papers 8. International Statistical Institute, Voorburg, The Netherlands.

Goldstone, J. 1986. The demographic revolution in England: A re-examination. *Population Studies* 40: 5–33.

Jencks, C. and S.E. Mayer. 1990. The social consequences of growing up in a poor neighborhood, in L. Lynn and M. McGeary (eds.), *Inner-city poverty in the United States*, National Academy Press, Washington, DC, pp. 111–86.

Lee, J. and C. Campbell. 1997. *Fate and Fortune in Rural China: Social Organization and Population Behavior in Liaoning, 1774–1873*. Cambridge University Press, Cambridge.

Lee, J. and C. Campbell. 1998a. Getting a head: Headship succession and household division in three Chinese banner serf communities, 1789–1909. *Continuity and Change* 13(1): 117–41.

Lee, J. and C. Campbell. 1998b. Getting a head in Northeast China: Household succession in four banner serf populations, 1789–1909, in A. Fauve-Chamoux and E. Ochiai (eds.), *House and stem family in Eurasian perspective*, International Research Center for Japanese Studies, Kyoto, pp. 403–30.

Lee, J.Z. and C. Campbell. 2005. Living standards in Liaoning: Evidence from demographic outcomes, in R.C. Allen, T. Bengtsson, and M. Dribe (eds.), *Living standards in the past. New perspectives on well-being in Europe and Asia*, Oxford University Press, Oxford, pp. 403–26.

Lee, J.Z. and F. Wang. 1999. *One Quarter of Humanity: Malthusian Mythology and Chinese Realities 1700–2000*. Harvard University Press, Cambridge, MA.

Levine, D. 1987. *Reproducing Families: The Political Economy of English Population History*. Cambridge University Press, Cambridge, MA.

Liu, Hui-chen Wang. 1959. *The Traditional Chinese Clan Rules*. J.J. Augustin, New York.

Plakans, A. 1984. *Kinship in the Past: An Anthroplogy of European Family Life 1500–1800*. Blackwell, Oxford.

Rosero-Bixby, L. and J.B. Casterline. 1993. Modeling diffusion effects in fertility transition. *Population Studies* 57: 147–67.

Sampson, R. and S. Raudenbush. 1999. Systematic social observation of public spaces: A new look at disorder in urban neighborhoods. *American Journal of Sociology* 105(3): 603–51.

Sampson, R., S. Raudenbush, and F. Earls. 1997. Neighborhoods and violent crime: A multilevel study of collective efficacy. *Science* 277(5328): 918–24.

Sampson, R., J. Morenoff, and T. Gannon-Rowley T. 2002. Assessing 'neighborhood effects': social processes and new directions in research. *Annual Review of Sociology* 28: 443–78.

Sastry, N. 1996. Community characteristics, individual and household attributes, and child survival in Brazil. *Demography* 33(2): 211–29.

Schofield, R. 1985. English marriage patterns revisited. *Journal of Family History* 10: 2–20.

Tsai, L. 2004. The Informal State: Accountability and Public Goods Provision in Rural China. Ph.D. dissertation, Harvard University, Department of Government.

Tsui, A.O., D.P. Hogan, J.D. Teachman, and C. Welti-Chanes. 1981. Community availability of contraceptives and family limitations. *Demography* 18: 615–25.

Watkins, S., J. Behrman, and H. Kohler. 2002. Social networks and changes in contraceptive use over time: Evidence from a longitudinal study in rural Kenya. *Demography* 39(4): 713–37.

Weir, D. 1984. Rather late than never: Celibacy and age at marriage in English cohort fertility, 1541–1871. *Journal of Family History* 9: 340–54.

Wilson, W.J. 1987. *The Truly Disadvantaged*. University of Chicago Press, Chicago, IL.

Wrigley, E.A. and R. Schofield. 1981. *The Population History of England, 1541–1871: A Reconstruction*. Cambridge University Press, Cambridge.

Part II
The Importance of Family and Kin
over the Life Course

Chapter 4
The Presence of Parents and Childhood Survival: The Passage of Social Time and Differences by Social Class

Frans van Poppel[1] and Ruben van Gaalen[2]

Abstract This study focuses on the effects on survival of children of growing up in a family with or without both biological parents and/or stepparents. We use data from a representative sample of births from cohorts born in the Netherlands between 1850 and 1922. We first describe the long-term trends in the presence of fathers, mothers, and stepparents in families of children between birth and age 15. We then study the impact on survival of children of (a) the permanent absence of one of the parents, and (b) the entrance of a stepparent, focusing on changes in the effect over time and social class. Our analysis confirmed the more important role of the mother for survival, and showed that more durable effects of parental absence grew in importance over time, and revealed hardly any observed social class differences on mortality effects.

Keywords survival, family structure, Netherlands, social class

1 Changing Living Arrangements of Children

From the 1970s on, the living arrangements of children in Western societies have undergone a fundamental change. As a consequence of the rise in nonmarital fertility, the increase in union disruption and higher proportions of men and women remarrying or entering a new union after the break-up of an earlier one, more and more children have been raised in one-parent families, or spent their childhood with a stepfather or stepmother (Andersson 2002; Hernandez and Myers 1993; Heuveline and Timberlake 2002). These changes in the Western family generated popular and scholarly concern over their impact on children. Researchers were led to consider the implications of this change in the family structure with regard to a variety of outcomes for children such as school drop-out, drug use, and occupational attainment (Aughinbaugh, Pierret, and Rothstein 2005).

---

[1]Netherlands Interdisciplinary Demographic Institute (NIDI), The Hague, The Netherlands

[2]Netherlands Interdisciplinary Demographic Institute (NIDI), The Hague, The Netherlands, and Statistics Netherlands (CBS), Voorburg, The Netherlands

Demographers and epidemiologists have in particular focused on the direct and later-life effects on the survival of children experiencing divorce or growing up in a single-parent family. A series of studies in a variety of Western countries has shown that parental divorce and living in a one-parent household has striking effects on mortality risks of children over various stages of the life course (see, e.g., Preston, Hill, and Drevenstedt 1998; Östberg 1997; Blakely et al. 2003; Modin 2003; Martin et al. 2005; Hansagi, Brandt, and Andréasson 2000; Weitoft et al. 2003).

In the debate over the consequences for children of growing up in these specific family situations, various authors have pointed to the similarity between the experiences of children in present-day families and those that started their life in the nineteenth century (Griffith 1980). It is suggested that the new era of familial instability that many Western countries entered after the mid-1960s confronted children born in the 1970s and 1980s with a degree of family instability and family complexity that was similar to the experiences of their great-grandparents when they were young. Reference is made to the fact that up until the cohorts born early in the twentieth century, family disruption due to high mortality and remarriages following the loss of a spouse were very common. A complex family structure in which children were coresiding with stepparents and stepsiblings and were affiliated with three different families was the result (see the contributions in Dupâquier et al. 1981). In addition, until 1880, in particular in the cities, high proportions of children were born out-of-wedlock (Shorter 1971).

The parallel between the present-day and the historical situation has been a source of inspiration for many scholars. Historians and demographers have tried to find out whether growing up in an unstable and complex household in the nineteenth century had consequences for children that are comparable to those in contemporary Western societies. The attention was in particular directed at the survival prospects for children who had lost their mother or father in early childhood (see Persson and Öberg 1996; Bengtsson 1996; Högberg and Bröström 1985; Åkerman, Högberg, and Andersson 1996). The publication of Derosas and Oris' book *When Dad Died* (2002) provided a stimulus to research in this area. In various contributions, the consequences of the death of a father or mother on the mortality level of children were studied (see in particular the contributions by Derosas 2002; Beekink, van Poppel, and Liefbroer 2002; Breschi and Manfredini 2002; Campbell and Lee 2002; Tsuya and Kurosu 2002). In *Life under Pressure* (Bengtsson, Campbell, Lee et al. 2004), the same authors presented updated versions of these studies (Breschi et al. 2004; Tsuya and Kurosu 2004; Campbell and Lee 2004; Lee, Campbell, and Feng 2004).

Most of the historical studies mentioned above have exclusively focused on one, often small, community. Historians of mortality have recently stressed the fact that until the first decades of the twentieth century, the "disease environment" and economic circumstances varied enormously from place to place, leading to regional differences in the expectation of life at birth in the order of 15–30 years (Johansson and Kasakoff 2000). Given the strong dependence of infant and childhood mortality on the disease environment, it is important to analyze in a variety of contexts the effect of the family situation of children on their survival.

A second characteristic of the historical studies is that they rarely study variation over time in the consequences for children of growing up in a broken family. The changes in the role that family members, the state, and social institutions played for the well-being of family members—changes in particular visible from the last quarter of the nineteenth century—might have had an effect on the survival of children growing up in a mother-headed or father-headed family. A longer time-perspective on survival prospects might help to improve our understanding of the consequences for children of growing up in a specific living arrangement and of the role that parents played.

A third characteristic of many of the studies on survival of children growing up in various family situations is that they hardly ever try to find out whether there are any variables that mediate or moderate the effect of parental loss. Several present-day studies have shown that the effects of parental loss on survival are different for individuals living in different socioeconomic positions (Martin et al. 2005; Blakely et al. 2003; Östberg 1997). It is therefore important to study whether and how the child's parent's position in the social structure had an effect on the change in survival prospects of the child associated with the loss of one of the parents.

Finally, most of the historical studies in which the effect of parental absence on survival of children is studied make use only of vital registration data. In principle, these sources allow the researcher to find out whether or not the father or mother was still alive at consecutive ages of the child. They do not, however, positively confirm that a father or mother actually lived with his or her children. Willful desertion, labor migration, and other factors could lead to short- or long-term absences that could create difficulties for the family's economy and, in a later stage, the child's health and survival. Only by collecting data on actual living arrangements of children on a day-by-day basis can this problem be solved.

The purpose of this paper is to study *historical changes* in the effect that presence of parents—the narrowest kin—had for the survival prospects of children. In doing that, we will try to do justice to the suggestions given above. We will analyze data that cover changes in living arrangements of children born in the Netherlands between 1850 and 1922. We study not one single community but three (of the 11) Dutch provinces, each with its particular social and economic structure. We focus on a time period from the middle of the nineteenth century to WWII, a period in which the regions underwent radical changes in their economic, social, and family structure. The sample includes one large city, and four smaller cities and rural areas, clearly differing in levels of mortality. The dataset that we use allows for a child-centered perspective on the type, number, and characteristics of persons with which the child lived during the first stage of its life; the analysis is made on a day-by-day basis, and for different social classes.

2 Explaining Effects of Parental Loss and Absence on Mortality of Children: The Role of Time, Social Class, Gender, and Age of the Child

A range of factors has been suggested to explain why unstable families and disruptive home environments can be damaging to children, both at the time they occur and later in life (Martin et al. 2005). In some cases, the association between loss of a parent and health damage, or death, of a child is a statistical artifact (Martikainen and Valkonen 1996). One might think of a common risky event shared by one parent and one or more children such as a vehicle accident, fire, or infectious disease (Over et al. 1992). Many such events lead to the death of the child during the same day as the parent or within days or weeks, and incorrectly create an impression of an effect of having lost a parent. Similarly, when a common unfavorable environment is shared by parents and children, both run a risk of early death. In other cases, however, the loss of a parent through death or divorce is a stressful life event that directly or indirectly may precipitate the onset of a disease. The absence of a parent could have consequences for the lives of the remaining spouse and his or her children that endanger the health of the children and increase their mortality risks. It is mainly in this domain that historical studies have located the origin of increased health risks of children that experience the loss or the continuous absence of one of their parents.

As Reher and González-Quinones (2003) so aptly expressed, families that lost one of the parents (or, one might add, from their start included only one parent) were to a certain degree emotionally, socially, and economically dysfunctional families. The loss or absence of a parent endangered the smooth operation of the family for shorter or longer periods, and could produce dramatic changes in the economic and physical situation of the household and that of the children (Blom 1991). The effect that this absence had on the survival of the children living in the household depended on a range of factors: whether it was the father or the mother that was absent; the age of the child at the time the absence started; the options available to the remaining parent; and the role that other interested parties, including the society at large, were able and willing to play, etc.

Historically, in Western societies, women were almost entirely responsible for the nourishment of newborn children and the implementation of feeding practices afterwards. When breast-feeding was the only safe nourishment for newborn children, the mother's absence was practically fatal for children. Mothers performed most housekeeping tasks, spent more time with their children, and were the primary caregivers to children. When the mother was away, the level of contamination in the household easily increased, and nutritional deficiency and risks of injuries and accidents to children grew. The mother usually maintained connections with extended kin and neighbors and was therefore better able to acquire support from family and friends in times of need. The father's role was mainly economic: families were dependent on the father for the provision of goods and services. The absence of the father could lead to reduced consumption possibilities, forced moves to lower standard housing, and could require mothers to take up paid labor, thereby reducing the time they could spend on the care of their children. Almost all studies, therefore, find that the absence of the mother had a stronger negative effect on survival of the child than did the loss of the male breadwinner.

The age of the child was also a key factor for the child's survival prospects after the loss or absence of a parent. In particular, during the first weeks after delivery, maternal death could lead to infant death within hours or days, due to the lack of adequate feeding of the child. If resources were few, pathogens abundant, and sanitation a luxury, finding substitute food for the newborn was practically impossible. The strong age-dependency was not only related to the availability of breast-feeding. During the first 6 months of a child's life, the time the mother spent on food preparation, laundry, bathing the child, housecleaning, and nursing of sick children had a direct influence on the survival of her child. It is thus the absence of the mother— almost always through death—directly after the birth of a child that is assumed to have had strong effects on the survival of the child.

Historical research has paid a lot of attention to the social class differences in infant and child mortality. Social class determined the exposure and resistance to life-threatening factors for the child such as the availability and quality of food, water, clothing, housing, and knowledge of hygienic practices (van Poppel, Jonker, and Mandemakers 2005). The absence of a father usually resulted in a decline in the family's standard of living. By including the effect of social class on child mortality, it is possible to separate the economic effect of the father's absence from other changes initiated by the absence of the parent. It is also highly probable that the effects of parental loss or absence were stronger in some socioeconomic groups than in others.

Present-day research on this issue gives conflicting results. Martin et al. (2005), for example, showed that children from divorced homes of lower socioeconomic status lived shorter lives than those from homes of higher status. Blakely et al. (2003) found that increased mortality in children from one-parent families was due to correlated socioeconomic factors, but Weitoft et al. (2003) observed that children of single parents had increased mortality risks even after including socioeconomic circumstances. Of course the results of these studies cannot be generalized to a nineteenth- and early twentieth-century context. There are clear indications that the economic situation of one-parent households in the past was worse than that of complete families. The majority of unwed mothers had a proletarian background and the death of their children could primarily be a consequence of the poverty in which these women lived, and not of the absence of the father of the child. In general, one might expect that persons from the upper and middle classes were better able to protect their children against the negative health effects of parental loss or absence: they were well-off in their own right, had inherited property, or could take over ownership of their husbands' trade and business, and were sometimes supported by private or state pensions or widows' funds. Unmarried mothers, widows, and divorcées from lower social classes who did not own property were dependent on benefits from organized charity or had to find low-paid, home-based employment such as washing and sewing, which enabled them to combine work with childcare and domestic duties. Female wages were often insufficient to support the existence of mother and child. By introducing the social class to which families belonged, we will try to find out how socioeconomic position mediated or moderated the effect of the absence of the parent on the survival of the child. To study the influence of the socioeconomic situation of the family on the living arrangements of children, we will use information about the occupation of the father of the child at the time of birth of the child.

Many children lived with just one parent for a limited time only. Often, unmarried mothers married either the father of their child or a man who was not the biological father (Kok, van Poppel, and Kruse 1997). Widowed persons, especially widowers and divorced people who were left with very young children, tried to mitigate the effect of the loss of the spouse by finding a substitute nurse, housekeeper, or breadwinner.[1] Entry into the stepchild status in one sense normalized the child's situation, but the outcome was not always positive: selective neglect (medical, nutritional, physical, or emotional) in comparison to children living with both their biological parents could place the stepchildren at greater risk. Parents tend to invest more in biological children than in stepchildren (Zvoch 1999), and this could result in excess mortality when stepparents entered the household. Research has shown that stepchildren are more vulnerable to fatal child maltreatment (Kornin 1987; Stiffman et al. 2002). Studies in historical populations and in developing countries, however, provide mixed results. Bledsoe (1990) showed with data for Sierra Leone that children had the greatest chance of survival when they were being cared for by a parental union of their biological mother and father. Where only one member of that union was their parent, that parent could not provide them with as much care and affection as was given to the children of the new union for fear of jeopardizing that union. Voland (1988), using data on infant and child mortality for Ostfriesland (Germany) in the period 1668–1879, argued that when through remarriage a genetically unre- lated reproducer was introduced within the family, investment deficits and risks for the stepchildren could be the result. On the other hand, Åkerman et al. (1996) showed with Swedish data that for children of remarried widows or widowers, death rates did not differ significantly from those of children in complete families. In a Dutch study Beekink et al. (1999) found that remarriage of widows or widow- ers did not result in a death rate that differed significantly from those of children in complete families. The conflicting results of these studies do not allow us to draw a firm conclusion regarding the effect of living with a stepparent on the mortality of stepchildren. We therefore take up this issue again and study whether the life chances of children increased or decreased after remarriage took place in compari- son with children living in complete families.

As has been stated in the introduction, many epidemiological studies are based on a restricted time perspective. Consequently, one cannot accurately study the importance of changes over time for specific stages of childhood, or the relative importance of the presence of the father or mother for child survival. What follows are some of the changes with potential effects on the survival of children in father- absent or mother-absent families. First of all, from the last quarter of the nineteenth century on, we point to the transformation of the role that mothers played compared to fathers in rearing their children, and to the decreasing importance of the role of the family in comparison to that of state and school. From the mid-1860s on, real wages in the Netherlands started to increase considerably. During a period of 40 years,

---

[1] A study of the Dutch city of The Hague showed that in the second half of the nineteenth century, 57 percent of divorced men, 42 percent of divorced women, 38 percent of widowers and 15 percent of widows remarried. Men remarried in general sooner than women, divorced men a bit less rapidly than widowers, and divorced women sooner than widows (van Poppel 1998).

between 1860 and 1900, real wages increased by more than 150 percent (van Zanden and van Riel 2000, 352–5). The rise in real wages after 1870 made it possible to harmonize ideals and reality regarding the division of labor between men, women, and children. The male breadwinner wage norm was already a normative standard long before the nineteenth century: whenever feasible, specialization took place in which the husband concentrated on earning an income while the wife focused on reproductive activities within the home. It was the rise in real income that made it possible for women to withdraw from the workforce and to restrict their role to that of housewife and mother, providing family members with valuable but unwaged personal care and support (Horrell and Humphries 1997). It made women wholly responsible for the organization of household affairs, for childcare and for arranging the family's social life. This loss of function on the father's part might have changed the relative importance of the parents for the survival of children and may have affected the chances of survival of children growing up in fatherless or motherless families. There were also changes in the economic and social position of one-parent families that may have had an effect on survival of children in these households. During a large part of the nineteenth century, children were strongly dependent on the presence of both parents in order to reach a decent level of living. As the economic role of the family became less important over time, and economic growth and public intervention in favor of the underprivileged diminished the adverse effects of the absence of one of the parents, the mortality risks for children from these families may have decreased. For divorced women with children, provisions for alimony were made in an increasing number of cases, and for widows with children there was a gradual extension of the system of widows' pensions, other financial resources, and the poor relief system. There were also technological advances that were very favorable for very young children confronted with the death of their mother: improved water quality, pasteurization of milk, and better artificial feeding made newborn children less dependent on the presence of their mother and may have decreased the mortality risks of motherless children. Cultural developments may have played a role as well. Particularly from the last quarter of the nineteenth century on, the state and private organizations assigned mothers an ever more important role in the health of their children, and that made survival of children more and more dependent on the presence of the mother. Sigle-Rushton, Hobcraft, and Kiernan (2005; see also Martin et al. 2005) pointed to another cultural change that may have played a role. Over time, growing up in a broken family became more commonplace. Alternative family structures became more widely accepted, divorce was accompanied by less stigma, and negative effects of community disapproval might have lessened. As a consequence, the average child of such a family came from a less troubled family, and the link between growing up in a particular living arrangement and subsequent well-being weakened over time.

It is hard to formulate specific hypotheses on the consequences of all these changes over time on the excess risks of children growing up in one-parent families. Reher and González-Quinones (2003) are the only ones who explicitly studied the changes over time on the effects of mother's absence (death) on survival of children. In the Spanish city of Aranjuez between 1870–1910 and 1911–1950, they observed a substantial enhancement of the importance of mothers for the health of their children. Orphaned children were substantially worse off in relative terms in the more recent period than in the earliest period: a development that Reher and González-Quinones attributed to improved maternal education, which gave mothers a much more central position for children's health. Reher and González-Quinones (2003) convincingly showed that during the period 1870–1950, mothers in particular became more important for children aged 1 year or more.

3   Data Sources on Living Arrangements and Mortality of Children in Historical Studies

Collecting information on the historical living arrangements of children and the associated mortality risks is a complicated task. Historical research often only has available registers of vital events linking together members of a conjugal family unit, but which do not inform us on actual coresidence of the members of that unit. Household or census listings, which do provide information about coresidence, might at the individual level detail the ages and relationships to the head of the household unit of all family or household members, but do not give information on death and survival of children living in such a household. These listings are cross-sectional in nature and give only a static picture of the situation of the child and thus cannot show the sequence of events that children are witnessing (Berkner 1972, 405; Kertzer 1985, 100–3; King 1990; Ruggles 1990).

Population registers as they exist in Belgium, the Netherlands, and parts of Italy allow us to overcome the problems discussed above. Population registers combine census listings with vital registration in an already linked format for the entire population of a municipality (Alter 1988). Population registers make it possible to focus on individuals within living arrangements and view these living arrangements from the perspective of the individual. By linking a series of registers over time, the familial experiences of the child can, in principle, be followed for a long period of time and can be related to changing historical situations (Janssens 1993, 50–1).

Continuous population registers in the sense of bound documents with nonremovable pages were enforced in the Netherlands by the Royal Decree of December 22, 1849. The registers had to record the population legally residing within the municipality. The starting point for the first registers was the census of 1849. The returns from this census were copied into the population register, and from then on all changes occurring in the population in the next decade were recorded in the register. In most municipalities, this procedure was repeated with each subsequent 10-year census, so that in principle every register covers a time span of 10 years between the censuses. For each individual, date and place of birth, relation to the head of the household, sex, marital status, occupation, and religion were recorded. New household members arriving after the registration had started were added to the list of individuals already recorded, and those moving out by death or migration were deleted with reference to place and date of migration or date of death.

Residents were required by law to report migration between communes at both the origin and destination. The registers thus present information on demographic events leading to changes in composition and size of households, including the characteristics of the person undergoing that event. In most municipalities, population registers remained in use until 1910 or 1920, after which date a new form of continuous registration was introduced, consisting of loose sheets, so-called *gezinskaarten* or family cards. The registration unit was then no longer the household but the family. This situation lasted until 1939.

It would be an illusion to think that the information given in the registers is always accurate (Knotter and Meijer 1995). In the first register, covering the period 1850–1859, a separate column stating the relationship of individuals to the head of the household was not included. However, inferences about the most likely relationship to the head of the household are in almost all cases relatively easy to make on the basis of characteristics such as order of registration, sex, and name and age of the person. In case of need, recourse can be made to the vital registration system (registration of births, deaths, and marriages). The registration system is not complete either. Some persons left their place of residence without a correct registration of their place of destination, and in several municipalities (parts of) the population registers have not survived WWII or other disasters. In general, one might say that the population registers were fairly accurate in reporting demographic events such as births, deaths, and marriages, but were less accurate in reporting migration.

The historical data on living arrangements of children that we use here were collected for the Historical Sample of the Netherlands (HSN), a national database with information on the complete life history of a 0.5 percent random sample (76,700 birth records) of men and women born in the Netherlands from 1812 until 1922. In all Dutch provinces a random sample of births was drawn which was stratified by period of birth (11 periods) and level of urbanization of the municipality (Mandemakers 2001). Information on the family situation relates only to a specific selected child. For this study, data are from children born between 1850 and 1922 in 3 of the 11 Dutch provinces—Zeeland, Utrecht, and Friesland—giving a total of 7,691 births rather evenly distributed over the three areas. The restriction to cohorts born in the period 1850–1922 is motivated by the fact that information on the family structure during childhood can only be collected by using the population register, available from 1850 on.[2]

The collection of information has progressed most for the three selected provinces. Zeeland as well as Friesland were for a long time rural areas, although both provinces had several old smaller towns with around 15–20,000 inhabitants by the middle of the 1850s. The economy of both regions started to change after 1900 when industrialization

---

[2] The children in the study were born in 234 different municipalities. They were all followed in the consecutive population registers from 1850 to 1939, and, in case of migration, in the population register of the new place of residence. As many of them spent part of their childhood in a municipality other than their municipality of birth, the total number of municipalities in our study for which we used the population registers is of course much higher.

Table 4.1 Demographic indicators for the three selected provinces and the Netherlands as a whole

	Zeeland		Utrecht		Friesland		Netherlands	
	Males	Females	Males	Females	Males	Females	Males	Females
Around 1850								
Probability of death (per 100) between								
– ages 0 and 15	45.8	44.3	42.2	40.2	30.3	28.7	38.4	36.2
– ages 25 and 55	42.5	39.9	34.5	33.3	37.4	36.0	36.8	35.2
Marital fertility (Ig)		0.898		0.896		0.816		0.828
Extramarital births (per 100 births)		4.2		5.6		2.8		4.7
Divorce rate (per 10,000 married couples)		1.32		0.15		0.43		1.23
Around 1900								
Probability of death (per 100) between								
– ages 0 and 15	22.9	19.4	27.3	24.5	18.5	16.9	24.9	22.4
– ages 25 and 55	19.3	18.6	20.7	18.7	20.6	21.5	22.3	21.0
Marital fertility (Ig)		0.746		0.799		0.647		0.753
Extramarital births (per 100 births)		2.9		3.4		2.0		2.6
Divorce rate (per 10,000 married couples)		4.72		5.83		3.29		6.33
Around 1930								
Probability of death (per 100) between								
– ages 0 and 15	8.3	6.7	8.2	6.9	8.1	6.3	9.5	7.6
– ages 25 and 55	10.2	12.6	11.9	12.8	12.1	13.5	13.4	14.0
Marital fertility (Ig)		0.391		0.448		0.330		0.452
Extramarital births (per 100 births)		1.5		1.9		1.4		1.8
Divorce rate (per 10,000 married couples)		5.3		14.3		5.8		19.2

took place. Utrecht, located in the center of the country, had a more urban character and its capital city grew from 48,000 inhabitants in 1850 to 155,000 in 1930.

As far as demographic factors affecting the living arrangements of children are concerned, the three provinces were heterogeneous enough to make them an interesting subject for comparative research. Grouped together, the three provinces might be considered more or less representative of the demographic situation of the Netherlands. Table 4.1 gives an overview of the differences between the provinces in mortality before age 15, mortality in adulthood, fertility, extramarital fertility and divorce, for three different periods.

4   Results

4.1   Long-Term Changes in One-Parent Families

Table 4.2 presents descriptive statistics for the relevant variables for two birth cohorts. The first one coincided more or less with the period before the decline in fertility and infant and childhood mortality (1850–1879), and the second one with the first stage of the demographic transition, characterized by decreases in fertility and mortality (1880–1922).

The probability that a child died before the age of 15 was 30 percent overall, but there were, as expected, clear differences by birth cohort. For children born before 1880, the probability of death was 39 percent (the unweighed average of Dutch national cohort life tables for birth cohorts 1850–1879 was 36 percent), and for children born between 1880 and 1922 it was 22 percent (national unweighed average for birth cohorts 1880–1922 was 21.1 percent). The large majority of the children in our sample were born in families of unskilled workers. Skilled workers in industry and agriculture came next. The proportions of farmers and middle class people were almost equal. The majority of the children were born in rural areas and belonged to a Protestant denomination.

Our main independent variable was the permanent absence of the father or mother from the family. We determined the exact date (and age of the child) at which the father or mother permanently left the household. For some families, this was already the case at the time of birth of our sampled child (unwed mothers, not living with the judicial father of the child). For the large majority, it happened when the father or mother died. For some fathers and mothers, permanent absence was initiated by divorce or migration without return before the index child was 15 years old. We calculated the proportion of children for whom the father or mother was absent at the age of death of the child or (if surviving) at age 15. Before age 15, 29 percent of the children experienced the absence of their father, and the same percentage was confronted with the loss of their mother. Only a very small percentage (a total of 4 percent of all children) lived with a stepparent at the time of their death or at age 15.

Table 4.2 Description of dependent and independent variables by birth cohort

Variable	All	Born 1850–1879	Born 1880–1922
Deceased <15 years	0.30	0.39	0.22
Before 1880	0.46	–	–
After 1880	0.54	–	–
Sex of child			
Male	0.52	0.52	0.51
Female	0.48	0.48	0.49
Father's social class			
Class unknown	0.04	0.05	0.03
Upper class	0.06	0.06	0.06
Middle class	0.11	0.10	0.12
Farmers	0.12	0.13	0.11
Skilled workers	0.26	0.24	0.27
Unskilled workers	0.41	0.42	0.39
Father's religion			
Protestant	0.68	0.69	0.68
Catholic	0.23	0.21	0.24
No religion/no info	0.09	0.10	0.08
Character of birthplace			
Rural	0.67	0.69	0.66
Urban	0.33	0.31	0.34
Age of mother at birth			
Age <20	0.01	0.01	0.01
Age 20–35	0.69	0.68	0.70
Age >35	0.30	0.31	0.29
Presence of parents			
Mother absent at age of death of child or at age 15	0.29	0.28	0.30
Father absent at age of death of child or at age 15	0.29	0.29	0.30
Stepmother present at age of death of child or at age 15	0.03	0.03	0.02
Stepfather present at age of death of child or at age 15	0.01	0.01	0.01
N	7,691	3,509	4,182

Table 4.3 gives the same information for various social classes. The occupations of the father of the child were classified into a social class scheme proposed by van Leeuwen and Maas (van Leeuwen, Maas, and Miles 2002).[3] This scheme distinguishes 12 classes, but because of small numbers, we merged these into 3 classes with more or less comparable living conditions: *Upper/middle class and farmers*, *Workers (skilled and unskilled in- and outside agriculture)*, and *Social class unknown*.

The probability of dying was clearly higher for children for whom the social class was unknown and for the children of workers than for children from the

[3] Most farmers in the regions studied here owned their relatively large holdings. We wish to thank Dr. Andrew Miles (University of Birmingham), Dr. Bart Van de Putte (University of Louvain), Dr. Marco van Leeuwen (International Institute for Social History, Amsterdam), and Dr. Ineke Maas (Utrecht University) for invaluable help with coding and classifying these occupations.

Table 4.3 Description of dependent and independent variables by social class

Variable	All	Unknown	Upper	Middle	Farmers	Skilled workers	Unskilled workers
Deceased <15 years	0.30	0.35	0.27	0.27	0.26	0.29	0.33
Period of birth							
Before 1880	0.46	0.53	0.46	0.40	0.49	0.42	0.48
After 1880	0.54	0.47	0.54	0.60	0.51	0.58	0.52
Sex of child							
Male	0.52	0.55	0.50	0.50	0.53	0.51	0.52
Female	0.48	0.45	0.50	0.50	0.47	0.49	0.48
Father's religion							
Protestant	0.68	0.67	0.67	0.66	0.68	0.65	0.71
Catholic	0.23	0.24	0.20	0.23	0.25	0.27	0.20
No religion/no info	0.09	0.09	0.13	0.11	0.07	0.08	0.09
Place of birth							
Rural	0.67	0.54	0.60	0.47	0.91	0.50	0.79
Urban	0.33	0.46	0.40	0.53	0.09	0.50	0.31
Age of mother at birth							
Age <20	0.01	0.11	0.00	0.01	0.01	0.01	0.01
Age 20–35	0.69	0.73	0.73	0.68	0.68	0.68	0.70
Age >35	0.30	0.16	0.27	0.31	0.31	0.31	0.29
Presence of parents							
Mother absent <15	0.09	0.11	0.08	0.08	0.10	0.09	0.08
Father absent <15	0.08	0.05	0.09	0.08	0.09	0.08	0.08
Stepmother <15	0.04	0.01	0.03	0.05	0.03	0.04	0.03
Stepfather <15	0.01	0.04	0.01	0.01	0.02	0.01	0.01
N	7,691	312	488	862	917	1,990	3,122

upper/middle classes and farmers. The group with unknown social class was mainly children born out-of-wedlock.[4] Illegitimate children were usually the first born of very young mothers and ages at birth were therefore much lower for the group with unknown social class.[5] Differences between social classes in the percentage of absent parents were only visible for the group with unknown social class.

Figures 4.1 and 4.2 describe for each exact age of the child what percentage of *surviving* children in a birth cohort were living with only one of their biological parents, or with a stepparent.[6] The data only indicate whether at least one of the parents was present and they do not imply that no other persons were present in the family. The birth cohort 1880–1922 is split into two groups in these presentations; one coinciding with the first stage of the demographic transition (1880–1899), the other with the last stage (1900–1922). By way of comparison, we also included information on children born during the period 1965–1985.[7]

---

[4] The fact that information on the social class of the father is missing is often due to the absence of the father in the first place.

[5] It is important to take this factor into account in the analysis as death risks are *always* higher among children with parity one and born of mothers under the age of 20.

[6] These percentages therefore differ from those presented in Table 2 where data are given for all children whether deceased or alive before age 15.

[7] These data are derived from retrospective information on the childhood of the main respondents of the Netherlands Kinship Panel Study (NKPS) (Dykstra et al. 2005), which is a random sample of more than 8,000 individuals within Dutch households.

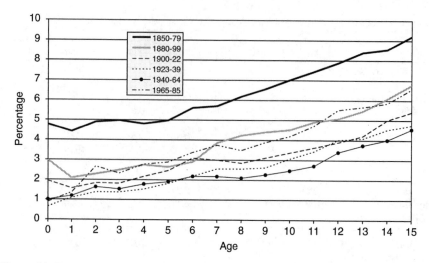

Figure 4.1 Percentage of children coresiding without a (step)father, by age of the child and birth cohort

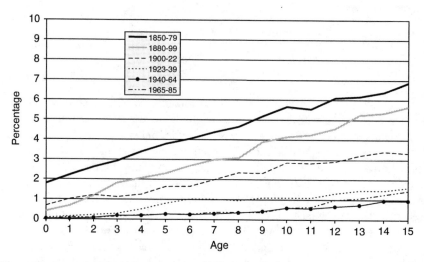

Figure 4.2 Percentage of children coresiding without a (step)mother, by age of the child and birth cohort

Figure 4.1 shows that in the middle of the nineteenth century, a considerable percentage of the children grew up with their mother but without father or stepfather. At birth, this applied to almost 5 percent of the children, and at age 15 to about 9 percent. At younger ages, these were for the most part children of unmarried mothers but as the children grew older, it was mostly due to the fact that women lost their spouse and did not remarry. As can be seen in Figure 4.2, in the nineteenth century a much smaller percentage of children lived without their biological mother or stepmother. In the older generations, living without a mother was mainly due to the death of the biological mother.

It was not very common for a child to coreside with its biological mother and a stepfather or its biological father and a stepmother: even among 15-year-old children born in 1850–1879, this applied to only 2 percent and 7 percent of the children respectively.

5 Method: Event History Analysis

In studying the effect of parental absence on survival of children, we have tried to follow as closely as possible the approach that was applied in an earlier Dutch study by Beekink et al. (1999). Compared to that study, we have a larger number of cases and data that are more or less representative for children born in the Netherlands in the period between 1850 and 1922. This allows us, in particular, to run models for consecutive historical periods and for two social classes (and for social class unknown). We did not make a distinction between reasons for the absence of parents as almost all absence was due to the death of one of the parents.

Our aim is to analyze the interdependence between the presence of parents and the survival of their offspring in a dynamic way by including time-dependent information. We estimate the mortality risk of children, taking into account the impact of independent variables that change their value during childhood, focusing on changes in the family structure.[8] This will be done by using event-history analysis (Blossfeld and Rohwer 1995). One of the advantages of this method, compared to ordinary least squares (OLS), is that it allows us in the analysis to include right-censored cases, that is, children of which we only have life course information until a certain point in time. As we were mainly interested in the effects of changing covariates on the death rate, and not in the effect of the age of the child as such, we applied the Cox model (Cox 1972). The Cox model is a proportional hazard model and can be written as:

$$r(t) = h(t)\exp(A(t)\infty)$$

The transition rate $r(t)$ is the product of an unspecified baseline rate $h(t)$ and a second term specifying possible influences of a covariate vector $A(t)$ on the transition rate. This rate is not a probability—it can have a value higher than one—and cannot be empirically measured as such. In this case, it is a local description of the possible development of the survival process of children under varying structural conditions, with the proviso that the event has not yet occurred.

For all children we have a complete window of observation from birth to death, or right censoring, which gives us at least one *episode* per child. As we were primarily

---

[8] The data file constructed for this analysis contains information on one observation per family only (see data description).

interested in the effects of the loss of the parents during the period that the child was still dependent on its parents, we only studied mortality of children during the first 15 years of life. For each child, age at death was calculated in days. Where this age was not available, information on age at date of departure was available.

We can also use the change of the values of our dependent variable—"child alive"—and the time-varying independent variables of interest, like "mother present" or "father present", but also "arrival stepfather" and "lives with mother only". Every time a variable of interest changes its value, we update this information in our observation window using the method of episode splitting, creating an additional episode. In this way, we are not only able to investigate the effect of the absence of a parent, but also the duration effect, assuming that the impact of this event is stronger shortly after it occurred. Lastly, time-independent variables like birth cohorts, gender of the child, social class, religious denomination of the parents, level of urbanization, and age of the mother at birth are held constant in every single record or episode. We used significance tests to compare the outcomes for each category with that of the reference category. In addition to that, we performed Wald tests (Holm's method) to investigate whether the outcomes of two categories were statistically different.

The assumption that the baseline rate does not change with age of the child is tested by estimating different models for the period between birth and age 15 (Model 1), and separately for the most vulnerable phase in the life of the child, that is, the first 6 months after birth (Model 3). We also model the age range between 6 months and 4 years (Model 4), and between 4 and 15 years (Model 5). In addition to that, for the whole age range (ages 0–15), we also estimate the effect on survival of the child of time elapsed since the absence of the parent (less or more than 1 month) (Model 2). As a consequence of the small number of cases, we had to concentrate the multivariate analysis for Models 2 to 5 on the effects of the presence of the parents, taking into account birth cohort and social class, and leaving out the effect of the presence of stepparents. In Models 3 to 5, we only focus on the effect of the survival of the biological parents.

6   Outcomes

Model 1 in Table 4.4 examines the effects of the death of a parent on the mortality of children between birth and age 15. In addition to birth cohort and social class, we also included the variables religion of the father of the child, urban/rural character of the place of birth of the child, and age of the mother at birth. The entries in the table are relative risks.

The first column in Table 4.4 shows, as expected, decreases in childhood mortality over time (risks were almost halved after 1880), rather strong social class differences (with children of workers and of unknown social class background showing much higher mortality than children of families of the upper and middle classes and farmers), and higher mortality among children of old mothers. Column 2 adds

Table 4.4 Estimated relative risks of dying between birth and age 15, full model

Variable	t-value		t-value		t-value	
Birth cohort						
1850–1879	1.92**	(15.27)	1.88**	(14.79)	1.89**	(14.79)
1880–1922 (Ref.)	1.00		1.00		1.00	
Sex						
Male	1.07*	(1.66)	1.07*	(1.68)	1.07*	(1.68)
Female (Ref.)	1.00		1.00		1.00	
Social class father[a]						
Unknown	1.42***	(3.28)	1.30**	(2.16)	1.30**	(2.11)
Upper, middle and farmers (Ref.)	1.00		1.00		1.00	
Workers	1.24***	(4.44)	1.24***	(4.48)	1.24***	(4.49)
Religion[b]						
Protestant	0.74***	(4.37)	0.75***	(4.21)	0.75***	(4.20)
Catholic	0.72***	(4.28)	0.73***	(4.15)	0.73***	(4.15)
No religion/info (Ref.)	1.00		1.00		1.00	
Character birthplace						
Rural	0.97	(0.56)	0.98	(0.56)	0.98	(0.55)
Urban (Ref.)	1.00		1.00		1.00	
Age of mother at birth						
Age mother <20	0.78	(1.16)	0.79	(1.04)	0.79	(1.08)
Age mother 20–35	0.89***	(2.62)	0.88**	(2.87)	0.88**	(2.89)
Age mother >35 (Ref.)	1.00		1.00		1.00	
Absence of mother						
Mother absent <15			1.53***	(4.65)	1.53***	(4.33)
Mother present (Ref.)			1.00		1.00	
Absence of father						
Father absent <15			1.01	(0.15)	1.05	(0.46)
Father present (Ref.)			1.00		1.00	
Presence stepparent						
Mother absent × Stepmother					0.89	(0.48)
Father absent × Stepfather					0.27*	(1.86)
N (subjects)	7,691		7,691		7,691	
N (observations; incl. split episodes)	14,980				14,980	
Events	2,302		2,302		2,302	
Log likelihood	−20046.29		−20035.16		−20032.25	

*Significant at 10%; **significant at 5%; ***significant at 1%; absolute value of *z* statistics in parentheses.
[a]Coefficients of "unknown" and "workers" do not statistically differ (Wald test $\chi^2 = 0.14$; $p = 0.71$).
[b]Coefficients of Protestants and Catholics do not statistically differ (Wald test $\chi^2 = 0.48$; $p = 0.49$).

information on the absence of the parents. The outcomes suggest that over the whole historical period and during the whole childhood period, the absence of the mother increased the mortality rate of children with a factor 1.53, i.e., it caused a more than 50 percent increase in the child's death risks. The effect of the loss of the father was not significant and much weaker than that of the mother. In nineteenth-century Western societies, it was the mother who was the main keeper within the home and had almost complete responsibility for childcare. She was available as primary caregiver, dealt with the affective life of the family, and had closer ties to the children than the father had. The death of the mother therefore could lead to an increase of the level of environmental contamination, higher nutritional deficiency, greater risks of injuries and accidents, and fewer preventive measures for, and later medical treatment of, the child. Usually, mothers maintained connections with extended kin and with friends and were therefore more able, as surviving parent, to acquire support from family and friends. Continuity in the child's daily life could more often be secured after the death of the father, as compared to after the death of the mother. When very young children were present in the house, an important consequence of the mother's death was that no one was available to breast-feed the child or that the child had to be weaned prematurely.

In column 3 in Table 4.4 we studied what happened with the mortality risks of children when a stepparent arrived in the household. It appeared that the arrival of a stepmother after the death or leaving of the biological mother brought some improvement in the living conditions of children who had lost their mother: the relative risk decreased from 1.53 to 1.36 ($0.89 \times 1.53 = 1.36$), but was still higher than for those children who still had their biological mother (reference = 1.00). The effect of the arrival of a stepfather was positive as well. In fact, the effect was extremely large, leading to such an improvement in the living conditions of children that they were better-off than children who lived with their own biological father ($0.27 \times 1.05 = 0.28$ versus 1.00) (Table 4.4). Part of this effect might be due to the mortality-decreasing effect that marriage of the unwed mother had on the survival prospects of the illegitimate child (Kok et al. 1997); and part of it might be due to the small number of events, combined with unexplained heterogeneity. We estimated a separate model (results not shown here) selecting only those children who experienced the death of their biological father during childhood and estimated the effect of the arrival of a stepfather. The effect was more positive for children from the upper social class, and it was more positive before 1880. In any case, growing up in a stepfamily appeared not to be as harmful as often is suggested by folk belief: at least as far as survival prospects are concerned, children who got a stepparent were better-off than children living in a one-parent family.

In Table 4.5 we estimated separate models for birth cohorts and for social classes, controlling for the other selected variables.

The table reveals that the positive "father effect" on child survival increased after 1880 whereas that of the mother decreased. This last result is contrary to the findings of Reher and González-Quinones and it is hard to find an explanation for this outcome. Only in the first cohort did the entrance of a stepmother lead to a decrease in the mortality effect of the loss of the biological mother. In both cohorts, children living with a stepfather were better-off than children living with their mother only, but the effects of the stepfather's entrance never reached statistical significance.

Table 4.5 also shows the differences between social classes in the effect of the parent's absence on children's mortality. Losing one's mother had a mortality-increasing effect both for children of the upper and middle classes and among children of workers. These effects are comparable with the results of the full model (the main effect of the mother's absence), and do not point to large additional class

Table 4.5 Estimated relative risks of dying between birth and age 15, for birth cohort and social class (controlled for sex of the child, religion, character of birthplace, and age of mother)

	Birth cohort		Social class		
	1850–1879	1880–1922	Upper/Middle/ Farmers	Workers	Unknown
Mother absent	1.56***	1.36	1.81***	1.68***	0.79
	(3.94)	(1.48)	(3.14)	(4.16)	(0.85)
Father absent	0.88	1.66**	1.09	0.93	1.18
	(1.07)	(2.57)	(0.41)	(0.54)	(0.73)
Mother	0.71	1.41	0.47	0.90	3.82**
absent × Stepmother	(1.21)	(0.76)	(1.42)	(0.36)	(1.76)
Father	0.19	0.37	0.00	0.54	0.00
absent × Stepfather	(1.64)	(0.98)	(0.00)	(0.85)	(0.00)
N (subjects)	3,505	4,186	2,269	5,111	311
N (observations; incl. split episodes)	6,948	8,032	4,533	9,728	719
Events	1,372	930	600	1,594	108
Log likelihood	−10839.81	−7622.78	−4511.75	−13207.06	−583.87

*Significant at 10%; **significant at 5%; ***significant at 1%; absolute value of z statistics in parentheses.

differences above the main effect of social class in the full model. The effect of losing one's father hardly varied between social classes and was rather small. The entrance of a stepmother had a statistically not significant decreasing effect on mortality risks of children in father-only families of the upper/middle class and among workers, but a strong increasing effect on child mortality in father-only families of unknown social class. However, the number of cases was very restricted here. The entrance of a stepfather had a reducing effect on the mortality risks of children in all social classes, but the effects never reached statistical significance.

In Table 4.6 separate models are presented for combinations of birth cohort and social classes.

The absence of the mother had a strong mortality-increasing effect on children from both the upper/middle class and from workers in the first birth cohort. Compared to that cohort, risks for children in the more recent cohort decreased. There were, in fact, in both periods no strong differences between the two main social classes in the negative effects of the loss of the mother on the child's survival prospects. The effects of the father's absence increased over time and changed from being positive (decreasing mortality risks of children) to negative (increasing the child's mortality), for both the upper/middle class and for workers. Leaving aside the very small group of children for which the social class was unknown, the entry of a stepmother generally had a buffering effect on the death risks of children who had lived in a motherless family. The same applied for fathers but effects never reached statistical significance.

In a second stage, we investigated whether the effects of parental loss differed according to the time elapsed since the absence of the parent. We tested a model in which we differentiated mortality risks of children according to two durations of

Table 4.6 Estimated relative risks of dying between birth and age 15, for birth cohort and social class combined (controlled for sex of the child, religion, character of birthplace, and age of mother)

	Social class					
	Upper/Middle/Farmers		Workers		Unknown	
Birth cohort	1850–1879	1880–1922	1850–1879	1880–1922	1850–1879	1880–1922
Mother absent	1.90***	1.49	1.70***	1.58*	0.81	0.47
	(2.95)	(1.04)	(3.73)	(1.71)	(0.67)	(1.09)
Father absent	0.85	2.04*	0.82	1.49	1.09	1.34
	(0.64)	(1.94)	(1.28)	(1.43)	(0.30)	(0.73)
Mother absent × 28.45*** Stepmother	0.13**	1.58	0.87	0.75	1.71	
	(1.97)	(0.66)	(0.44)	(0.38)	(0.51)	(2.62)
Father absent × Stepfather	0.00	0.00	0.47	0.50	0.00	0.00
	(0.00)	(0.00)	(0.74)	(0.68)	(0.00)	(0.00)
N (subjects)	1,016	1,253	2,319	2,782	166	145
N (observations; incl. split episodes)	2,123	2,410	4,446	5,282	377	342
Events	347	253	951	643	74	34
Log likelihood	−2324.93	−1771.71	−7110.11	−5005.47	−353.18	−156.29

*Significant at 10%; **significant at 5%; ***significant at 1%; absolute value of z statistics in parentheses.

loss of the parent: families in which the parent had been absent for less than 1 month, and families in which the mother or father was absent already for more than 1 month. We present here the results first for birth cohorts and social class separately (Table 4.7), and next for social class and birth cohort combined (Table 4.8).

Table 4.7 makes clear that at both durations of absence, the loss of the mother had increasing effects on the mortality of children. Yet, when less than 1 month had elapsed since the absence of the mother, the death risks of children were higher than when more than 1 month had passed (2.28 vs. 1.43). The extreme vulnerability of the child in the first month after the loss of the mother was especially visible before 1880; after 1880, mortality risks of children in such families still differed from those of children in complete families but the strength of that effect was halved. The absence of the mother after 1880, however, had stronger effects after the first month of the child's life.

Children in the first cohort who had lost their father did not run any additional mortality risks during the first month after the loss of the father, nor in the period after that first month: these effects both became noticeable in the more recent cohort. In general, one might say that over time, the mortality effects of parental absence were stronger after a longer period of time had elapsed since the absence of the father and mother. For children from the upper classes, there were hardly any differences in the effects of the mother's absence during and after the first month following the loss of the mother. Children of workers experienced a reduction of life chances if the mother had died less than 1 month ago, compared to if she had died more than 1 month ago ($\chi^2 = 4.98$; $p = 0.03$). As regards absence of fathers, the differences in the effect were rather limited.

Table 4.7 Estimated relative risks of dying between birth and age 15, for birth cohort and social class by time elapsed since the death of the parent (controlled for sex of the child, religion, character of birthplace, and age of mother)

	Birth cohort			Social class		
	All	1850–1879	1880–1922	Upper/ Middle/ Farmers	Workers	Unknown
Mother absent <1 month	2.28***	2.79***	1.28	2.48**	2.95***	0.77
	(3.67)	(4.13)	(0.46)	(2.02)	(3.99)	(0.41)
Mother absent >1 month	1.43***	1.35***	1.51**	1.53**	1.52***	0.90
	(3.63)	(2.62)	(2.06)	(2.25)	(3.33)	(0.36)
Wald test χ²	*3.59** *	*7.12*** *	*0.08*	*0.97*	*4.98** *	*0.05*
p-value	*0.05*	*0.00*	*0.78*	*0.32*	*0.03*	*0.82*
Mother present (Ref.)	1.00	1.00	1.00	1.00	1.00	1.00
Father absent <1 month	0.98	0.75	2.06*	0.89	0.69	0.91
	(0.09)	(0.97)	(1.85)	(0.19)	(0.91)	(0.20)
Father absent >1 month	1.02	0.89	1.47*	1.15	0.95	1.21
	(0.20)	(1.01)	(1.93)	(0.65)	(0.41)	(0.74)
Wald test χ²	*0.03*	*0.28*	*0.69*	*0.15*	*0.53*	*0.28*
p-value	*0.86*	*0.60*	*0.41*	*0.70*	*0.46*	*0.60*
Father present (Ref.)	1.00	1.00	1.00	1.00	1.00	1.00
N (subjects)	7,691	3,505	4,186	2,269	5,104	311
N (observations; incl. split episodes)	21,166	9,749	11,417	6,443	13,661	1,062
Events	2,302	1,372	930	600	1,594	108
Log likelihood	−20033.34	−10839.79	−7623.37	−4513.69	−13205.36	−587.37

*Significant at 10%; **significant at 5%; ***significant at 1%; absolute value of z statistics in parentheses.

Table 4.8 combines social class and birth cohort. We observe that children of workers during the period 1850–1879 had lower life chances if the mother had died less than 1 month ago. After 1880, the immediate effect of the loss of the mother had become much less important in both social classes, in particular in the upper/ middle class where risks for children decreased to less than half of what they had been in the first cohort. After 1880, the short- and longer-term effect of the mothers' absence became *less* important. For fathers, the tendency was that short-term and more durable effects of the father's presence increased in importance, but the effects were never statistically significant. It thus appears that in the more recent birth cohort, the absence of parents in general had a less durable effect on the survival of children; whereas before 1880, this effect was much more restricted to the first month after the loss of the parent.

As stated before, we expected that the effect of parental loss on child mortality was not only dependent on the duration elapsed since the absence of the parent, but also on the age that the child had reached when experiencing this loss. In a series of models, we distinguished three age ranges of children at the time of absence of the parents: children aged less than 6 months (Model 3, Table 4.9), children aged

Table 4.8 Estimated relative risks of dying between birth and age 15, for birth cohort and social class combined, by duration elapsed since the death of the parent (controlled for sex of the child, religion, character of birthplace, and age of mother)

	Social class					
	Upper/Middle/Farmers		Workers		Unknown	
	Birth cohort					
	1850–1879	1880–1922	1850–1879	1880–1922	1850–1879	1880–1922
Mother absent <1 month	3.19**	1.25	3.42***	2.02	1.07	0.00
	(2.32)	(0.21)	(4.12)	(1.08)	(0.10)	(0.00)
Mother absent >1 month	1.39	1.75	1.48***	1.51	0.81	0.85
	(1.45)	(1.63)	(2.78)	(1.53)	(0.62)	(0.27)
Wald test χ^2	*3.33**	*0.09*	*6.45****	*0.17*	*0.14*	*0.00*
p-value	*0.10*	*0.76*	*0.01*	*0.68*	*0.71*	*1.00*
Mother present (Ref.)	1.00	1.00	1.00	1.00	1.00	1.00
Father absent <1 month	0.69	2.30	0.48	2.12	0.94	0.89
	(0.47)	(0.78)	(1.38)	(1.15)	(0.10)	(0.16)
Father absent >1 month	0.95	1.83	0.86	1.32	1.06	1.59
	(0.20)	(1.60)	(0.98)	(0.98)	(0.18)	(0.96)
Wald test χ^2	*0.15*	*0.04*	*1.10*	*0.44*	*0.03*	*0.44*
p-value	*0.70*	*0.84*	*0.30*	*0.51*	*0.87*	*0.50*
Father present (Ref.)	1.00	1.00	1.00	1.00	1.00	1.00
N (subjects)	1,016	1,253	2,319	2,782	166	145
N (observations; incl. split episodes)	3,013	3,430	6,188	7,473	548	514
Events	347	253	951	643	74	34
Log likelihood	−2328.62	−1772.06	−7107.69	−5005.39	−355.57	−157.35

*Significant at 10%; **significant at 5%; ***significant at 1%; absolute value of z statistics in parentheses.

between 6 months and 4 years (Model 4, Table 4.9), and children aged between 4 and 15 years (Model 5, Table 4.9). As mentioned earlier, we excluded the presence of stepparents. We again looked at differences between birth cohorts and at overall social class differences.

Remarkably enough, the negative effects of the absence of the mother were almost the same at all ages of the child: mortality risks were around 50 percent higher when the mother was absent. A negative effect of the absence of the father was only visible when the child was between 4 and 15 years old: for younger children mortality risks of children decreased when the father was absent. Over time, the effect of the loss of the mother very early in the child's life hardly diminished; the effect at ages 6 months to 4 years and 4–15 years increased a little bit. For all ages of the child, the mortality effect over time of the father's absence increased.

Losing one's mother was highly risky for very young children and for children from the upper/middle classes, and a little less so for working class children. The

Table 4.9 Estimated relative risks of dying, for birth cohort and social class combined, by duration elapsed since the death of the parent (controlled for sex of the child, religion, character of birthplace, and age of mother)

Children aged less than 6 months at the time of death of the parent

		Birth cohort		Social class		
	All	1850–1879	1880–1922	Upper/Middle/Farmers	Workers	Unknown
Mother absent	1.47**	1.53**	1.08	2.42***	1.58**	0.60
	(2.34)	(2.33)	(0.21)	(3.04)	(2.10)	(1.24)
Mother present (Ref.)	1.00	1.00	1.00	1.00	1.00	1.00
Father absent	0.92	0.75	1.73	0.95	0.63	1.44
	(0.50)	(1.38)	(1.63)	(0.14)	(1.61)	(1.15)
Father present (Ref.)	1.00	1.00	1.00	1.00	1.00	1.00
N (subjects)	7,691	3,505	4,186	2,269	5,111	311
N (observations; incl. splitted episodes)	14,449	6,643	7,806	4,361	9,392	696
Events	1,051	616	435	268	725	58
Log likelihood	−9262.33	−4942.51	−3596.25	−2041.12	−6085.74	−322.37

Children aged from 6 months up to 4 years at the time of death of the parent

		Birth cohort		Social class		
	All	1850–1879	1880–1922	Upper/Middle/Farmers	Workers	Unknown
Mother absent	1.55***	1.47**	1.72*	1.23	1.75***	1.24
	(2.95)	(2.21)	(1.93)	(0.61)	(3.14)	(0.54)
Mother present (Ref.)	1.00	1.00	1.00	1.00	1.00	1.00
Father absent	0.91	0.79	1.26	0.62	0.94	0.97
	(0.57)	(1.26)	(0.73)	(1.10)	(0.30)	(0.08)
Father present (Ref.)	1.00	1.00	1.00	1.00	1.00	1.00
N (subjects)	6,624	2,885	3,739	2,001	4,374	249
N (observations; incl. splitted episodes)	13,289	5,951	7,338	4,074	8,630	585
Events	950	550	400	233	677	40
Log likelihood	−8213.49	−4309.20	−3258.18	−1743.46	−5576.41	−212.13

(continued)

Table 4.9 (continued)

| | Children aged 4–15 years at the time of death of the parent | | | | | |
| | Birth cohort | | | Social class | | |
	All	1850–1879	1880–1922	Upper/Middle/ Farmers	Workers	Unknown
Mother absent	1.53**	1.49**	1.62	1.47	1.62**	1.47
	(2.57)	(2.15)	(1.41)	(1.33)	(2.35)	(0.48)
Mother present (Ref.)	1.00	1.00	1.00	1.00	1.00	1.00
Father absent	1.30	1.15	1.81*	1.74**	1.18	0.55
	(1.49)	(0.70)	(1.70)	(1.97)	(0.74)	(0.81)
Father present (Ref.)	1.00	1.00	1.00	1.00	1.00	1.00
N (subjects)	5,593	2,299	3,294	1,750	3,641	202
N (observations; incl. splitted episodes)	12,140	5,283	6,857	3,803	7,836	501
Events	301	206	95	99	192	10
Log likelihood	−2526.49	−1576.59	−760.64	−716.92	−1526.02	−49.10

*Significant at 10%; **significant at 5%; ***significant at 1%; absolute value of z statistics in parentheses.

mortality-increasing effect of the absence of the mother was maintained among workers at higher ages of the child: for children in these age groups, mortality was still around 60 percent higher when the mother was absent. Children who had passed the age of 4 years and whose fathers belonged to the working class mainly felt the consequences of their mother's absence.

7 Conclusion and Discussion

It is generally agreed that for the healthy development of the child, the presence of parents is highly beneficial. To capture the effects of the strengths and weaknesses that parents pass on to their children longitudinal, intergenerational study designs are essential (Seltzer et al. 2005). In following such designs, it is important to realize that there has been a process in which many of the functions that families served in the past have been transferred to nonfamilial modes of organization, and that the remaining roles for fathers and mothers have changed. The relevant contexts influencing families, thus, have changed over time, but have done so in differing degrees for various social classes.

By using data from Dutch population registers for birth cohorts 1850–1922, we had the opportunity to study changes over time in the family situation of children and to analyze effects of the presence of the father and the mother on the child's life prospects. This allowed us to shed some light on how the role of fathers and mothers has changed over time in response to economic, political, cultural, and social change, and how this has affected the mortality of children.

Our reconstruction of the day-by-day living situation of children taught us that growing up in an incomplete family was much less common in cohorts of children born after 1900 than it was in cohorts born in the middle of the nineteenth century. For children born between 1850 and 1964, there has been a continuous decrease in the percentage living without their biological father or mother.

We started with the hypothesis that the role of fathers was much less important for a child's survival than the role of mothers and this hypothesis was clearly confirmed. A key issue in light of the current high incidence of divorce and nonmarital childbearing and childrearing is the role of nonbiological parents for children's welfare. The role of quasi-kin such as stepparents with their ambiguous rights and obligations was studied with our data as well. We observed that the arrival of a stepmother brought some improvement in the living conditions of children in motherless families and the same applied to the arrival of a stepfather in fatherless families.

Our main idea was that over time the effect of the father's and mother's absence would change, but we did not have a clear idea in which direction. Our analysis revealed that over time, the role of the father seemed to grow in importance whereas that of the mother decreased. The improvement in the position of the child after remarriage of the father was no longer visible in the more recent birth cohorts. Our analysis made clear that children in all social classes were in an unfavorable position after the loss of their mother. We also found that over time, the absence of parents had a more durable effect on the survival of children; whereas earlier on, this effect had been much more restricted to the first month after the loss of the parent. Remarkably, we observed no difference in the negative effects of the absence of the mother according to the age of the child; whereas the father's absence only had an impact on older children. Over time, the effect of the loss of the mother and the father at higher ages of the child increased slightly.

The outcomes of our study do not lend themselves to firm conclusions regarding the main hypotheses with which we started. Undoubtedly, this is partly caused by the small number of cases on which our analysis is based. We observed only 1,372 children's deaths in the first cohort and 930 in the second. Because of the small numbers, we could not use a refined social class classification. This had much to do with our decision to use only information on our sampled persons and not on their siblings present in the household at the same time.

Our study explicitly focused on the presence of father and mother in the household, and not on their death; that may have resulted in outcomes that are not in line with earlier studies of this issue.

Nonetheless, we find some confirmation of the trends observed by Reher and González-Quinones (2003) in their study on Spain in the late nineteenth and early twentieth centuries. We observe that over time mothers became increasingly important for their children's health, not during the first year of life but at higher ages—a development that can be linked to the central role that mothers were assigned and actually started to play for the health of their children. Particularly from the last quarter of the nineteenth century and onwards did members of the learned middle classes, in close cooperation with church and state organizations, begin efforts to educate the masses and to drive them to adopt the moral standards of the middle classes. In this civilizing offensive, the necessity of changes in the division of labor between men and women and the need for improvement in domestic hygiene played a very important role (De Regt 1984). Married women were expected to concentrate their energy, attention, and labor on the home and the family, caring for their husbands and children and maintaining the household in a material sense. This civilizing offensive also encouraged more attention to be devoted to the improvement of hygiene in the household. It found fertile ground as women now had more time for such activities, primarily because of the increase in household incomes (van Zanden and van Riel 2000, 402–8). The sanitary movement accorded a major role to deficient household arrangements in the spread of serious diseases. It recognized voluntary reforms within the private sphere as one of the most direct and effective means of improving public health. This information concentrated on the proper construction of the house itself, especially ventilation and plumbing to ensure the circulation of clean air, careful home nursing of patients with contagious diseases to prevent the spread of infections, special hygiene in the nursery, and general housekeeping measures designed to ensure cleanliness. The concern about the high rate of infant mortality inspired Dutch campaigners to propose "maternal" rather than material solutions. A reduction in infant deaths was expected to follow from the re-education of the mother who would be persuaded not to work outside the home, to improve her domestic hygiene, and to bathe, clothe, and tend her infants properly. The mother was to be educated by means of supervision at the new and expanding health care facilities directed at women and children and through propaganda, courses, books, and pamphlets (Marland 1992). In such a situation, infant and child survival became more and more dependent on the efforts of the mother.

Acknowledgments We gratefully acknowledge a grant to Frans van Poppel from the National Institute on Aging (1P01AG18314), which supported the research project *Health Inequalities in Life Course Perspective (Early-life Conditions, Mortality and Longevity)* of which the results are reported here. We want to thank Dr. Aart Liefbroer (NIDI/Free University Amsterdam) for his support in preparing the HSN data.

References

Åkerman, S., U. Högberg, and T. Andersson. 1996. Survival of orphans in nineteenth-century Sweden, in L.-G. Tedebrand (ed.), *Orphans and foster-children. A historical and cross-cultural perspective*, Umeå University, Umeå, pp. 83–103.

Alter, G. 1988. *Family and the Female Life Course: The Women of Verviers, Belgium, 1849–1880.* University of Wisconsin Press, Madison, WI.

Andersson, G. 2002. Children's experience of family disruption and family formation: Evidence from 16 FFS countries. *Demographic Research* 7(2): 343–64.

Aughinbaugh, A., C.R. Pierret, and D.S. Rothstein. 2005. The impact of family structure transitions on youth achievement: Evidence from the children of the NLSY79. *Demography* 42(3): 447–68.

Beekink, E., F. van Poppel, and A.C. Liefbroer. 2002. Parental death and death of the child: Common causes or direct effects? in R. Derosas and M. Oris (eds.), *When dad died. Individuals and families coping with distress in past societies*, Peter Lang, Bern, pp. 233–61.

Beekink, E., F. van Poppel, and A.C. Liefbroer. 1999. Surviving the loss of the parent in a nineteenth-century Dutch provincial town. *Journal of Social History* 32(3): 641–70.

Bengtsson, M. 1996. *Det hotade barnet. Tre generationers spädbarns- och barnadödlighet i 1800-talets Linköping.* Linköpings universitet, Linköping.

Bengtsson, T., C. Campbell, J.Z. Lee et al. 2004. *Life Under Pressure. Mortality and Living Standards in Europe and Asia, 1700–1900.* MIT Press, Cambridge, MA.

Berkner, L. 1972. The stem family and the developmental cycle of the peasant household: An eighteenth-century Austrian example. *The American Historical Review* 77(2): 398–418.

Blakely, T., J. Atkinson, C. Kiro, A. Blaiklock, and A.D'Souza. 2003. Child mortality, socioeconomic position, and one-parent families: Independent associations and variation by age and cause of death. *International Journal of Epidemiology* 32(3): 410–18.

Bledsoe, C. 1990. Differential care of children of previous unions within Mende households in Sierra Leone, in J.C. Caldwell, S. Findley, P. Caldwell, M.G. Santow, W.H. Cosford, J. Braid, and D. Broers-Freeman (eds.), *What we know about health transition: The cultural, social and behavioural determinants of health*, The proceedings of an international workshop, Canberra, May, 1989, Health Transition Series No. 2, Australian National University, Canberra, pp. 561–83.

Blom, I. 1991. The history of widowhood: A bibliographic overview. *Journal of Family History* 16: 191–210.

Blossfeld, H.-P. and G. Rohwer. 1995. *Techniques of Event History Modeling. New Approaches to Causal Analysis.* Erlbaum, Mahwah, NJ.

Breschi, M. and M. Manfredini. 2002. Parental loss and kin networks: Demographic repercussions in a rural Italian village, in R. Derosas and M. Oris (eds.), *When dad died. Individuals and families coping with distress in past societies*, Peter Lang, Bern, pp. 369–88.

Breschi, M., R. Derosas, and M. Manfredini. 2004. Mortality and environment in three Emilian, Tuscan, and Venetian communities, 1800–1883, in T. Bengtsson, C. Campbell, J.Z. Lee et al.

(eds.), *Life under pressure. Mortality and living standards in Europe and Asia, 1700–1900*, MIT Press, Cambridge, MA, pp. 209–52.

Campbell, C. and J. Lee. 2002. When husbands and parents die: Widowhood and orphanhood in late Imperial Liaoning, 1789–1909, in R. Derosas and M. Oris (eds.), *When dad died. Individuals and families coping with distress in past societies*, Peter Lang, Bern, pp. 301–34.

Campbell, C. and J. Lee. 2004. Mortality and household in seven Liaoning populations, 1749–1909, in T. Bengtsson, C. Campbell, J.Z. Lee et al. (eds.), *Life under pressure. Mortality and living standards in Europe and Asia, 1700–1900*, MIT Press, Cambridge, MA, pp. 293–324.

Cox, D. 1972. Regression models and life tables (with discussion). *Journal of the Royal Statistical Society* Series B, 34: 187–220.

De Regt, A. 1984. *Arbeidersgezinnen en beschavingsarbeid. Ontwikkelingen in Nederland 1870–1940, een historisch-sociologische studie.* Meppel, Bonn.

Derosas, R. 2002. Fatherless families in 19th-century Venice, in R. Derosas and M. Oris (eds.), *When dad died. Individuals and families coping with distress in past societies*, Peter Lang, Bern, pp. 421–52.

Dupâquier, J., E. Helin, P. Laslett, M. Livi-Bacci, and S. Sogner (eds.). 1981. *Marriage and Remarriage in Populations of the Past.* Academic Press, London.

Dykstra, P.A., M. Kalmijn, T.C.M. Knijn, A.E. Komter, A.C. Liefbroer, and C.H. Mulder. 2005. *Codebook of the Netherlands Kinship Panel Study: A multi-actor, multi-method panel study on solidarity in family relationships. Wave 1* (NKPS Working Paper No. 4). Netherlands Interdisciplinary Demographic Institute, The Hague.

Griffith, J.D. 1980. Economy, family, and remarriage. Theory of remarriage and application to preindustrial England. *Journal of Family Issues* 1: 479–96.

Hansagi, H., L. Brandt, and S. Andréasson. 2000. Parental divorce: Psychological well-being, mental health and mortality during youth and young adulthood. *European Journal of Public Health* 10: 86–92.

Hernandez, D. and D. Myers. 1993. *America's Children: Resources from Family, Government and the Economy.* Russell Sage Foundation, New York.

Heuveline, P. and J.M. Timberlake. 2002. Toward a child-centered life course perspective on family structures: Multi-state early life tables using FFS data, in E. Klijzing and M. Corijn (eds.), *Dynamics of fertility and partnership in Europe: Insights and lessons from comparative research* (Vol. II), United Nations, Geneva/New York, pp. 175–91.

Högberg, U. and G. Broström. 1985. The demography of maternal mortality: Seven Swedish parishes in the nineteenth century. *International Journal of Gynecology and Obstetrics* 23: 489–97.

Horrell, S. and J. Humphries. 1997. The origins and expansion of the male breadwinner family: The case of nineteenth-century Britain. *International Review of Social History* 42: 25–64.

Janssens, A. 1993. *Family and Social Change. The Household as a Process in an Industrializing Community.* Cambridge University Press, Cambridge.

Johansson, S.R. and A.B. Kasakoff. 2000. Mortality history and the misleading mean. *Historical Methods* 33: 56–8.

Kertzer, D. 1985. Future directions in historical household studies. *Journal of Family History* 10: 98–107.

King, M. 1990. All in the family? *Historical Methods* 23(1): 32–41.

Knotter, A. and A.C. Meijer. 1995. De gemeentelijke bevolkingsregisters, 1850–1920, *Broncommentaren*, Vol. 2, Instituut voor Nederlandse Geschiedenis, The Hague, pp. 79–118.

Kok, J., F. van Poppel, and E. Kruse. 1997. Mortality among illegitimate children in mid-nineteenth-century The Hague, in C.A. Corsini and P.P. Viazzo (eds.), *The decline of infant and child mortality. The European experience: 1750–1990*, Martinus Nijhoff Publishers, The Hague, pp. 193–211.

Kornin, J. 1987. Child maltreatment in cross-cultural perspective: Vulnerable children and circumstances, in R.J. Gelles and J.B. Lancaster (eds.), *Child abuse and neglect. Biosocial dimensions*, De Gruyter, New York, pp. 31–55.

Lee, J.Z., C. Campbell, and W. Feng. 2004. Society and mortality, in T. Bengtsson, C. Campbell, J.Z. Lee et al. (eds.), *Life under pressure. Mortality and living standards in Europe and Asia, 1700–1900*, MIT Press, Cambridge, MA, pp. 107–32.

Mandemakers, K. 2001. The historical sample of the Netherlands HSN. *Historical Social Research* 26(4): 179–90.

Marland, H. 1992. The medicalization of motherhood: Doctors and infant welfare in the Netherlands, 1901–1930, in V. Fildes, L. Marks, and H. Marland (eds.), *Women and children first. International maternal and infant welfare 1870–1945*, Routledge, London/New York, pp. 74–96.

Martikainen, P. and T. Valkonen. 1996. Mortality after death of spouse in relation to duration of bereavement in Finland. *Journal of Epidemiology and Community Health* 50: 264–8.

Martin, L.R., H.S. Friedman, K.M. Clark, and J.S. Tucker. 2005. Longevity following the experience of parental divorce. *Social Science and Medicine* 61(10): 2177–89.

Modin, B. 2003. Born out of wedlock and never married—It breaks a man's heart. *Social Science and Medicine* 57: 487–501.

Östberg, V. 1997. The social patterning of child mortality: The importance of social class, gender, family structure, immigrant status and population density. *Sociology of Health and Illness* 19(4): 415–35.

Over, M., R.P. Ellis, J.C. Huber, and O. Solon. 1992. The consequences of adult ill-health, in G. Richard and A. Feachem et al. (eds.), *The health of adults in the developing world*, Oxford University Press, Oxford, pp. 161–208.

Persson, B. and L. Öberg. 1996. Foster-children and the Swedish state 1785–1915, in L.-G. Tedebrand (ed.), *Orphans and foster-children. A historical and cross-cultural perspective*, Umeå University, Umeå, pp. 51–81.

Preston, S.H., M.E. Hill, and G.L. Drevenstedt. 1998. Childhood conditions that predict survival to advanced ages among African-Americans. *Social Science and Medicine* 47(9): 1231–46.

Reher, D.S. and F. González-Quinones. 2003. Do parents really matter? Child health and development in Spain during the demographic transition. *Population Studies* 57: 63–76.

Ruggles, S. 1990. Family demography and family history. *Historical Methods* 23(1): 22–31.

Seltzer, J.A., C.A. Bachrach, S.M. Bianchi, C.H. Bledsoe, L.M. Casper, P.L. Chase-Landale, T.A. DiPrete, V.J. Hotz, S.P. Morgan, S.G. Sanders, and D. Thomas. 2005. Explaining family change and variation: Challenges for family demographers. *Journal of Marriage and Family* 67: 908–25.

Shorter, E. 1971. Illegitimacy, sexual revolution and social change in modern Europe. *Journal of Interdisciplinary History* 2: 237–72.

Sigle-Rushton, W., J. Hobcraft, and K. Kiernan. 2005. Parental divorce and subsequent disadvantage: A cross-cohort comparison. *Demography* 42(3): 427–46.

Stiffman, M.N., P.G. Schnitzer, P. Adam, R.L. Kruse, and B.G. Ewigman. 2002. Household composition and risk of fatal child maltreatment. *Pediatrics* 109(4): 615–21.

Tsuya, N.O. and S. Kurosu. 2002. The mortality effects of adult male death on women, and children in agrarian households in early modern Japan: Evidence from two Northeastern villages, 1716–1870, in R. Derosas and M. Oris (eds.), *When dad died. Individuals and families coping with distress in past societies*, Peter Lang, Bern, pp. 261–301.

Tsuya, N.O. and S. Kurosu. 2004. Mortality and household in two Ou villages, 1716–1870, in T. Bengtsson, C. Campbell, J.Z. Lee et al. (eds.), *Life under pressure. Mortality and living standards in Europe and Asia, 1700–1900*, MIT Press, Cambridge, MA, pp. 253–92.

van Leeuwen, M.H.D., I. Maas, and A. Miles. 2002. *HISCO: Historical International Standard Classification of Occupations*. Leuven University Press, Leuven.

van Poppel, F. 1998. Nineteenth-century remarriage patterns in the Netherlands. *Journal of Interdisciplinary History* 28(3): 343–83.

van Poppel, F., M. Jonker, and K. Mandemakers. 2005. Differential infant and child mortality in three Dutch regions, 1812–1909. *Economic History Review* 58(2): 272–309.

van Zanden, J.L. and A. van Riel. 2000. *Nederland 1780–1914. Staat, instituties en economische ontwikkeling*. Uitgeverij Balans, Amsterdam.

Voland, E. 1988. Differential infant and child mortality in evolutionary perspective: Data from late 17th to 19th century Ostfriesland (Germany), in L.L. Betzig, M. Borgerhoff Mulder, and P.W. Turke (eds.), *Reproductive behaviour: A Darwinian perspective*, Cambridge University Press, Cambridge, pp. 253–61.

Weitoft, G.R., A. Hjern, B. Haglund, and M. Rosen. 2003. Mortality, severe morbidity, and injury in children living with single parents in Sweden: A population-based study. *Lancet* 361 (9354): 289–95.

Zvoch, K. 1999. Family type and investment in education: A comparison of genetic and stepparent families. *Evolution and Human Behavior* 20(6): 453–64.

Chapter 5
When Do Kinsmen Really Help? Examination of Cohort and Parity-Specific Kin Effects on Fertility Behavior. The Case of the Bejsce Parish Register Reconstitution Study, 17th–20th Centuries, Poland

Krzysztof Tymicki

Abstract The present study aims to investigate the parity specific effect of kin help on the transition between births among natural and controlled fertility birth cohorts of the Bejsce parish. The hypothesis states that kin help should be of particular importance in the case of higher order births. Thus, kin effects understood as reduction in the costs of childbearing (direct childcare, provision of the resources) or nutritional effects should be of particular importance at higher parities. The analyses are based on the multilevel hazard models of parity transition with kin effects represented by time-constant and time-varying covariates. The data used for the estimation of the models come from the reconstitution of the registers from Bejsce parish located in south-central Poland. The reconstitution covers the period between 1730 and 1968. The results suggest that there was a strong kin effect especially at higher parities. These effects were mostly associated with the presence of nongenerative relatives (grandparents). The analyses reveal only weak differences in the kin effect between natural and controlled fertility regimes.

Keywords kin, fertility, parity transition, parish registers

1 Introduction

In traditional agricultural societies, family life was strongly influenced by the extended kinship network which determined the economic and social well-being of the household (Laslett 1988). A broad system of kinship and the multigenerational nature of the traditional family was frequently a safety net against uncertainty associated with agricultural production as well as with various unforeseen events. Therefore, the economic system of agriculture and the kinship network provided a substantial increase in certainty about the future by diversifying risk among family members (Kohler and Hammel 2001). This paper explores one aspect of the influence

Institute of Statistics and Demography, Warsaw School of Economics, Poland

T. Bengtsson and G.P. Mineau (eds.), *Kinship and Demographic Behavior in the Past.*
© Springer Science+Business Media B.V. 2009

of kin on family life, namely, the influence of kin on rates of reproduction within households.

Many studies concerning traditional populations have shown that the existence of kin networks strongly enhances the reproductive performance of individuals by providing them with additional childcare or material resources (Burnstein, Crandall, and Kitayama 1994; Dunbar and Spoors 1995; Hill and Hurtado 1996; Sear, Mace, and McGregor 2003; Tymicki 2004). A theoretical framework that explains the ultimate causes of such kin-oriented altruism is related to kin selection theory. This theory predicts that individual actions should be oriented toward enhancement of the reproduction of close relatives (Grafen 1984).

The theory of kin selection originates in the work of Hamilton (1964). Basic evolutionary reasoning states that each organism during its life strives for an optimal allocation of resources in order to maximize its lifetime reproductive success. The fact that the human life span consists of reproductive ages (15–49) and nonreproductive ages (childhood and postmenopausal period), creates an opportunity to distribute investments between self-reproduction (*direct investments*) and reproduction of relatives (*indirect investments*). Therefore, the overall lifetime reproductive performance of an individual could be divided between *direct* and *indirect reproductive efforts*.

Hamilton (1964) reflected on the role of indirect reproduction as a potential explanation of altruistic behavior. He pointed out that organisms could also contribute to the genetic pool of the population by investing in the reproduction of relatives. Such a genetic contribution could explain why genetically related organisms show altruistic behavior towards each other.

Hence, the kin selection framework provides a point of reference for the analysis of kin influence on individual reproductive performance. However, applications of this framework to any historical or traditional population must be made carefully. This is due to the fact that kin-oriented altruistic behavior should be considered as a product of an evolutionary process. Therefore, it cannot be assumed that there is an evolutionary force that selects traits associated with kin-oriented altruism in the studied population. Thus, the issues of interest are short-term social and demographic consequences of kin-oriented help, rather than the long-run evolutionary consequences of such behavior. Moreover, one must be fully aware that altruistic behavior towards relatives is not merely "genetically programmed"; rather, it is enhanced and maintained by social norms and the rules of reciprocity (Gintis et al. 2003).

Several authors have investigated kin effects on female reproductive behavior (Sear et al. 2003; Tymicki 2004). The results show that there is a strong influence of selected kin groups on the rates of progression to the next birth, resulting in higher completed fertility. However, these investigations were not concerned with birth order, which might be considered a simplification, since it is unrealistic to assume that kin help had an equal effect over the whole life span of the recipient. It is more plausible to suppose that the intensity of the kin effect on reproduction differed with respect to the parity of the recipient. Therefore, the present analysis focuses on the hypothesis that kin help has a differential parity specific component among its effects.

If there is a differential kin effect manifest over the reproductive life span of an individual, it should be observable as a positive relationship between the presence of various kin groups and an increased proportion of higher order births. This reasoning is based on the assumption that help provided by kinsmen should lower costs associated with childbearing and thus facilitate the achievement of higher completed fertility. This argument is based on an economic analysis of supply and demand for children (Becker 1998; Becker and Barro 1988; Easterlin and Crimmins 1985). Within this framework, the growing costs of children are one of the main factors that reduce demand for children, thus causing reduction of completed fertility. Similarly, reduction in costs should stimulate demand for children and therefore lead to higher fertility. From this perspective, those households that receive help from kin groups should exhibit higher fertility due to reduced costs of having children. This reduction in costs could be associated with direct childcare (time spent on helping behavior), provision of resources (both for mother and child), and improving the nutritional status of the children.

It has to be noted that the forms of help and their effect on reproductive behavior could have different meaning in the context of controlled and natural fertility regimes. In the latter case, help could primarily concern provision of nutritional resources both to the mother and child, whereas among controlled fertility groups, help could reduce alternative costs of having children, like foregone wages or time costs. Moreover, the kin effect in the case of both fertility regimes should be of particular importance for the transition to above-average birth orders. That is, the kin effect should be significant in the case of birth orders that exceed the average for a given population or cohort. This implies that individuals receiving help from their families achieved above-average reproductive success in their groups, which converges with the above-mentioned evolutionary reasoning. In order to understand these relationships, we have to throw some light on the pathways of kin influence on female reproduction.

1.1 Pathways of Kin Influence on Reproduction

As described extensively elsewhere (Crognier 2003; Crognier, Baali, and Hilali 2001; Tymicki 2004), in order to account for the positive relation between kin-oriented help and reproductive success of the recipient, both components of reproductive success have to be considered: the number of produced offspring and the number of surviving offspring. The hypothesis concerning the kin effect on reproduction assumes that this effect operates through both components. Kin help leading to higher completed fertility is understood as provision of resources that increases survival of newborn children and lowers costs of additional children. Theoretically, these two factors constitute an extensive list of potential influences. Kinsmen can both contribute to increased offspring survival and facilitate progression to the next birth.

Kin effects on the number of surviving offspring or survival of newborn infants have been investigated in many studies (Beise and Voland 2002; Sear et al. 2003; Sear et al. 2000; Tymicki 2004), though the relationship between the presence of relatives and the risk of transition to next birth, with few exceptions, has not been of particular interest to demographers so far (Sear et al. 2003; Tymicki 2004). Previous studies were primarily interested in the effect of kin on the rates of transition to subsequent birth, whereas the current study focuses on the distribution of kin effects over the life span of the recipient. As noted earlier, using the demand–supply framework, it can be shown that kin help lowers the costs of childbearing and promotes higher completed fertility. However, it should be noted that there could be different pathways of kin influence on reproductive behavior before and after the transition from natural to controlled fertility.

In human populations without deliberate fertility control, the pace of conceptions and deliveries is regulated by the set of factors known as proximate mechanisms (Bongaarts 1978). These factors, like duration of lactation, postpartum ammenorhea, irregularities in the menstrual cycle (higher frequency of anovulatry cycles), and coital frequency were responsible for the probability of transition between successive births and thus lifetime reproductive outcome. Therefore, the possible pathways of kin influence on the reproductive rates of women among natural fertility populations are associated with the provision of resources and reduction of workload. Improvement in the nutritional status of women thanks to provision of resources may lead to better biological conditions and thus to shorter birth intervals and higher transition risks (Cumming, Wheeler, and Harber 1994; Ford and Huffman 1993; John 1993; Mosley 1979; Pebley, Hermalin, and Knodel 1991). On the other hand, kin support might reduce women's workload, which in turn could increase the amount of time spent in the household and possibly affect their reproductive behavior. However, it might be difficult to capture these effects and separate them from the physiological rhythm of reproduction in natural fertility populations. As shown by Sear et al. (2003), we cannot rule out kin effects on the rates of reproduction in populations without deliberate fertility control, although it could be argued that these effects might be much stronger in populations in which fertility was a controlled process and families were limiting their reproductive behavior consciously (Easterlin and Crimmins 1985; Galloway, Hammel, and Lee 1994; Tymicki 2004).

If we consider the above-mentioned theory, we may suppose that a shift in the demand–supply schedule might create a possibility for kinsmen to affect the fertility rates of their relatives. In the pretransitional period (natural fertility), members of the kin group contributed mostly to reproductive behavior of relatives by increasing infant survival and nutritional status of the mother. In the posttransitional period, however, kinsmen lowered the costs associated with childbearing and thus led to higher fertility of their relatives. Existing evidence suggests that this could be associated with both the provision of resources to the recipient's household and childcare (Turke 1988; Weisner and Gallimore 1977). On the one hand, provision of resources lowered the costs of children and, on the other hand, childcare was helpful because it changed the opportunity structure for parents.

1.2 Heterogeneity and Fertility

Heterogeneity with respect to individual fecundability is one of the major problems in research focused on the correlates of reproductive behavior in traditional or historical populations with natural fertility levels. The issue of heterogeneity basically refers to underlying differences between women in the levels of their fecundability (Larsen and Vaupel 1993). Some women might be more fertile due to factors that we cannot observe directly, such as, better health status or genetic endowment. Therefore, unobserved heterogeneity might obscure true relationships between studied variables and cause severe difficulties in isolating proper causal relationships between them (Vaupel and Yashin 1985). For that reason, it is necessary to control for heterogeneity in models of kin effect on reproduction.

Heterogeneity is not the only problem that might obscure true relationships between kin effects and reproductive rates. We have to be aware of the fact that phenotypic and environmental effects might trigger a positive relationship between presence of kin and reproductive rates (Sear et al. 2003). For instance, due to intergenerational inheritance of fertility, women from large families might have many offspring, but this does not necessarily imply that there was kin-oriented help from the families' many potential helpers. For that reason, we apply methodology that minimizes potential heterogeneity and confounding of phenotypic or environmental effects.

1.3 The Groups of Potential Kin Helpers

In the present study, we use identical definition of the kin groups as in the previous study (Tymicki 2004). The first group consists of a woman's older children, also called *helpers-at-the-nest*. Older children are considered to relieve the mother from burdens associated with childbearing and thus enhance the mother's reproduction. Analyses of the influence of *helpers-at-the-nest* on maternal fertility has proven this effect to be significant (Bereczkei 1998; Crognier et al. 2001; Hill and Hurtado 1996), although in some cases results have been quite ambiguous (Sear et al. 2003). Generally, it can be assumed that the presence of older children indeed enhances the woman's parity transition risk, although there is a differential effect with respect to the sex of helpers.

The second group of potential helpers, called *out-of-the-nest* helpers, consists of individuals who have terminated their reproductive span (a woman's mother and mother-in-law). This group can also include other kinsmen, for instance a woman's sisters and brothers (*mother's kin helpers*), her husband's brothers and sisters, and the husband's and wife's parents. Although some of these individuals are still able to reproduce (for instance, the woman's siblings), this does not necessarily exclude them from the group of potential helpers.

The effect of grandparents can be divided between the effect of *reproductive* and *postreproductive* helpers. The effect of *reproductive* helpers is rather straightforward since the presence of a young and reproductive grandmother inhibits reproductive performance of a daughter. This is due to the fact that a young grandmother prefers to contribute to her own reproduction rather than to the reproduction of her daughter. Moreover, a young mother might be expected to contribute to the reproductive effort of the young grandmother rather than to her own. Quite the opposite effect could be attributed to the presence of a *postreproductive* (nonreproductive) grandmother.

Females who have terminated their reproduction are able to devote their time and resources to helping relatives. The relationship between the presence of *postreproductive* females in the household and individual reproductive behavior has been widely analyzed under the so-called *grandmother hypothesis* (Beise and Voland 2002).

The magnitude of the grandparent's effect could be reinforced by the economic system and rules of inheritance among Polish peasant families. Usually, newly married couples moved to the husband's parents' farm and were dependent up to the moment when the parents passed on the farm to the son (Kopczynski 1998; Stys 1959). Depending on the inheritance system, the oldest or youngest son usually became head of the family after the death of the father. Therefore, the development of a man's own family was strictly related to economic independence, which was attained after his father's death. These explanations could be useful in understanding the hypothesis concerning a positive relationship between absence of the paternal grandfather and higher completed fertility.

Some studies have found the group of *out-of-the-nest* helpers to be an important source of help for mothers among traditional hunter-gatherers (Hill and Hurtado 1996; Sear et al. 2003). It could be assumed that the help provided by this group is associated both with provision of resources and direct childcare. For instance, a woman's male siblings and father would be concerned with provision of goods, and her mother with direct childcare. Women in postreproductive stages turned out to be an important group, affecting the survival of children, and thus leading to higher fertility.

2 Data

2.1 The Study Site

The present analysis of kin effects on reproductive outcomes of females are based on data from the reconstitution of registers from Bejsce parish located in south-central Poland. This reconstitution study was initiated by the Institute of Anthropology, Polish Academy of Science, in the year 1965 under the supervision of Professor Edmund Piasecki. The research team aimed at collecting demographic and anthropometric data using the technique of parish register reconstitution. For the study site, the researchers chose Bejsce parish located in the south-central part of Poland (100 km northeast of Cracow). The search criteria restricted the choice to large, rural parishes, located on fertile soils, with a long and continuous settlement history, and well-preserved parish registers from the seventeenth to the twentieth centuries. The Bejsce parish fulfilled each of these criteria and, moreover, was homogeneous with respect to nationality and the religion of its inhabitants. Also, it was not exposed to any dramatic depressions like wars or plague. The whole parish was founded in the year 1313, and throughout its history has relied on agricultural production. Unfortunately, information on the size of owned land was missing or incomplete and thus could not be included in the database. For that reason, it was also impossible to reconstruct any information about socioeconomic status (SES) of the inhabitants. Due to data collection obstacles, researchers finally decided to reconstruct only data that allowed the tracing of the demographic history of the whole population and particular families covering the period from 1690 to 1968. These data were published and described in a monograph by Piasecki (1990). The research team reconstructed the books of baptisms, burials, and marriages; and linked obtained data into one database containing around 40,000 cases. These data allowed the reconstruction of families and genealogies for the whole period under investigation. Estimates of data accuracy show that the registers were rather complete from 1740 onwards (Piasecki 1990). Therefore, the present analyses were conducted only for cohorts born after the year 1740. As already mentioned, inhabitants of the parish were quite homogenous with respect to social status, which at least partially compensates for the lack of information on SES. The majority of the population were small landholders or leased the land from the manor house. Only a minority (around 5–10%) were landless and worked as hired labor force.

2.2   Shortcomings of Reconstitution Data

Although parish register data offer interesting research material, they are not free from limitations. One main issue concerning the use of parish register reconstitution databases is the problem of selectivity. There are two major sources of distortions that might lead to selectivity of the data. First, parish registers were not run very strictly. Thus, not all individuals had the same chance of being registered. Second, migration was not recorded (for a detailed description of the shortcomings of parish reconstitution data, see Kasakoff and Adams 1995; Saito 1996; Voland 2000).

In the case of the Bejsce database, these problems are fortunately a minor concern since, as noted earlier, the parish books were run in a quite strict way after the year 1740 due to the introduction of civil laws (connected with the tax system) that required accuracy in the entering of records into the registers. In addition, migration in Bejsce parish could be divided between temporal and permanent processes. Temporal migration was associated with labor migration of teenage boys and girls (around ages 14 to 18). This process does not constitute a major problem since after this period these individuals returned home and stayed in the parish for the rest of their lives. Permanent migration of individuals or whole families was rather rare (less than 3% of the total database) and could not have any impact on the quality of the data (Piasecki 1990). Nor does in-migration to the parish represent a major problem due to its low rate (around 1% of the total database).

2.3   Sample Selection and Preparation

The requirements of multilevel event-history analysis guided the construction of the database to analyze parity specific kin effects. This analysis of the intensity of transition to next birth with respect to kin variables and parity was designed to capture the differential kin effect in cohorts experiencing natural and controlled fertility. Therefore, it was necessary to distinguish between women who gave birth in these two different reproductive regimes. Such a distinction is somewhat arbitrary; however, in the Bejsce parish a drop in the fertility rates could be noticed around the turn of the twentieth century. Cohorts born before the year 1900 experienced relatively high fertility with a total fertility rate (hereafter TFR) between 5.5 and 6.0. Cohorts born after 1900 were characterized by significantly lower TFRs, ranging from 4.0 for the birth cohort 1900–1920 to 3.0 for the birth cohort 1941–1960. Thus, the year 1900 was chosen as a threshold between high and low fertility in this population and we have named them as the *natural* and *controlled* fertility periods. These terms refer to general concepts that are useful from a theoretical point of view. Thus, what is meant by using the terms *natural* and *controlled* hereafter, with respect to fertility in Bejsce parish, is the separation of high and low fertility rather than reference to the fact of fertility control.

In order to account for differential kin effects in these two groups, a dummy variable was created indicating whether a woman belongs to the natural fertility or controlled fertility cohort. Therefore, the model for each birth was calculated separately for natural and controlled fertility birth cohorts.

The models for natural fertility birth cohorts were calculated for the transition from first birth to second birth and for up to the 10th birth and higher (calculated jointly for transition 9–10 and higher). For the controlled fertility birth cohorts, models were calculated for the transition from first to second birth and for up to the fifth birth (jointly for transitions to fifth birth and higher). The samples sizes are presented in the Table 5.1.

The transition to first birth was excluded from the analysis. There were two reasons for exclusion of the first parity transition. First, transition to first birth and transition to higher order births involve different durations. In the case of this model, the

Table 5.1 Number of studied events (births) by fertility regime (birth cohort of women) and birth order in the population of Bejsce parish

Birth order	Natural fertility	Controlled fertility	Total
2	1,639	483	2,122
3	1,533	405	1,938
4	1,398	296	1,694
5	1,254	163	1,417
6	1,062	88	1,150
7	848	43	891
8	670	23	693
9	462	14	476
10	282	8	290
11	144	3	147
12	58	1	59
13	27	0	27
14	11	0	11
15	2	0	2
Total	9,390	1,527	10,917

basic duration was modeled as the number of months since last birth. This basic duration could be essentially the same for all parity transitions higher than transition to first birth. The second reason, which is theoretical in nature, argues that it is plausible to assume that there is a difference between a set of correlates responsible for transition to first birth and transition to higher order parities. It is known that transition to first birth in historical populations to a large extent was determined by the transition to first marriage (Goody 1983; Livi-Bacci 1999). First marriage was closely followed by first birth and therefore it could be assumed that there was a different set of determinants responsible for entering into first marriage that are not included in the models.

The hazard model consists of basic duration, which is the transition to subsequent birth, a set of variables responsible for the kin effect, and a set of control variables. Most of the kin effect on the risk of parity transition is captured by the following time-varying covariates: (i) presence of the *helpers-at-the-nest* (male and female siblings of an index child at least 10-years old), (ii) presence of maternal grandmother in reproductive age vs. presence of maternal grandmother in postreproductive age, (iii) presence of maternal grandfather, and (iv) presence of paternal grandmother and grandfather. The only kin variable represented by a time-constant covariate is the presence of the mother's younger sisters and brothers.

The group of control variables, which may be responsible for a delayed or faster transition to the next birth, are as follows: (i) whether previous birth was multiple or single, (ii) age of mother at previous birth, and (iii) fate of the previous child (whether previous child died within 1 year after birth). Among these variables, the age of the mother at previous birth is of particular importance since it could influence interbirth intervals and therefore completed fertility.

The individuals in the analysis were censored in the following cases: (i) death, (ii) lost to follow-up (presumably migration), (iii) reaching limit of reproductive age (45 years of age), (iv) lack of next parity transition, and (v) birth interval longer than 72 months. In the last case, it was assumed that a birth interval lasting more than 72 months was related to some irregularities in reproductive functions probably caused by sterility or miscarriage (compare similar assumption in Sear et al. 2003).

Other censoring events have little significant influence on the studied sample. As already mentioned, the process of migration applies to a marginal fraction of the sample. Reaching the age of 45 and the death of an individual constitutes a case of natural censoring and does not influence the sample structure and size. Censoring due to lack of transition to subsequent birth could be caused by deliberate stopping of reproduction (in the case of controlled fertility cohorts).

3 Methods

The event-history approach was applied in order to model the risk of transition to next birth with respect to kin effects as the major explanatory variables. Event-history models are quite useful when we want to account for time dependency and for the fact of censoring in the data. Moreover, recently produced software allows us to account for unobserved heterogeneity (Lillard and Panis 2000). The mathematical representation of the transition rate in the multilevel model containing unobserved heterogeneity can be given by the following formula:

$$\ln \mu_{ij}(t) = y(t) + \sum_k \beta_{jk} x_{ijk} + \sum_{k'} \gamma_k, v_{jk}, + \delta_i \tag{1}$$

where μ_{ij} is the intensity and (t) stands for basic duration, here time since last birth. Thus, the whole term $\mu_{ij}(t)$ refers to the rate of occurrence of an event at time t (the birth of jth infant) for the ith woman. The component $y(t)$ captures the baseline hazard (i.e., the effect of duration on the intensity of the studied event). The x_k represents kth time constant covariate specific to the child level with β as the respective regression parameter. The γ_k, represents the k'th covariate on the mother's specific level. The last parameter, δ_i, is responsible for the mother-specific heterogeneity.[1]

In comparison with a previous study (Tymicki 2004), there was no need to calculate a multilevel model since each model has been calculated separately with respect to a given birth. In the previous analyses, it was necessary to build a multi-level model since all parity transitions for each woman were merged into one data-base. Therefore, it required a hierarchical structure of the database since one woman could contribute with several children to the analysis.

On the other hand, as mentioned above in the theory section, the main source of distortions in the model is unobserved differences in fecundability between women and phenotypic and environmental confounds. That was the reason for including a mother-specific heterogeneity factor and a set of time-varying and time-constant covariates that characterize the groups of mother-kinsmen. All of these kin-related covariates were coded as dummy variables.

As already discussed in the previous section, each model has been calculated separately for birth cohorts exhibiting natural and controlled fertility. This distinc-tion was based on the TFR presented earlier in this paper. In order to estimate the multilevel hazard regression model of the influence of kin variables on transition to subsequent parities, the aML software has been used (Lillard and Panis 2000).

4   Results

The models of the parity specific kin effects were calculated with respect to fertility regime, i.e., natural vs. controlled fertility, and therefore are presented in two sepa-rate tables (compare Tables 5.2, 5.3). Generally, the results presented in the form of the relative risks reveal patterns similar to those shown in earlier analyses (Tymicki 2004). The kin influences on the risk of transition between successive births are

---

[1] It is assumed that the heterogeneity parameter δ_i is normally distributed.

Table 5.2 Kin influence on parity transition risks among natural fertility birth cohorts of women form Bejsce parish. Parameters refer to the relative risks—exp(β); standard errors in parentheses

	Transition						
	1–2	2–3	3–4	4–5	5–6 & 6–7	7–8 & 8–9	9–10 and higher
Female helpers-at-the-nest (ref. category-present)	0.95 (0.049)	0.97 (0.057)	0.97 (0.064)	1.01 (0.071)	0.90* (0.058)	0.96 (0.076)	0.99 (0.154)
No female helpers-at-the-nest							
Male helpers-at-the-nest (ref. category-present)	1.02 (0.050)	0.99 (0.057)	0.93 (0.065)	0.95 (0.072)	1.11* (0.058)	1.12 (0.073)	1.10 (0.150)
No male helpers-at-the-nest							
Mother's younger brothers (ref. category-present)	1.14** (0.023)	0.79 (0.204)	0.85 (0.165)	1.08 (0.095)	1.32*** (0.061)	1.58*** (0.074)	1.42*** (0.094)
No younger brothers							
Mother's younger sisters (ref. category-present)	1.04 (0.023)	1.40* (0.203)	1.28 (0.165)	1.03 (0.095)	1.47*** (0.063)	1.51*** (0.074)	1.45*** (0.139)
No younger sisters							
Maternal grandmother at reproductive ages (ref. cat.-alive)	1.12*** (0.032)	1.23*** (0.037)	1.12** (0.045)	1.17*** (0.054)	1.35*** (0.046)	1.08* (0.037)	2.29*** (0.059)
Dead							
Maternal grandmother at postreproductive ages (ref. cat.-alive)	0.79*** (0.040)	0.81*** (0.046)	0.82*** (0.054)	0.78*** (0.062)	0.70*** (0.051)	0.82*** (0.041)	0.32*** (0.091)
Dead							
Maternal grandfather (ref. category-alive)	1.01 (0.048)	1.03 (0.053)	1.07 (0.065)	0.96 (0.071)	0.90 (0.067)	0.81** (0.092)	0.63*** (0.135)
Dead							
Paternal grandmother (ref. category-alive)	1.15*** (0.052)	1.17*** (0.059)	1.03 (0.071)	1.09 (0.076)	0.85** (0.073)	0.69*** (0.106)	0.54*** (0.158)
Dead							

(continued)

Table 5.2 (continued)

	Transition						
	1–2	2–3	3–4	4–5	5–6 6–7	7–8 & 8–9	9–10 and higher
Dead							
Paternal grandfather (ref. category-alive)	1.23*** (0.052)	1.25*** (0.061)	1.37*** (0.071)	1.47*** (0.078)	1.10 (0.079)	1.56*** (0.103)	1.96*** (0.153)
Dead							
Single vs. multiple birth (ref. category-single birth)	0.86 (0.483)	0.87 (0.273)	0.67 (0.251)	0.60* (0.295)	0.99 (0.258)	1.20 (0.234)	0.23 (1.013)
Multiple birth							
Age of mother at given transition (ref. category 14–19)							
19–25	1.26*** (0.048)	1.31*** (0.061)	1.32*** (0.081)	1.21 (0.138)	1.09 (0.278)	1.00 (0.000)	1.00 (0.000)
25–30	1.02 (0.061)	1.01 (0.065)	1.04 (0.068)	1.06 (0.077)	1.13 (0.083)	1.49 (0.307)	1.34 (1.732)
30–35	0.77*** (0.096)	0.75*** (0.082)	0.86* (0.081)	0.79*** (0.079)	0.90 (0.064)	1.05 (0.089)	2.90*** (0.250)
35+	0.51*** (0.141)	0.37*** (0.118)	0.32*** (0.115)	0.34*** (0.101)	0.44*** (0.067)	0.42*** (0.077)	0.41*** (0.126)
Fate of the previous child (ref. cat. Previous child survived until first birthday)							
Previous child died within 1 year after birth	3.51** (1.143)	0.97 (0.065)	0.89 (0.081)	0.93 (0.085)	0.97 (0.074)	0.86 (0.093)	1.11 (0.137)
ln-L	−77305.2	−77290.7	−77314.7	−77314.0	−77177.2	−77212.1	−77210.8

* = 10%
** = 5%
*** = 1%

Table 5.3 Kin influence on parity transition risks among controlled fertility birth cohorts of women form Bejsce parish. Parameters refer to the relative risks—exp(β); standard errors in parentheses

	Transition							
	1–2		2–3		3–4		4–5 and higher	
Female helpers-at-the-nest (ref. category-present)	0.99	(0.0894)	0.97	(0.1205)	0.77	(0.1780)	1.07	(0.1625)
No female helpers-at-the-nest								
Male helpers-at-the-nest (ref. category-present)	0.94	(0.0895)	0.92	(0.1197)	0.93	(0.1614)	1.11	(0.1593)
No male helpers-at-the-nest								
Mother's younger brothers (ref. category-present)	1.94***	(0.1826)	1.09	(0.1347)	2.64***	(0.3511)	1.80**	(0.2425)
No younger brothers								
Mother's younger sisters (ref. category-present)	3.19***	(0.0466)	1.11	(0.1825)	1.07	(0.1143)	2.49***	(0.2628)
No younger sisters								
Maternal grandmother at reproductive ages (ref. category-alive)	0.74*	(0.1612)	1.46**	(0.1527)	0.97	(0.3683)	2.84***	(0.3564)
Dead								
Maternal grandmother at postreproductive ages (ref. category-alive)	0.78**	(0.1089)	0.72***	(0.1215)	0.61***	(0.1673)	0.40***	(0.1603)
Dead								
Maternal grandfather (ref. category-alive)	0.95	(0.0896)	0.90	(0.1156)	0.83	(0.1612)	0.57***	(0.1547)
Dead								
Paternal grandmother (ref. category-alive)	0.81**	(0.0952)	0.81*	(0.1177)	0.86	(0.1745)	0.84	(0.1958)
Dead								
Paternal grandfather (ref. category-alive)	0.96	(0.1010)	1.22	(0.1415)	1.13	(0.1985)	0.98	(0.2136)

(continued)

Table 5.3 (continued)

	Transition			
	1–2	2–3	3–4	4–5 and higher
Dead				
Single vs. multiple birth (ref. category-single birth)	1.26 (0.5586)	2.10* (0.4352)	1.14 (0.6124)	0.58 (0.7559)
Multiple birth				
Age of mother at given transition (ref. category 14–19)				
19–25	1.03 (0.1034)	0.58*** (0.1482)	0.41*** (0.2278)	0.40 (0.6128)
25–30	0.94 (0.1367)	0.49*** (0.1481)	0.31*** (0.1879)	0.38*** (0.2666)
30–35	1.17 (0.2380)	0.41*** (0.1987)	0.30*** (0.2265)	0.37*** (0.2233)
35+	0.22*** (0.4399)	0.19*** (0.3565)	0.19*** (0.3371)	0.28*** (0.2561)
Fate of the previous child (ref. category Child survived until first birthday)				
Previous child died within 1 year after birth	2.09 (0.6843)	1.63*** (0.1359)	0.88 (0.2226)	1.26 (0.2536)
ln-L	–14738.8	–14831.2	–14825.9	
–14841.6				

* = 10%
** = 5%
*** = 1%

much stronger and clearer in the case of the natural fertility birth cohorts than in the case of controlled fertility cohorts.

Both for women born before and after the turn of the twentieth century, there is no effect of the number of brothers or sisters of a woman on her risk of transition between parities.

Also the absence of younger siblings of an index child tends to have the reverse effect to that expected (Murphy and Knudsen 2002). However, this relationship has an intuitive explanation: women who did not have any children prior to the index child, run a higher risk of experiencing the next birth.

On average, women from natural fertility birth cohorts who did not have any children at least 10 years older than the index child, revealed around 40 percent higher risk of transition to the sixth birth and higher. Thus, we may wonder whether the presence of young caretakers had any positive influence in the case of parity-specific transition risks.

The results suggest that there is a positive effect of the absence of a reproductive grandmother at each of the studied birth transitions. A woman whose mother was alive and still reproductive had a lower risk of progression to subsequent birth. On the other hand, reproductive women whose mother had died had, on average, a 25 percent lower risk of transition to next birth at each of the parities. This effect was particularly profound in the case of the highest parities (transition to ninth birth and higher). Those women whose mothers were dead had an almost 70 percent lower risk of transition to the ninth birth and higher. A similar pattern could be noticed in the case of the influence of a maternal grandfather and paternal grandmother. Absence of a mother's father and father's mother decreased the risk of transition to higher order births, although these effects were much weaker than in the previous case. On the contrary, the absence of the paternal grandfather seemed to enhance the risk of transition at each of the parities.

In the case of women who entered motherhood after the turn of the twentieth century, the patterns of kin influence are similar to the case of natural fertility birth cohorts. The results are presented in Table 5.3. Again, the most important effect could be attributed to the effect of grandparents. Absence of the maternal grandmother decreased chances for transition at each of the parities. This effect was also present in the case of the maternal grandfather and paternal grandparents although it was much less clear.

As in the case of natural fertility birth cohorts, there was no parity specific effect of the *helpers-at-the-nest*. There was also a positive effect of the absence of the mother's younger sisters or brothers at given parity transition. Generally, the patterns of kin influence in the case of controlled fertility birth cohorts are much less clear, which might be due to the lower number of cases under analysis.

The effects of the included control variables are similar or both models. There is practically no effect of twin births on subsequent parity transition. In the case of the natural fertility cohorts, twin births have a rather inhibiting effect on the transition to subsequent conception. This effect is much less clear in the case of controlled fertility birth cohorts, which might be a consequence of some spurious effects due to an insufficient number of cases.

The estimated effect of the mother's age reveals quite a predictable pattern. Both for natural and controlled fertility birth cohorts, women from Bejsce parish exhibit a decreasing risk of parity transition with age.

There is also a significant replacement effect at lower parities. Women who have lost their previous child experience higher transition risks in comparison with women whose child survived the first 12 months of life. This effect is particularly strong in the case of death of the first or second child (cf. Tymicki 2005).

5 Discussion

The present paper analyzed parity specific kin effects among women from the population of Bejsce parish. The analyses of parity specific kin effects were designed to answer questions about the relative importance of help provided by closest kin across an individual's reproductive history. The results reveal only weak support for the original hypothesis that kin help should be of crucial importance at higher parities.

Generally, the results overlap with the findings of the previous analyses of the effect of closest kin on the transition to next birth without regard to parity (Tymicki 2004). Surprisingly, selected groups of family members did not have an effect on the increased risk of transition to higher birth orders. An exception here is the group of so-called *nongenerative helpers* (grandparents). The most spectacular is the effect of the maternal grandmother, both in the case of natural and controlled fertility birth cohorts. Absence of a maternal grandmother decreases the risk of transition to the 10th birth by 70 percent in comparison to those women whose mother was still alive (among natural fertility cohorts). It has to be noted that the absence of a maternal grandmother decreases the risk of each parity transition by, on average, 30 percent.

Interestingly, there is also a significant effect due to the presence of a maternal grandfather at higher parities. Absence of a mother's father decreases chances of transition beyond the seventh birth by 30 percent (on average). The effect on the transition to subsequent births was rather constant across individual reproductive history in the case of the maternal grandmother. Contrary to this, the effect of the maternal grandfather was concentrated at higher order births. This might be evidence for direct help obtained by the mother from her parents, which possibly enabled the couple to attain a higher number of births.

The shape of the parity-specific effect of maternal grandmothers who were under the age of 45, seems to be quite opposite from the previously described effects. The absence of a reproductive grandmother increased the risk of transition at each of the parities.[2]

---

[2] Extremely high results for the 10th and higher parity transition are probably due to the insufficient number of cases under analysis and therefore should be interpreted very cautiously.

This, however, might be explained by the fact that daughters of those women who became grandmothers relatively early, under the age of 45, started their own reproduction early and therefore progressed to higher parities slower than the reference category. This effect is present both among natural and controlled fertility cohorts.

Another effect worth mentioning is associated with the presence of paternal grandparents among natural fertility birth cohorts. The nature of the relationship between the presence of a paternal grandmother and the risk of transition to subsequent parities is mixed. The absence of the husband's mother (paternal grandmother) increases the risk of transition to parity 2 and 3 and decreases the risk at higher parities. On the other hand, the absence of the husband's father (paternal grandfather) increases the risk of transition at each of the parities. As already noted, such an effect could be attributed to the economics and the inheritance system among Polish peasant families. Therefore, the positive relationship between the absence of the paternal grandfather and the higher risk of transition to subsequent births could be partially explained by the economic foundations of the peasant family formation process.

A similar explanation could be assumed in the case of the effect of a paternal grandmother at lower parities. Moreover, the results reveal a positive relationship between the presence of a husband's mother and transition to higher parities. This was probably related to the fact that a nonreproductive paternal grandmother could still be used as a caretaker for the children in the household.

As can be noticed, these effects are missing among cohorts born after the turn of the twentieth century as a result of the increasing importance of sources of income other than agriculture. Although the process of industrialization progressed much more slowly in Poland than in the rest of Western Europe, it finally led to changes in the family formation process.

As already noted, on the basis of the current and past results, the theoretically predicted positive effect of *helpers-at-the-nest* can be questioned. The results obtained here suggest the opposite conclusion. The presence of children at least 10 years older than the index child inhibited rather than promoted the reproductive performance of the mother. Certainly, the possibility that those children were helpful in the household cannot be completely ruled out. However, on the basis of the current data and analysis such an effect cannot be isolated in a satisfactory way. The only significant pattern shows that the presence of older children in the household inhibited transition to higher order births by a purely demographic effect of lower parity progression ratios.

There was also no effect of a mother's siblings, which could be a sign of weak support between the family members. Of course there might be some flow of goods and services between the households of siblings, but apparently it did not have an effect on the rates of reproduction.

The present analysis is by no means exhaustive and leaves room for further investigations. Since the working database is a pure register of demographic events, we cannot rule out the possibility that more detailed data would bring more comprehensive and consistent results. As shown by other anthropological studies investigating kin effects, the use of small but richer databases or a narrower focus of the analysis might bring results that converge with the theoretical predictions (Bereczkei

1998; Turke 1988; Weisner and Gallimore 1977). Moreover, the present models did not aim to reveal causal relationships between the analyzed variables, but rather to show interdependence between the presence of kin and rates of reproduction.

Since, at present, there is no suitable benchmark for the present analysis, the results obtained cannot be compared. However, analyses based on existing parish register reconstitution data from other countries might bring comparable results. Therefore, it seems highly desirable to conduct a comparative analysis using other sources of parish data. This might involve other methods like estimation of parity specific birth probabilities or parity transition ratios with respect to the described kin variables. This might bring some new evidence to suggest that at least some kin variables had a profound effect on the rates of reproduction in historical European populations. Therefore, the present study is just a first step towards comprehensive description of these effects and opens a new perspective on the understanding of reproductive behavior in the past.

Acknowledgments I would like to acknowledge my advisors, Professor Janina Jozwiak (Warsaw School of Economics) and Professor Hans-Peter Kohler (Population Studies Center, University of Pennsylvania) for their help and advice. I also would like to thank Professor Tadeusz Bielicki (Director of the Institute of Anthropology, Polish Academy of Science) for providing me with the database.

References

Becker, G.S. 1998. *A Treatise on Family*. Harvard University Press, Cambridge, MA.

Becker, G.S. and R.J. Barro. 1988. A reformulation of the economic theory of fertility. *Quarterly Journal of Economics* 103: 1–25.

Beise, J. and E. Voland. 2002. A multilevel event history analysis of the effects of grandmothers on child mortality in a historical German population (Krummhorn, Ostfiesland, 1720–1847). *Demographic Research* 7: 470–94.

Bereczkei, T. 1998. Kinship network, direct childcare, and fertility among Hungarians and Gypsies. *Evolution and Human Behavior* 19: 283–98.

Bongaarts, J. 1978. A framework for analysing the proximate determinants of fertility. *Population and Development Review* 4: 105–32.

Burnstein, E., C. Crandall, and S. Kitayama. 1994. Some neo-Darwinian decision rules for altruism: Weighing cues for inclusive fitness as a function of the biological importance of the decision. *Journal of Personality and Social Psychology* 67: 733–89.

Crognier, E. 2003. Reproductive success: Which meaning? *American Journal of Human Biology* 15: 352–60.

Crognier, E., A. Baali, and M-K. Hilali. 2001. Do helpers at the nest increase their parents' reproductive success? *American Journal of Human Biology* 13: 365–73.

Cumming, D.C., G.D. Wheeler, and V.J. Harber. 1994. Physical activity, nutrition, and reproduction, in K.L. Campbell and J.W. Wood (eds.), *Interactions of environment, fertility and behavior, human reproductive ecology*, New York Academy of Science, New York, pp. 55–76.

Dunbar, R.I.M. and M. Spoors. 1995. Social networks, support cliques, and kinship. *Human Nature* 6: 273–90.

Easterlin, R.A. and E. Crimmins. 1985. *The Fertility Revolution. A Supply Demand Analysis*. University of Chicago Press, Chicago, IL.

Ford, K. and S. Huffman. 1993. Maternal nutrition, infant feeding and post-partum amenorrhea: Recent evidence from Bangladesh, in R. Gray, H. Leridon, and A. Spira (eds.), *Biomedical and demographic determinants of reproduction*, Calderon, Oxford, pp. 383–90.

Galloway, P.R., E.A. Hammel, and R.D. Lee. 1994. Fertility decline in Prussia, 1875–1910: A pooled cross-section time series analysis. *Population Studies* 48: 135–58.

Gintis, H., S. Bowles, R. Boyd, and E. Fehr. 2003. Explaining altruistic behavior in humans. *Evolution and Human Behavior* 24: 153–72.

Goody, J. 1983. *The Development of Family and Marriage in the Europe*. Cambridge University Press, Cambridge.

Grafen, A. 1984. Natural selection, kin selection and group selection, in J.R. Krebs and N.B. Davies (eds.), *Behavioral ecology*, 2nd edition, Blackwell, Oxford, pp. 5–31.

Hamilton, W.D. 1964. The genetical evolution of social behavior: Part I and Part II. *Journal of Theoretical Biology* 7: 1–52.

Hill, K. and M. Hurtado. 1996. *Ache Life History. The Ecology and Demography of Foraging People*. Aldine de Gruyter, New York.

John, A.M. 1993. Statistical evidence on links between maternal nutrition and post-partum infertility, in R. Gray, H. Leridon, and A. Spira (eds.), *Biomedical and demographic determinants of reproduction*, Calderon, Oxford, pp. 372–82.

Kasakoff, A.B. and J.W. Adams. 1995. The effect of migration on ages at vital rates events: A critique of family reconstitution in historical demography. *European Journal of Population* 11: 199–242.

Kohler, H-P. and E.A. Hammel. 2001. On the role of families and kinship networks in pre-industrial agricultural societies: An analysis of the 1698 Slavonian census. *Journal of Population Economics* 14: 21–49.

Kopczynski, M. 1998. *Studia Nad Rodzina Chlopska w Koronie w XVII-XVIII Wieku. Studies on the Peasant Family in the Central Districts of Poland in 17th to 18th Century*. Wydawnictwo Krupski i S-ka, Warszawa.

Larsen, U. and J.W. Vaupel. 1993. Hutterite fecundability by age and parity: Strategies for frailty modeling of event histories. *Demography* 30: 81–102.

Laslett, P. 1988. Family, kinship and collectivity as systems of support in pre-industrial Europe: A consideration of the 'nuclear-hardship' hypothesis. *Continuity and Change* 3: 153–75.

Lillard, L.A. and C.W.A. Panis. 2000. *AML Multilevel Mulitprocess Statistical Software, Release 1.0*. EconWare, Los Angeles, CA.

Livi-Bacci, M. 1999. *The Population of Europe. A History*. Blackwell, Oxford.

Mosley, H.W. 1979. The effects of nutrition on natural fertility, in H. Leridon and J. Menken (eds.), *Natural fertility: Patterns and determinants of natural fertility; Proceedings of a seminar on natural fertility*, Ordina Editions, Liege, pp. 85–105.

Murphy, M. and L.B. Knudsen. 2002. The intergenerational transmission of fertility in contemporary Denmark: The effects of number of siblings (full and half), birth order, and whether male or female. *Population Studies* 56: 235–48.

Pebley, A.R., A.I. Hermalin, and J. Knodel. 1991. Birth spacing and infant mortality: Evidence for eighteenth and nineteenth century German villages. *Journal of Biosocial Science* 23: 445–59.

Piasecki, E. 1990. *Ludnosc Parafii Bejskiej w Swietle Ksiag Metryklanych z XVIII–XX W. Studium Demograficzne (Population of the Bejsce parish [Kielce voivodeship, Poland] in the light of parish registers of the 18th–20th centuries. A demographic study)*. PWN, Warsaw.

Saito, O. 1996. Historical demography: Achievements and prospects. *Population Studies* 50: 537–53.

Sear, R., R. Mace, and I. McGregor. 2000. Maternal grandmothers improve nutritional status and survival of children in rural Gambia. *Proceedings of the Royal Society of London* Series B 267: 1641–7.

Sear, R., R. Mace, and I. McGregor. 2003. The effects of kin on female fertility in rural Gambia. *Evolution and Human Behavior* 24: 25–42.

Stys, W. 1959. *Wspolzaleznosc rozwoju rodziny chlopskiej i jej gospodarstwa (The interdependence between family development and peasant economy)*. Wroclawskie Towarzystwo Naukowe, Wroclaw.

Turke, P.W. 1988. Helpers at the nest: Childcare networks on Infaluk, in L. Betzig, M. Borgerhoff-Mulder, and P.W. Turke (eds.), *Human reproductive behavior*, Cambridge University Press, Cambridge, pp. 173–88.

Tymicki, K. 2004. The kin influence on female reproductive behavior. The evidence from the reconstitution of Bejsce parish registers, 18th–20th centuries, Poland. *American Journal of Human Biology* 16: 508–22.

Tymicki, K. 2005. The interplay between infant mortality and subsequent reproductive behavior. Evidence for the replacement effect from historical population of Bejsce parish, 18th–20th centuries, Poland. *Historical Social Research* 30(3): 240–64.

Vaupel, J.W. and A.I. Yashin. 1985. Heterogeneity's ruses: Some surprising effects of selection on population dynamics. *The American Statistician* 39: 176–85.

Voland, E. 2000. Contributions of family reconstitution studies to evolutionary reproductive ecology. *Evolutionary Anthropology* 9: 134–46.

Weisner, T.S. and R. Gallimore. 1977. My brother's keeper: Child and sibling caretaking. *Current Anthropology* 18: 169–90.

Chapter 6
Places of Life Events as Bequestable Wealth: Family Territory and Migration in France, 19th and 20th Centuries

Lionel Kesztenbaum

Abstract Previous studies have shown that the family influences migration decisions in various ways, but very few of them take into account past migrations among the kinship group. In this study, we take advantage of new historical data, based on the TRA survey, to discuss the extent to which kinship influences migration. We use the concept of spatial capital to capture all the knowledge families possess about geographical locations. We are then able to show how this knowledge is—or is not—handed down from one generation to another. This is a key point of the analysis of migration as it means that migration decisions are not only influenced by individual characteristics or economic or historical context, but also by the past migration behavior of the family. As such, migration is not only an investment for the migrant or for his close relatives but can be seen as a long-term investment of the kinship group.

Keywords Migration, spatial capital, family, France 19th century

1 Introduction

Scholars who study migration usually emphasize macroregularities underlying human mobility. In particular, economists, sociologists, and demographers focus on the age pattern of migrations. In this view, the life cycle hypothesis appears as an important and useful tool of analysis (see, e.g., Courgeau 1984; Sandefur and Scott 1981). Migrations follow a "bell-shaped curve", decreasing after a peak around the age of 20. Although the peak can occur earlier or later, depending on historical and geographical contexts, the shape of the curve seems extremely general over time and space, and nineteenth century France is no exception (Courgeau 1993). More precisely, age can be seen as a proxy for vital events that happen during the life cycle (see Courgeau and Lelièvre 2003) because mobility evolves by age as people leave their parental home, get married, have children, and so on.

L'Institut National de la Recherche Agronomique (INRA), Laboratoire d'économie appliquée, and Institut National d'Études Démographiques (INED), Université d'Evry France

However, these empirical regularities do not necessarily provide a good framework for fully understanding the migration process. Among the various mechanisms underlying migration decisions,[1] this chapter focuses on the precise influence of kinship. Two recent studies have made important efforts to reconsider kinship determination in mobility choices. The first one (Gribaudi 1987) analyzes the making of the working class in Turin and shows how integration into urban places relied strongly on kinship. The second study (Rosental 1999) concentrates on nineteenth century France and highlights family mechanisms that produce a migration decision, in particular by relating them to the various opportunities available at a given moment. Both studies agree on the central importance of kinship in migration and on the importance of the timing of individual mobility within a family life cycle. The birth rank of the child, for instance, appears as an essential determinant of mobility because it affects the possibility that an individual will move or not, given his family needs and offers.

From this point of view, migration seems to be best understood as a family undertaking and very strongly related with the kinship network. At the opposite position is Lesger, Lucassen, and Schrover's (2002) article, significantly entitled "Is there life outside the migrant network?", which criticizes the excess of "chain migration" studies in the literature, and not only the ones on family chain migration.

In this study, we will take advantage of new historical data based on the TRA survey, to discuss precisely the extent to which kinship influences migration. We focus on two central aspects of migration; the decision to migrate and the choice of place to move to. One may think that family forms (for example, number of siblings, type of professional orientation, and nuclear family) as well as individual factors (birth rank, gender) have a particular influence on mobility. But it is also clear that these forms depend on the historical conditions and the socioeconomic background in which they fit, and so we need to investigate further how the context shapes the mobility decision. Families rely on external factors such as socioeconomic, legal, and cultural conditions. Our purpose here is not to measure all these factors and take them into account in the decision to migrate, but only to evaluate the family territory and observe its influence on migration decisions. For each individual, we produce an estimation of the places where members of his family live or have lived, which represents, in some way, the spatial capital he inherited. We then assess the link between this family portfolio of places and the migration comportment of the heir.

The purpose of this chapter, then, is to reassess the influence of kinship on geographic mobility by taking into account past migrations within the family. We use the concept of spatial capital to capture all the knowledge families possess about

---

[1] A complete description is to be found in Greenwood (1997). For the case of nineteenth-century France, see Ogden and White (1989), especially Chapter 1 (Migration in later nineteenth- and twentieth-century France: the social and economic context) by P. Ogden and P. White, and Chapter 2 (Internal migration in the nineteenth and twentieth centuries) by P. White.

geographical locations. In practical terms, this capital is estimated by the spatial distribution of places that were once visited by any member of the family. This capital is seen as investments made by the family in certain locations from generation to generation. We are able to show how this knowledge is, or is not, handed down from one generation to another. This is a key point of the analysis of migration as it means that migration decisions may not only be influenced by individual characteristics or economic and historical context, but also by the past migration behavior of the family. In this way, migration is not only an investment for the migrant or for his close relatives but can also be seen as a long-term investment of the kinship group. The first part will present the database and the key hypotheses we made in reconstructing families and localizing them in space and time. We then provide a description of the family territory and give some clues to the geographical dispersion of French families. From this geographical observation, we next observe individual mobility; first, what is the influence of the family territory on migration decisions and, second, whether individuals stay in or leave this territory.

2   The Military Registers and the TRA Survey

Historical studies of kinship are often constrained by the sources available, which only record households or discontinuous changes in family organization. The TRA survey offers efficient observations of French families over one and a half centuries for vital events such as marriages or deaths. Military records help to overcome these limited data as conscripts were very precisely traced by the army during an important part of their life cycle. We start by describing our database, focusing on the hypothesis we use to reconstitute families and to observe geographical mobility.

Our sample is based on the TRA survey (also known as "3000 familles" survey). Initiated by Jacques Dupâquier and Denis Kessler, this survey aims to reconstitute the patterns of French families whose ancestors were born in the beginning of the nineteenth century. It is based on a patronymic method: all people whose surname begins with the letters T, R, and A are recorded from various sources. Apart from the classical "État-civil",[2] the two main sources are wedding and fiscal records. The first source gives information on TRA people at the time of their marriage, especially their place of birth, the residence of the groom and his bride, and the residence of both their parents.[3] The second source is the TSA ("Table de successions et absences"). Created after the 1799 law (22 *frimaire* year VII), the TSA is used by the French administration in order to tax inheritance. For every deceased person, the

---

[2] From the French Revolution onwards, the État-civil records births, marriages, and deaths in all French communes. It was also used in the TRA survey but mainly for family reconstitution.

[3] A more accurate description and usage of the TRA sample, especially the wedding records, can be found in Dupâquier and Kessler (1992).

TSA notes whether he or she left an inheritance.[4] Both these sources are used to reconstitute the families of the TRA people. They also give us some information on their places of residence but only at fixed moments in the life cycle, that is, mainly at births, weddings, and deaths.

Military records are the core of our sample. Contrary to the other sources involved in the TRA survey, they provide a continuous record of residences between the ages of 20 and 46.[5] Just before and after Germany's defeat in the war of 1870, the French army was completely transformed. Replacement[6] was abolished and replaced by a conscription army. Military duty now applied to everyone, except for those excused for medical reasons. The second major change concerned the length of military service. Before the war of 1870, the French army was a semiprofessional army. Military service lasted 7 years, but people were fully discharged from military duty after leaving the forces. Beginning with the 1872 law, military service was divided into a short portion of active service and a longer portion in the reserve army. Thus, people stayed in the army for 26 years in a combination of active and reserve service. While in the reserve, training periods were held and individuals could be recalled at any time in case of war. In this process, individuals had to declare their successive residences, or risk penalties or even jail sentences. The army created a complete and efficient system to monitor all conscripts, in order to locate them at any time. The military registers ("les registres matricules") were the centre of this system, where all persons were recorded and followed until discharged.[7]

The military records were collected for all TRA people born between 1847 and 1900, but only for a sample of "departements" (French territorial division). The choice of the "departements" collected was oriented by the desire to balance some of the main geographic and socioeconomic characteristics of France at that time. We sought to find an equilibrium between Paris and the "provinces", between North and South France (mainly for the differential in inheritance custom), and between rural and urban areas. Therefore, we collected the whole Parisian area ("le bassin parisien"), which consists of three "departements": Seine (with Paris itself), Seine-et-Marne, and Seine-et-Oise. We also collected from ten other "departements" within the country.

---

[4] A complete description of the fiscal data is to be found in Bourdieu, Postel-Vinay, and Suwa-Eisenmann (2004).

[5] Age at end of observation varies in the sample as the military law changes.

[6] Before 1872 people could draw to escape military duty, and those who were enrolled could pay someone else to take their place (replacement).

[7] More details on this particular source are to be found in the original texts of the laws (law of "27 juillet 1872 sur le recrutement de l'armée" and law of "15 juillet 1889 sur le recrutement de l'armée") or in the army manuals ("Code-manuel..." 1873). An excellent summary is provided in Farcy and Faure (2003, 14–22). On the general organization of the army and the consequences of the changes of the 1872 law on this organization, see the study by Odile Roynette (2000).

Wedding records were collected for all weddings that included a TRA individual and that occurred in the nineteenth century. TSA records have been collected for all TRA persons who died between 1800 and 1940. Both these sources are exhaustive for the whole of France, with certain exceptions due to accidental source destruction (e.g., war, fire). These two main databases have been used to reconstitute the families of the conscripts collected in the military records. Conscripts are located at the end of the TRA survey because they were born in the second part of the nineteenth century; we can therefore link them without much difficulty.

The TRA survey is representative of the French population at the time of the survey.[8] Nevertheless, it has some shortcomings. The most important one is surely the absence of women, both in the military records and in the family reconstruction. Indeed, we lose all women after the first generation because their children take the name of the father and, therefore, they are no longer TRA.[9] Thus, while we are still able to consider the life course of TRA women as they keep their birth name until their death, we cannot follow their children. By using the genealogy from the bottom to the top, we lose the matrimonial branch when considering the ancestors of a TRA individual. We can find the father and his relatives (uncles and aunts) but not the mother's. In the same way, we can find information on the father of the father and follow it along the patriarchal branch, but at each step we lose both parents of the mother. We can, however, still obtain some information on the family-in-law through the wedding records, which give us the residence at time of marriage of the parents of the mother (the matrimonial grandparents). This can compensate somewhat for the lack of data and give us indications, if only partially, on the residence of this part of the family.

So, the main, and perhaps the most difficult, assumption is the neutrality of the matrimonial lineage. It does not mean that this branch does not play any role in the migration, but only that this role is by no way different or particular from the role of the patrimonial lineage. This is of course debatable, but at this stage the matrimonial lineage cannot be evaluated in our study. We analyze inheritance only from the point of view of the patrimonial lineage that we reconstitute from the TRA.

3   Defining Kinship with Historical Sources

Conscripts are the main focus of our analysis and we complete the data from the military records by considering the family networks given by the TRA. The immediate family members that we consider here are the brothers and the father of a given conscript. For each TRA person recorded in the military registers, we also

---

[8] See, for instance, Bourdieu and Kesztenbaum (2004).

[9] Except for the very few weddings that involve two TRAs, groom and bride; however, as underlined in (Rosental 2002), there are not enough TRA names in the French population to make this kind of wedding frequent by chance (i.e., most of these weddings are endogenous).

have all brothers who survive to age 20, as they are all recorded by the army, except at the margin of our sample.[10] We also have some information on his father and mother directly from the military records, as the military system was based on the responsibility of the father if his son did not attend at the army. Table 6.1 describes precisely the construction of the database and the linkage between military records and other sources. Using these data, we are able to link 79 percent of the fathers to the wedding records and 60 percent to the TSA. On the whole, almost 90 percent of the military sample can be linked with the TRA survey, either by the wedding or by the fiscal records.[11] Thus, we were able to reconstitute the family for an important part of the sample.

Whereas wedding and fiscal records only identify where someone lives at a given moment (marriage, death, and so on), the military records compile all residences during the period between the end of active military service (around the age of 23) and the end of all military duty (around 46 years of age). In this chapter, we use both discrete and continuous records of residence, but we do not give equal weight to these two kinds of places. We study mobility only for people listed in the

Table 6.1 The military sample and its links to the TRA survey

Generation	Source	N	Proportion (%)	Proportion of conscripts (%)
Conscript	Total	2,896		
	TSA	1,166	40.26	
	Wedding	948	32.73	
	TSA and wedding	537	18.54	
	TSA or wedding	1,577	54.45	
Father	Total	1,982		
	TSA	1,172	59.13	60.19
	Wedding	1,513	76.34	79.28
	TSA and wedding	1,014	51.16	53.21
	TSA or wedding	1,671	84.13	86.98
Grandfather	Total	1,794		
	TSA	675	37.63	42.96
	Wedding	820	45.71	51.38
	TSA and wedding	568	31.66	36.29
	TSA or wedding	927	51.67	58.05
Great-grandfather	Total	1,735		
	TSA	277	15.97	20.65
	Wedding	260	14.99	18.65
	TSA and wedding	171	9.86	12.57
	TSA or wedding	366	21.10	26.73

[10] People born at the beginning (around 1850) or at the end (just before 1900) of our sample may, respectively, have an older or younger brother who escapes from our sample.

[11] People who could not be linked to either of the two sources are not randomly selected as they are usually foreigners who married or died abroad and so cannot be found in the TRA sources, which cover only Metropolitan France. In most cases, these people are thrown out of our study (as we do not have any of their family information). We are aware of this limitation, but it is one that is inherent in our sample.

military records and for whom we have continuous records of residence. We use the rest of the family, i.e., their parents and grandparents, as a background of some of the main characteristics of the family in terms of geographic and socioeconomic behavior. This family background helps us to explore the potential links between migration and family network.

Another important aspect of our research is how to characterize the places in our sample. We use the basic unit in the French administrative organization, the "commune". We then consider communes as the main reference for places. This choice is debatable since this administrative unit is not perfectly constant over time. Yet, thanks to the reference dictionary of communes (Motte, Seguy, and There 2003), we can identify the places listed in our database. On the basis of the various sources of the TRA survey, we are able to locate each person in a commune at different moments of his life cycle. We thus have a precise measure of the individual trajectories since the commune is a very small administrative unit (France is divided into no less than 36,000 communes).

We first characterize a commune by its geographical localization. We have coordinates of all French communes which allows us both to locate them in the territory of France and to calculate distances between them. All distances we use are "as the crow flies". This simplification does not take into account natural elements that may considerably limit mobility, such as mountains or rivers, but we choose "as the crow flies" distances as a convenient way to approximate the real distance between two places and argue that the bias is not too heavy on the whole sample.

We also take into account some characteristics of the commune. Each commune is defined as urban or rural at a given moment in time; thus, our definition of urbanity is dynamic. We consider a commune to be urban if it has more than 2,500 inhabitants at the census directly preceding the moment of residence. For the conscript, as we know the exact time of mobility this measure is almost perfectly in accordance with reality. For the rest of the sample, there can be quite a long time between the moment an individual moved to a commune and the time at which he is recorded in this commune (e.g., at his wedding or the time of birth of one of his children); but this should not be an important bias as few communes became urban before the end of the nineteenth century.[12]

4 The Spatial Capital of Families

For each individual we make an inventory of all places of residence within his family. We consider that these define a family territory which can be seen as "spatial capital" and as such matters in the mobility decisions of family

---

[12] A more accurate description of French urbanization is provided in Dupâquier (1988) and Lepetit (1988).

members.[13] Let us first summarize the characteristics of this territory by a few indicators.

To constitute the family territory of a given conscript in our sample, we compile the locations of his ancestors, from both the TSA and wedding records, including the places of residence of both spouses at the time of marriage (before they moved in together), the habitations of both their parents, all his grandparents (if they are still alive), and all his great-grandparents on his father's side. We assume that both parents are living in the same place after their marriage even though that is not always the case,[14] so by default we use the place of residence of the father at the time of the marriage of his children. It is only when the father's residence appears to be missing (in most cases because he is not alive any more), that we use, when available, the place of residence of the mother.

Table 6.2 shows all the locations available in the TRA database and how we use them. We construct two different indicators of the family in terms of genealogic profoundness: one from the parents' habitations, the second from the grandparents and great-grandparents' habitations. The former is based on the mobility of the parents. Firstly, mobility before marriage is estimated with the birth place and the residence at the time of marriage for both spouses—that is, for the father and mother of a given conscript. We then complete it by using the places of birth of the children of the family (the conscript and his siblings)[15] as a measure of the post-marital mobility of the parents. We can obtain up to 15 places, as the maximum number of children in our sample is 11. This pool of places is heavily dependent upon the number of children, but it gives us a good estimation of the parent's mobility, except for mobility before marriage. This first estimate of the family territory is not constrained by family reconstitution but by the size of the family itself. Nevertheless, it gives an approximation of parental mobility and consequently defines a territory that is a reference for the children's generation. We will refer to this definition of family as "parental family".

We then use a second definition by compiling a family as large as possible, but only in the ascending branch. We use both grandparents and great-grandparents, but not the residence of the parents after their wedding (i.e., the successive places of

---

[13] "Spatial capital" is used here as a special kind of both human and social capital at an individual scale. It is then relatively close to the definition given by Levy (2003) in the dictionary of geography, under the article on *capital spatial*: "Le capital spatial est un capital, c'est-à-dire un bien social cumulable et utilizable pour produire d'autres biens sociaux". For us, it is a way to capture social networks but also links with places in various dimensions. For more details, see Levy (2003) and the references given. We use social capital as defined in Lin (2001): "as resources embedded in social networks and accessed and used by actors for actions". For a more accurate description of social capital, see the recent survey by Durlauf and Fafchamps (2005).

[14] In the whole TRA database, roughly 5 percent of the marriages with both places of the parents recorded show a different place of residence for the father and for the mother of the bride or groom.

[15] As we also use the TRA database to find the sisters of the conscripts; in this case, siblings can be either men or women.

birth of their children), to provide an estimation of the territory that is independent from the number of children in the last generation. We obtain up to 18 places, depending mostly on the success of family reconstitution. In contrast to the first definition, we refer to these as "ancestral families".

These two different approximations of the family territory are almost completely independent. They express two different views of the family's residences. One, ancestral families, is the memory of past places where ancestors lived, even if nobody lives there any more. It is a vision of place as a patrimony or an inheritance

Table 6.2 Construction of the spatial capital

Individual	Nature of the place	N	(%)	Parental family	Ancestral family	Source
ALL		2,896				
Ego	Birth place	2,865	98.9	X		M
Siblings	Birth place first sibling	1,904	65.7	X		MTW
	Birth place second sibling	1,154	39.8	X		MTW
	Birth place third sibling	678	23.4	X		MTW
	Birth place fourth sibling	378	13.1	X		MTW
	Birth place fifth sibling	205	7.1	X		MTW
	Birth place sixth sibling	107	3.7	X		MTW
	Birth place above sixth sibling	121	4.2			
Father	Birth place	2,380	82.2	X	X	TW
	Residence at his wedding	2,200	76.0	X		W
	Residence of his parents at his wedding	1,997	69.0		X	W
Mother	Birth place	2,190	75.6	X	X	W
	Residence at her wedding	2,122	73.3	X		W
	Residence of her parents at her wedding	1,968	68.0		X	W
Grandfather	Birth place	1,502	51.9		X	WT
	Residence at his wedding	1,394	48.1		X	W
	Residence of his parents at his wedding	1,234	42.6		X	W
	Residence at death	1,261	43.5		X	T
Grandmother	Birth place	1,328	45.9		X	W
	Residence at her wedding	1,273	44.0		X	W
	Residence of her parents at her wedding	1,215	42.0		X	W
Great-grandfather	Birth place	595	20.5		X	WT
	Residence at his wedding	490	16.9		X	W
	Residence of his parents at his wedding	415	14.3		X	W
	Residence at death	609	21.0		X	T
Great-grandmother	Birth place	451	15.6		X	W
	Residence at her wedding	439	15.2		X	W
	Residence of her parents at her wedding	448	15.5		X	W

which has been influenced by the mobility of ancestors, but also influences, as any inheritance, the generation who receives it. In ways we are unable to define precisely, people are linked to these places. The residences of the parents, however, are more proximate. In most cases, the parents are still living there, unless they moved after the birth of their last child, and even if they do not live there anymore, they did so not long ago and they probably still have some links to the place.

We implicitly consider all these places as places where the family has some ties. We do not know whether these ties are still up-to-date, but we may suppose that a commune in the family territory is in some way related to the family's history and can still play a role in family choices. Note that, unlike some recent studies based on interviews (Bonvalet, Gotman, and Grafmeyer 1999), which reveal real links identified by the respondents and which use quantitative and qualitative analysis of family territory, we only have theoretical links recorded by the successive living places of the people we are studying. As a result, we have an approximate image of the past—the trace people left by living somewhere. Hence, we must not forget that our family territory is only a partial and reduced one.

5   The Family Territory

Table 6.3 gives a quantitative summary of the family territory constructed in terms of number of residences for parental families. In theory, there are a maximum of 15 different places available, but most families have around three children and so only six places are available. In fact, very few families have more than eight places (5% of the sample). For ancestral families (Table 6.4), the theoretical maximum is 18 places. In contrast to the parental family, a significant portion of the sample reaches this upward limit. Two thirds of the sample has four or more places available, and one third has 10 or more. However, some conscripts have not been successfully linked with the TRA survey and have no ancestral family approximation. Thus, a little more than 20 percent of our sample has only one or fewer places available. To avoid problems with sample size, we choose to limit our analysis to people with at least two places. Respectively, 15% and 23% of the sample is lost in parental and ancestral families by removing these data.

This loss does not produce an important bias as people who could not be identified in our sources are not much different from the others, according to the main characteristics. We perform a probit regression (not shown here) to estimate the effects of these variables on the probability of linking a conscript in the TRA database. Although sons of a wealthy father have greater chances of being linked, other individual characteristics, such as occupation or place of residence, do not change this probability. It seems then that linked people constitute a representative sample of all conscripts we collected.

The distribution of places for the two kinds of families is relatively close to what we might expect after family reconstitution. Unsurprisingly, parental families are concentrated around five places, which corresponds exactly to families having only

Table 6.3 Frequency distribution of parental families according to the total number of places

Number of places	N	(%)
0	11	0.55
1	291	14.59
2	92	4.61
3	74	3.71
4	120	6.02
5	613	30.74
6	354	17.75
7	210	10.53
8	104	5.22
9–10	89	4.46
11 or more	36	1.81
All families	1,994	100.00

Table 6.4 Frequency distribution of the ancestral families according to the total number of places

Number of places	N	(%)
0	375	20.79
1	54	2.99
2	39	2.16
3	116	6.43
4	320	17.74
5	53	2.94
6	41	2.27
7	33	1.83
8	58	3.22
9	102	5.65
10	140	7.76
11	136	7.54
12–15	180	9.98
16 or more	157	8.70
All families	1,804	100.00

one child whose father's wedding has been found. Except for this concentration, the sample is relatively heterogeneous with the distribution decreasing as the number of places rises. Ancestral families are more equally distributed, though we can see some concentration points reflecting the success or failure of linkage with the TRA. The high percentage of 4-place-families corresponds to a father's wedding without any information on the grandparents, while 10 or more places are related with data on both parents and grandparents.

The number of different places within a family gives a first estimation of the diversity of its territory. We calculate the number of different communes among all the communes available. In other words, we are trying to measure the size of the spatial capital in each family. Table 6.5 gives the detailed results of these calculations, both for parental and ancestral families. The first line of the the tables shows "stable" families or families with only one location in their "pool" of places. As we can

Table 6.5 Number of different places according to the number of places available, by family

Parental family	Total number of places available									
	2	3	4	5	6	7	8	9–10	11 or more	All
Number of different places 1	58.70	40.54	19.17	17.13	16.10	21.43	21.15	17.98	27.78	21.39
2	**41.30**	45.95	40.00	37.19	33.90	35.71	30.77	28.09	13.89	35.76
3		**13.51**	30.83	30.34	29.66	23.33	26.92	31.46	30.56	26.83
4			**10.00**	14.03	15.82	11.90	11.54	11.24	8.33	12.06
5				**1.31**	4.24	5.25	5.77	7.86	13.88	3.07
6					**0.28**	2.38	3.85	3.37	5.56	0.89
N	92.00	74.00	120.00	613.00	354.00	210.00	104.00	89.00	36.00	1,692.00

Ancestral family	Total number of places available												
	2	3	4	5	6	7	8	9	10	11	12–15	16 or more	All
Number of different places 1	28.21	19.83	17.81	18.87	9.76	6.06	12.07	9.80	10.00	8.82	6.11	4.46	12.22
2	**71.79**	58.62	43.13	33.96	34.15	33.33	22.41	22.55	25.71	21.32	10.56	5.10	29.45
3		**21.55**	33.13	33.96	21.95	27.27	32.76	22.55	20.71	21.32	21.67	16.56	24.15
4			**5.94**	11.32	12.20	21.21	25.86	22.55	15.71	25.74	20.56	14.65	13.96
5				**1.89**	17.07	9.09	3.45	14.71	15.00	15.44	18.89	23.57	10.25
6					**4.88**	3.03	1.72	3.92	7.86	5.15	9.44	12.74	4.58
7							1.72	3.92	3.57	1.47	8.33	12.10	3.35
8 or more									1.43	0.74	4.44	10.83	2.04
N	39.00	116.00	320.00	53.00	41.00	33.00	58.00	102.00	140.00	136.00	180.00	157.00	1,375.00

see, the proportion of these families is remarkably constant, whatever the total number of places, if we exclude families with only few (two or three) whereabouts available. This proportion is around 20% in parental families and 10% in ancestral families. This suggests that there are very concentrated families for whom migration between communes seems to be nonexistent or very rare. The diagonal gives us the opposite situation, i.e., families whose places were all different. In contrast to stable families, this indicator seems to be dependent on the number of places available. These families totally disappear when we consider enough locales, suggesting that diversity is quantitatively limited among families. Between these two extremes stands an important part of the sample, in which place diversity is relatively limited, with about half of the sample having only two or three different locations. This reveals a dispersion of the families among a small number of residences. This number seems to increase regularly from one generation to another (as the number of different places increases with the number of places available, i.e., with the number of generations we consider).

So these two distributions suggest various forms of family distribution among communes, with a core of very stable families, and a dispersion of family members that is rather limited. Parental families are less concentrated than we expected, suggesting a quite high postmarital mobility—which is consistent with other studies showing high levels of mobility in this part of the life cycle (see Bourdieu et al. 2000; Moch 1992). On the contrary, ancestral families are more concentrated than we expected, suggesting that there is some kind of maximum size of the spatial capital of families.

We estimate the diversity of the places that constitute the spatial portfolio of a given individual by measuring the number of communes in this portfolio. Whatever their number, these communes can be either (very) close or (very) distant in terms of spatial distribution. We now try to measure the spatial concentration of family as it may influence migration. A very concentrated family, even one living in many different places, should restrain mobility, or at least limit long-distance moves, whereas a family with fewer residences that are more spread out in terms of geographic distance might promote more mobility. We then estimate the barycentre of the family territory, i.e., the theoretical point that is the centre of all places within the family territory. Clearly, this point is a theoretical one, and acts as a shortcut to help us estimate the concentration (or the dispersion) of the family. We then distinguish between relatively concentrated families, for whom all places are close in geographical space, and dispersed families that have a large family territory. To do so, we calculate the average distance from each place in the territory to the barycentre. We do not weight places: each commune where a member of the family is living or has ever lived is considered with the same weight for the calculation of the barycentre. We then obtain a measure of dispersion among families.[16] Figure 6.1 shows the division of families according to this measure of dispersion. The graph

---

[16] This measure is thought to be a simple, if not perfect, summary of the dispersion of places among a given family.

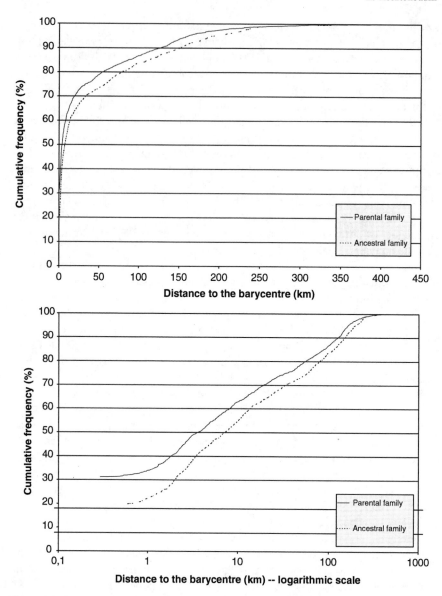

Figure 6.1 Cumulative frequency of the mean distance to the barycentre (kilometer—as the crow flies). Normal and logarithmic scale

in logarithmic scale shows a very regular increase in the mean distance to the bary-centre between approximately 4 and 250 km. Between these two limits, distance to the barycentre is rather equally distributed among the families. We find very con-centrated families as half of the sample has a mean distance below 4 km. There is also a very small group of dispersed families, for whom distance to the barycentre equals several hundred kilometres.

The last indicator we use to describe family territory is related to urbanization. As rural or urban status is linked to mobility decisions, we wish to measure a degree of "urbanity" (or "rurality") for each family. We then calculate the ratio between urban places and all places available. From this ratio, we can distinguish families that are completely rural or urban (for one generation or more) from families in which some members are living in an urban area.

6 Migrants as Heirs

After having highlighted various forms of kinship, defined in terms of their relation to space, we now wish to explore the links between these family forms and the mobility of their members. Our aim is twofold. First, we look at the influence of family forms on the decision of mobility itself. Second, we observe how individuals use the family pool of places they inherited and, in particular, in which cases they extend this patrimony or stay within it. We focus on the men of the last generation who are recorded in the military registers. They are followed from the age of 20 until they die, are discharged for medical reason, or finish their military service at the age of 46. Thus, the mobility we observe is in some way particular as it occurred in the most active part of the life cycle when migration is mostly linked to job search or marriage mobility.

To explore the links between family forms and mobility, we separate migrants and nonmigrants. We then assume that the geographical dispersion of the family has an impact on whether its members choose to move or to stay. In other words, if the previous generations were stable, we could suppose the last generation was less prone to move. However, things are not that simple and it may be that different kinds of mobility are not influenced in the same way by family dispersion. In particular, relative stability in terms of communes—which is the only factor we are able to measure for family background—does not necessarily imply a lack of mobility. People could move within the same commune or could move only briefly—a very frequent phenomenon during this period of time when temporary migrations were common, especially in mountain areas.[17] In this case, family members may migrate even if we observe a high degree of sedentariness among the family. We cannot take into account temporary migration because, in general, it is not recorded in the military registers, but we do observe all other forms of mobility whether intra- or intercommune since we observe residential mobility within a commune. To be sure, the records are sometimes vague for rural areas but residential mobility is well recorded for cities and even small towns (the precise addresses

---

[17]On the historical evolution of seasonal or temporary migration, see the survey by Abel Chatelain (1976).

are often given which is never the case for someone living in a village). For these reasons, it is safe to say that data from military registers underestimate residential mobility by omitting rural mobility that occurred within the same commune.

One of the points at stake here is to see how different kinds of mobility are related to different family forms. We then consider migration between and within communes,[18] since both their meanings and consequences are very different for individuals, for example, in terms of social networks or integration in the labor market.[19] At the same time, we take advantage of the details of the military registers to consider the hazard of first migration in the observation period. In all cases, the reference point is the residence at the age of 20. We focus on the first migration after the age of 20, which is in some way particular as it distinguishes those who change their residence at least once in 26 years[20] from those who stay in the same place. We consider that the conscripts are observed from the end of their active military duty, a moment that varies from 20 years of age (no active military service) to 30 or even 40 years of age (professional soldiers), until the end of their military duty, a moment that varies from 41 years of age (under the 1872 law) to 51 years of age (under the 1905 law).

We then use Kaplan-Meier estimates to construct hazard rates and survival functions of the first migration during the observation period.[21] We consider separately the hazard rate of the first change of residence, the first change of commune, and the first change of residence within the same commune, the last one being estimated only for people living in an urban dwelling.

The other main point of our analysis is the differential role of places during the life cycle. Places we consider as references for family background are collected at particular moments of time, e.g., weddings or deaths. They are places of reference related to such vital events. On the other hand, we study continuous mobility in the last generation and so we have information on places that are not directly related to a vital event. The qualitative difference between these two kinds of mobility may

---

[18] However, migration within communes is only available for cities; therefore, we consider it only for communes with more than 2,500 inhabitants.

[19] However, it is only a simple way to characterize geographic mobility. To be precise, we should also have taken migration distance into account as it strongly affects migrants through selection process (see discussion in Courgeau and Baccaïni (1989), Adams, Kasakoff, and Kok (2002) or Bourdieu et al. (2000) for the same historical period). Nevertheless, even though we here focus on the opposition between movers and stayers, without any consideration for the distance of migration, we control for other characteristics, e.g., wealth of the father, which could differ between short- and long-distance migrants.

[20] Twenty-six years is a shortcut to indicate the length of the observation period, which varies among individuals.

[21] The hazard rate of the first migration is defined for each period of time (for instance, a year) as the number of migrations in that period divided by the number of individuals at risk at the beginning of the period (a conscript is at risk of moving if he has not moved yet and is still under observation). This rate is expressed in person per unit of time (for instance, persons-per-year). On the statistical analysis of failure time data, see Kalbfleisch and Prentice (1980).

certainly influence the choice of places. In other words, we examine whether lifetime mobility involves the same places as vital events-related mobility.

Mobility before the age of 20 is surely a difficult point for our analysis as we do not observe continuous mobility before this age. Nevertheless, the military registers record the birth place of the conscript and two residences when he reaches the age of 20: his own residence and that of his parents. By comparing his birth place and his residence at 20, we estimate conscript mobility between birth and the age of 20. By comparing the residence of the conscript at the age of 20 and the residence of his parents at that moment, we assess whether his mobility was made alone or with his parents. We assume the conscript moved on his own before the age of 20 if he has a residence at 20 different both from his birth place and the residence of his parents.

We compute the estimated probability of at least one migration from the end of military service to the complete discharge of military duty, which means approximately from the age of 20 until the age of 46. We use Kaplan-Meier estimates to take into account the diversity of time under observation. We start by considering each variable independently to obtain an understanding of their influence on mobility decisions. The results shown in Tables 6 and 7 are expressed as the failure function (the opposite of the survival function) at the last age.[22] These tables show the probability of moving at least once, according to both the different definitions of mobility and the variables considered.

Mobility can be influenced by family forms but also by individual determinants, such as birth rank, or by the historical or geographical context. As such, we use some characteristics of the conscripts as control variables. Table 6 gives the probability of moving according to various individual characteristics. First, we use a birth rank indicator. We also consider some geographical indicators related to the habitation at the age of 20: whether this place is urban, rural, or Paris. Finally, we consider the year of birth to capture historical differences in mobility patterns, the length of active military service to estimate differences in the first time a conscript is at risk of moving, and the occupation at the age of 20, both as sector of activity and occupational status.[23]

For the family background, we take advantage of the TSA to estimate the father's wealth. We use it as a dichotomous variable, observing whether the father left an inheritance or not. We use the three indicators previously defined, i.e., diversity of places, dispersion of the family, and family urbanization to estimate the family territory. We divide these indicators into groups on the basis of the secondary analysis we conducted. Diversity of places is estimated by the number of different locations among the number of residences available. We then use three

---

[22] After, in fact, 26 years under risk. Some people are even followed after this date as military service was extended to 30 years after the First World War. However, the sample is very small after this date.

[23] For details on the way we construct individual indicators, especially occupations in the TRA survey, see Kesztenbaum (2006).

groups; "stable families" only have one different place in their family territory, whereas families with more than half of their places different (that is, approximately four places or more for parental families and five places or more for ancestral families) are characterized as "high diversity" families. The majority of the sample stands between these two groups. For ancestral families, the stable group is divided in two, separating out families with only one place in their portfolio as "very stable" families. Family dispersion is estimated in four groups; families with no dispersion at all (mean distance to the barycentre is equal to 0 km), low dispersion (between 0 and 4 km), medium dispersion (between 4 and 20 km), and high dispersion (above 20 km). And, finally, urbanization is estimated among the families in three categories; two extreme groups, i.e., when places in the family portfolio are all either rural or urban, and a "mixed" group where families have both urban and rural places in their portfolio.

These groups give a first estimation of the family territory as measured according to parental or ancestral families, and allow us to analyze the different family forms in studying mobility decisions.

As Table 6.6 shows, the results are significant and have the expected sign for the main individual variables. For example, conscripts born in a town have greater chances of intercommune migration than individuals born in the countryside, whereas conscripts born in Paris have a much higher probability of intracommune mobility. Part of these results come from our poor observation of intracommune mobility in the countryside, but it is also consistent with previous observations that show an important intracommune mobility and a quite reduced intercommune mobility in town, or at least in major cities (for the case of Paris, see Farcy and Faure 2003). Similarly, migration is smaller for farmers and is rather higher for industry and service workers and state employees. Finally, birth rank seems to have no effect.

The variables related to the spatial capital of the family also seem to influence mobility decisions (Table 6.7). In general, the probability of moving increases with the size and the scope of the spatial capital that is owned by the family. Thus, a greater diversity of communes in the portfolio, or a greater dispersion of the communes within the family, raises the probability of moving. These results are identical and significant both for parental and ancestral families. This may mean that the history of the family—observed here as the migrations of family members, as proxied by the portfolio of communes—plays an important role in determining present individual mobility. This may also mean that differences in the spatial distribution of the members of the families reveal both different resources (some local, some dispersed) and different ways of using these resources (e.g., local networks). These two explanations are not exclusive. Families with a lot of different places in their portfolio have more opportunities, i.e., more spatial resources to offer for future moves. In other words, migration generates migration (as family inheritance generates and constrains heirs). It is particularly clear when comparing intra- and intercommune mobility: the diversity of places does not have significant effects on the former but does increase the probability of the latter. This means that some families reproduce intercommune migration from one generation to another.

Table 6.6 Probability of at least one instance of mobility between 20 and 46 years of age according to individual characteristics

		All		Intercommune		Intracommune		
	N	Prob.	Khi²	Prob.	Khi²	N	Prob.	Khi²
Year of birth								
1850–1859	401	40.2	145.04***	31.7	82.71***	203	48.2	27.82***
1860–1869	520	66.7		55.2		330	53.7	
1870–1879	600	74.3		59.2		412	64.5	
1880–1889	541	77.2		54.4		389	68.7	
1890–1900	533	78.7		62.3		404	61.9	
Active military service								
None	423	56.8	58.27***	43.7	27.62***	232	52.8	12.21***
1–3 years	1,624	73.2		56.6		1,156	62.7	
4–8 years	525	65.0		52.0		332	59.3	
More than 8 years	23	88.4		73.1		18	38.9	
Place of living at the age of 20								
Rural	1,287	57.6	377.07***	50.5	10.63***	472	52.5	266.44***
Urban	521	64.0		60.9		732	39.3	
Paris	740	93.2		53.6		511	80.4	
Migration before the age of 20								
None	2,238	68.1	14.45***	52.7	21.37***	1,474	61.7	2.4
Migrant	266	75.9		64.3		207	54.5	
Sector of activity at the age of 20								
Farming	904	52.6	191.87***	46.5	39.99***	349	38.1	76.41***
Craft industry	430	70.2		53.9		308	63.8	
Industry	355	85.4		61.9		316	68.5	
Services	327	84.9		65.7		276	68.6	
Trading	374	75.0		52.7		313	67.7	
State employee	86	83.4		61.6		74	62.0	
Occupational status at the age of 20								
Unskilled worker	595	74.5	167.37***	56.3	37.14***	390	61.9	59.77***
Skilled worker	887	74.4		57.4		683	65.1	
Farmer	641	48.0		42.7		228	33.1	
White collar	355	85.3		62.4		337	69.8	
Birth rank, male only								
Only child	841	71.6	4.4	54.0	1.4	602	35.5	3.5
First born	932	67.4		53.3		609	41.4	
Second born	557	68.0		53.9		362	41.7	
Third or higher born	265	69.6		55.7		165	38.8	

Failure function after 26 years under observation ("Prob."). Khi² refers to log rank test of equality of survival functions.

*Significant at $p < 0.15$; **significant at $p < 0.10$; ***significant at $p < 0.05$.

Table 6.7 Probability of at least one instance of mobility between 20 and 46 years old according to family capital

				Migration				
		All		Intercommune		Intracommune		
	N	Prob.	Khi²	Prob.	Khi²	N	Prob.	Khi²
Parental family								
Wealth								
Father wealthy	890	59.7	42.66***	47.0	8.60***	518	53.0	14.29***
Father poor	628	75.7		55.2		490	66.7	
Diversity of places								
Stable	1,584	63.9	48.89***	49.6	32.56***	966	57.5	1.39
Medium	574	76.4		59.2		424	66.3	
High	179	83.9		68.3		150	58.6	
Dispersion								
None	572	60.5	95.93***	49.4	29.50***	337	52.6	35.31***
Low	608	58.6		49.6		291	48.2	
Medium	1,091	77.3		58.1		853	67.1	
High	62	85.8		71.5		55	55.5	
Urbanization								
Rural only	1,149	58.9	105.73***	51.0	3.24	468	48.8	24.94***
Mixed	926	77.0		56.2		816	64.0	
Urban only	262	80.8		54.3		256	64.4	
Ancestral family								
Wealth								
Wealthy	752	64.1	18.45***	52.3	1.26	240	68.5	9.02***
Mixed	109	59.7		49.2		63	49.0	
Poor	303	77.1		54.8		453	52.8	
Diversity of places								
Very stable	1,221	64.4	30.32***	50.1	9.47***	746	59.0	2.88
Stable	321	70.4		56.9		222	60.0	
Medium	426	75.0		57.9		324	59.8	
High	154	82.3		60.8		112	69.3	
Dispersion								
None	317	65.9	87.10***	51.7	17.17***	196	61.0	33.57***
Low	553	54.2		45.8		264	42.4	
Medium	1,157	75.0		57.3		856	64.0	
High	92	88.0		59.0		85	71.5	
Urbanization								
Rural only	1,179	60.8	74.66***	50.9	6.82***	578	52.9	14.47***
Mixed	864	77.9		57.2		749	64.4	
Urban only	79	83.7		52.3		77	65.6	

Failure function after 26 years under observation ("Prob."). Khi² refers to log rank test of equality of survival functions.

*Significant at $p < 0.15$; **significant at $p < 0.10$; ***significant at $p < 0.05$.

To go further, we control simultaneously for all variables, especially by considering the individual characteristics of the conscripts. To do so, we use a Cox proportional hazard regression (Table 6.8). We perform separate regressions when using the wealth of the father as the use of this variable significantly diminishes the size of our sample. We explore parental and ancestral families separately. The variables defining the territory of the family are entered as continuous for dispersion and urbanization whereas diversity of place is considered as three or four groups (parental or ancestral families, respectively). All other individual variables described in Table 6.6 are included in the regression even though their coefficients are not shown in the table. The total number of places available within each family is also included as a control variable.

Taken together, these regressions confirm the previous results. Family variables do affect the probability of migrating; in addition, most of the individual variables (not shown here) appear to be significant and have the expected sign.[24] Wealth of the father, for instance, always had a significant negative impact on mobility.

However, the size and scope of the spatial capital of a family has different influences depending on whether we consider intra- or intercommunal moves. Generally speaking, the spatial capital of the family has no influence at all (or even a negative, but not significant, influence) on intracommune mobility. Also, the level of urbanization of the family does not seem to matter in determining migration decisions. Yet there is one remarkable exception. Parents' level of urbanization reduces the hazard of intercommune migration. In other words, a child whose father presently lives in a town, or at an earlier point in time (at least during one period) lived in an urban setting, is less likely to change communes. This result suggests some kind of inertia: when part of the family has settled in an urban area, its heirs are in some way rooted there.

For intercommune mobility, the previous results are confirmed. Even after controlling for all other variables, including wealth of the father, diversity in the spatial capital of a family significantly increases the probability of moving. In other words, the more places an individual has in his family portfolio, the more likely he is to leave his birth place for another commune. As we previously explained, this suggests a positive influence of past migrations on present mobility. This can be seen in terms of resources (networks for instance) or in terms of habits (families of migrants, for example, who have a professional specialization). In both cases, it shows the importance of a history of migration in a given family in determining its members' mobility. Migration seems to be in some way bequestable goods.

The territorial scope of the family's members also plays an important role, again mostly for intercommune migration. This result holds for parental and ancestral families. Again, this suggests a determining influence of the kinship's places and

---

[24] The detailed results can be obtained on request from the author. They are rather similar to those given in Table 6.

Table 6.8 Effects of spatial capital on the hazard of first migration (Cox proportional hazard regression)

	Migration								
	All			Intercommune			Intracommune		
	Base model	Urban	Wealth	Base model	Urban	Wealth	Base model	Urban	Wealth
Parental family									
Observations	2,167	2,167	1,365	2,167	2,167	1,365	1,409	1,409	892
Years at risk	22,153	22,153	14,484	29,013	29,013	18,842	14,588	14,588	9,159
Failures	1,404	1,404	856	1,081	1,081	646	739	739	460
Log(likelihood)	−9243	−9242	−5276	−7283	−7282	−4095	−4522	−4522	−2603
Diversity of places									
Stable	Ref.	Ref.	Ref.	Ref.	Ref.	Ref.	Ref.	Ref.	Ref.
Medium	0.0594	0.0640	−0.0284	0.1986***	0.1944***	0.1711***	−0.0937	−0.0927	−0.1713*
High	0.1868**	0.1950**	0.0760	0.3460***	0.3380***	0.2792***	−0.1627	−0.1543	−0.2497
Dispersion	0.0011***	0.0010***	0.0009*	0.0013***	0.0014***	0.0010	0.0006	0.0005	0.0009
Urbanization		0.1051			−0.1855***			0.0499	−0.1347
Ancestral family									
Observations	1,958	1,958	1,068	1,958	1,958	1,068	1,277	1,277	682
Years at risk	20,007	20,007	11,515	26,216	26,216	14,697	13,210	13,210	7,193
Failures	1,271	1,271	675	980	980	525	674	674	342
Log(likelihood)	−8209	−8209	−3929	−6498	−6497	−3145	−4045	−4045	−1834
Diversity of places									
Very stable	Ref.	Ref.	Ref.	Ref.	Ref.	Ref.	Ref.	Ref.	Ref.
Stable	0.0817	0.0776	0.1909**	0.1160	0.1122	0.2791***	0.0397	0.0315	0.0886
Medium	−0.0387	−0.0409	−0.0716	0.0736	0.0726	0.0523	−0.1660**	−0.1717	−0.2856**
High	0.2262***	0.2222***	0.1626	0.1669	0.1630	0.2833	0.0785	0.0685	0.1748
Dispersion	0.0015***	0.0016***	0.0026***	0.0001	0.0007	0.0016***	0.0007	0.0008	0.0013*
Urbanization		−0.0801			−0.1188			−0.0893	

The numbers are the coefficients of the model and not hazard ratios. Separate regressions are used for parental and ancestral families respectively. All regressions included control for year of birth, length of active military service, place of living at the age of 20 (rural/urban/Paris), mobility before the age of 20 (as a dummy), sector of employment, and social status at the age of 20. Finally, standard errors are controlled for within family correlations.

*Significant at $p < 0.15$; **significant at $p < 0.10$; ***significant at $p < 0.05$.

of the transmission of spatial capital between generations. Spatial capital, whatever its form, is important when transmitted from father to son, but also when coming from more distant ancestors.

7 Pioneers or Followers?

In the previous section we highlighted how the spatial capital of families influences the migration decisions of their members. Let us now focus on migrants and explore the places to which they choose to move. All migrants are conscripts whose migrations are recorded between the ages of 20 and 46. Thus, the portfolio of places we observe is made up not only of the places where a given individual stays at birth, at marriage, and at death, but also of places where he lives during his working period. Conscripts enter adult life with a particular "spatial capital of places", provided either by their parents or by their larger kinship. If they choose to migrate, they may or may not stay within this family area. Whenever they choose not to stay with their familiar spatial capital, we call them "pioneers".

We use two separate definitions of pioneers. The first is a simple one, based on commune diversity at family level: a pioneer is someone who moves to a commune that does not belong to his family territory. In this case, the size of the family patrimony in terms of places is defined by a list of communes. Someone who moves outside of this list is a pioneer since he does not stay in his family territory, but instead discovers new places. This definition, however, has clear limitations. A migrant can go to a new place that is very close to his family territory. For instance, this would be the case for someone who married a woman from the closest village, just next to his birth place.[25] According to the second definition, we take into account the distance of the new place to the family territory. In this case, a pioneer is someone who has moved further than the maximum extension of the family territory. This maximal extension is estimated by the distance from the barycentre to the farthest commune of the territory.[26]

The main issue here is how to define new whereabouts and, as a result, how to define pioneers. The first definition is as large as possible and, even if some of these results are biased by the limits of our family reconstitution, we have an exhaustive observatory for the object we define here, that is, the places of the parents, and a more limited observatory of the places of the ancestors. We can see whether or not individuals restrained themselves to living in places where their ancestors have already moved, which may reveal some sort of stability of the latest generation. The second definition takes into account the scope of the territory of the family's members. It represents a more radical way to leave one's family as it means going far

---

[25] It may also be the case that one of his relatives whom we have not identified lives in that nearby place.

[26] It is equally determined by the greatest distance between the barycentre and a commune of the territory.

away from the family, at least the family as we define it. However, we should be cautious because moving away does not necessarily mean escaping from the family; rather, this distance may measure a larger separation from the family.

We then calculate the proportion of pioneers according to the two different definitions, but only for migrants, i.e., individuals who lived at least once in a commune different from their birth place. Thus, we observe the probability of a migrant to be a pioneer. We did this analysis using all previous variables. Table 6.9 gives the results for individual variables, and Table 6.10 gives the results for family variables, especially spatial capital.

The proportion of pioneers is strikingly high in the entire sample. A migrant who moves at least once from one commune to another has a more than 95 percent chance of moving at least once to a commune that does not belong to his family pool. More surprisingly, as Table 9 shows, the probabilities are very high both for parental and ancestral families. On the one hand, since ancestral families produce a more detailed description of the territory of the family's members, we might expect that the use of ancestral families would reduce the probability of being a pioneer. However, this is not the case. Ancestral families document a set of places that are in some way obsolete and thus we might expect an increase in the probability of being a pioneer. On viewing our results, it seems this last effect overcomes the extension of the territory: the spatial capital contributed by distant ancestors, grandparents for example, becomes quite useless.

Our results suggest that migrants always move to a new place at least once during their life cycle. This highlights a real gap between migrants and nonmigrants. While migrating from one commune to another means in some way escaping from the family, nonmigrating reveals not only stability but, even more, some attachment to the territory of the family. But, as mentioned above, we have only places of residence and not real links; hence, living in a place that does not belong to the territory of the other members of the family does not necessarily mean escaping from the family. For instance, migration can be a family decision which means the preservation of strong links between the migrant and his family.[27] Moreover, part of this result comes by construction of our data. As we consider all moves during the life cycle (at least part of it), we naturally increase the chance of having at least one commune different from the list of places that were already included in an individual's family pool of places. So, by estimating the proportion of individuals who migrated to another place at least once, and not, for example, the proportion who definitely left the family portfolio of residences, we overestimated the pioneer process.

But this point certainly does not explain all of these striking results. Another clue may be found in the qualitative specificity of the places we consider for the conscripts. We may wonder to what extent the use of places that do not rely on a specific event (for example, a wedding) produces a particular image of the influence

---

[27] For instance, see Lambert (1994) who developed a model of migration as a way to diversify risk within the family.

Table 6.9 Proportion of pioneers among migrants (change of commune)—individual variables

| | Parental families | | | | | Ancestral families | | | |
| | Communes pioneers | | | Distance pioneers | | Communes pioneers | | Distance pioneers | |
	N	Prop	Khi²	Prop	Khi²	Prop	Khi²	Prop	Khi²
All	994	92.6		57.0		93.7		49.8	
Year of birth									
1850–1859	123	91.1	1.95	56.1	4.54	89.7	10.25***	48.3	4.57
1860–1869	198	93.9		61.6		97.4		51.8	
1870–1879	243	91.8		58.4		94.7		54.3	
1880–1889	213	93.9		57.3		94.0		48.8	
1890–1900	217	91.7		51.6		91.3		45.0	
Active military service									
None	136	91.9	1.73	62.5	2.95	93.9	1.90	53.8	3.14
1–3 years	652	92.9		55.2		93.9		50.5	
4–8 years	194	92.3		59.3		93.4		45.5	
More than 8 years	12	83.3		58.3		84.6		38.5	
Place of living at the age of 20									
Rural	335	91.6	0.67	59.1	1.20	90.9	7.13***	49.9	0.00
Urban	412	93.2		54.5		94.5		50.2	
Paris	222	92.8		56.6		95.5		50.1	
Migration before the age of 20									
None	829	93.0	1.68	55.7	2.37*	94.1	0.35	49.4	0.78
Migrant	127	89.8		63.0		92.7		53.7	
Sector of activity at the age of 20									
Farming	295	92.9	3.77	65.1	17.80***	93.4	4.74	51.5	12.17**
Craft industry	172	92.4		59.3		94.7		47.6	
Industry	143	94.4		49.0		95.7		42.6	
Services	158	92.4		52.5		93.6		55.8	
Trading	147	91.2		53.1		92.1		55.0	
State employee	37	86.5		56.8		91.4		40.0	
Occupational status at the age of 20									
Unskilled worker	255	94.1	4.84	53.7	14.21***	95.5	3.81	56.6	7.15**
Skilled worker	361	93.6		56.8		94.8		48.9	
Farmer	180	91.7		68.3		91.6		48.2	
White collar	184	89.1		50.0		92.6		44.2	
Birth rank, male only									
Only child	248	92.3	3.52	57.3	0.44	93.3	1.79	45.6	2.70
First born	383	91.1		55.9		93.0		51.2	
Second born	246	95.1		58.5		95.5		51.2	
Third or higher born	117	92.3		57.3		93.0		52.2	

The table gives the proportion of intercommune migrants who lived at least once in a commune that does not belong to his family territory ("communes pioneers") or which is far away from that territory ("distance pioneers"); see text for details. "Khi²" refers to a khi² test of equality of the distribution for a given variable.

*Significant at $p < 0.15$; **significant at $p < 0.10$; ***significant at $p < 0.05$.

of the family on migration—a fact which complicates the use of places for vital events (residence at marriage or death, for instance) when studying migration. These places are by themselves related to the family and thus may exaggerate the role of the family in the migration process. By considering all places throughout the life cycle (before the age of 46), we show that the family is not the sole determinant of the migrants' choice of places.

And finally, one of our first concerns was the choice of place by the migrants compared to their original portfolio, i.e., the use individuals made of the places they inherited from their ancestors. On seeing our results, it seems that there is very little memory in migration as regards the choice of places: most of the migrants are not using the spatial investment made by their family. When it concerns migration for work (which is certainly the major determinant of mobility between ages 20 and 46), it seems that the places are, on the whole, chosen outside of the family network which, in fact, does not mean that this choice is completely independent from the family.

We go further and try to identify some gap between migrants by taking into account the distance of mobility. A pioneer must not only go to a place that is not in his family portfolio, but he must also go further than the scope of his family territory. In this case, parental and ancestral families produce different estimates. For parental families, we still observe an important proportion of pioneers among the migrants as migrants have an almost 60 percent chance of moving outside of the spatial capital of their family. This suggests that the territory defined by the successive living places of the parents is in some way too small for migrants, at least migrants in search of work. When considering ancestral families, we see a reduction of the probability for a migrant to be a pioneer according to the distance.

This can be explained in part by the definition of pioneers itself. As we extended the scope of the family territory by considering large families, we make it harder for an individual to move outside of this territory. A higher diversity of places or a higher dispersion of the family territory considerably reduces the probability of being a pioneer. This is not a surprise as it is more difficult to leave a large territory than a very small one.

These results also highlight the two different kinds of migration and two different uses of spatial resources by the family. The first kind of family focuses on local resources and therefore experiences mostly local mobility. In this case, we can speak of immobile mobility where migration occurs in a very concentrated area, even when involving different communes. On the other hand, there seem to be families among whom long-distance migrations are not exceptional, revealing a different use of their resources with, for instance, extended networks. These migrants do not need to move far away from the family. It is possible that these two different forms are completely disconnected and reveal two different types of families that use their resources differently. But it also might demonstrate two different parts of the same process, involving families that are not at the same stage of evolution. They might also be dependent on the changing needs of the family (for instance, larger or fewer numbers of children surviving to adult ages).

Table 6.10 Proportion of pioneers among migrants (change of commune)—family variables

	N	Communes pioneers		Distance pioneers	
		Prop	Khi²	Prop	Khi²
Parental family					
Wealth					
Father wealthy	328	91.8	0.84	92.5	3.24**
Father poor	286	93.7		95.9	
Diversity of places					
Stable	536	95.0	9.79***	67.2	50.18***
Medium	339	89.7		46.9	
High	119	89.9		40.3	
Dispersion					
Low	304	93.8	1.92	85.2	153.34***
Medium	630	91.6		44.4	
High	43	95.4		27.9	
Urbanization					
Rural only	427	95.1	6.94***	73.1	80.43***
Mixed	501	90.6		43.9	
Urban only	66	90.9		53.0	
Ancestral family					
Wealth					
Wealthy	337	93.9	3.61	49.0	0.07
Mixed	47	92.2		49.0	
Poor	138	89.0		47.7	
Diversity of places					
Very stable	488	93.7	0.72	51.8	3.82
Stable	177	94.9		46.9	
Medium	242	93.4		50.8	
High	93	92.5		41.9	
Dispersion					
Low	256	94.5	1.53	60.6	27.3***
Medium	659	92.9		44.8	
High	53	96.2		47.2	
Urbanization					
Rural only	511	94.7	1.98	55.4	15.49***
Mixed	470	92.6		44.7	
Urban only	19	94.7		26.3	

Same as Table 9 but only pioneers for parental families are considered here (that is, pioneers in comparison to the territory of their parental families).

8 Conclusion: Family and Migration

Defined in terms of their relation to space, families appear to be well diversified. Though purely theoretical, our concept of family territory gives us a background for studying migration. It measures the diversity between families in their relation to the places where they are living. We can thus observe how people use—or do not use—the spatial capital they inherited from their family. In order to observe this, we concentrate on a sample of French conscripts born in the second part of the nineteenth century.

Migration appears to be inherited because both the size and the scope of the family territory increase the probability of migration. But the effects of the spatial capital are different according to the kind of migrations we have considered. For instance, the size of the family territory influences intercommune migrations but not changes of residence within the same commune. So, it is clear that past migrations do influence mobility decisions of the last generation. The conscripts whose ancestors changed communes frequently have a higher probability of changing their commune. At this point we cannot determine whether this result is related to more resources and—as a consequence—more opportunities, or if it is related to migration habits that characterize "families of migrants".

On the other hand, places do not seem to be inherited by the migrants as many of them choose to migrate, at least once throughout their life cycle, to places that do not belong to the spatial capital of their family. We thus highlighted the importance of nonfamily habitations in the mobility of men in the most active part of the life cycle. On the whole, opportunities given by the family are more related to information on how to migrate than where to migrate. It seems that spatial capital is a matter of general skills that are helpful for migrating and is not related to specific place knowledge. These results weakened the influence of social networks in migration and the importance of chain migrations.

First, this chapter showed that studies of migration should take into account family history in explaining why people choose to migrate or not and, second, they must consider differently places related to life events and places affected by other factors. In other words, it seems as though people use different networks during their lifetime, depending on the stage of their life cycle, that is, the purpose of their migration—for instance, looking for work or for a spouse. This result concerning the adult part of the life cycle mirrors the use of migration as a survival strategy for children as described in Fontaine (1992).

We still need further investigations to determine precisely how migrants take advantage of the spatial investments made by their family. We must observe how the choice of places depends on both the particular circumstances of the individual and his family. For instance, choices of migration for a given individual can be constrained by the previous mobility of his siblings.

More importantly, not only does spatial capital refer to different uses of family spatial resources, but it also captures dissimilar behaviors between families, some investing more in social networks in a given place, some diversifying their spatial portfolio.[28] Spatial investments can be related to other family investments in different

---

[28] We may, for example, think of the kinship groups, described in Hontebeyrie and Rosental (1998), who stay in the same street (Wacquez-Lalo Street in Loos-lès-Lille) from one generation to the next.

manners. If we examine wealth, we can imagine some balanced decisions between investing in economic capital or in spatial capital. In some ways, differences in the size and the scope of the family territory refer to the different relationships to places within the groups of poor and wealthy. These remarks can be extended to investment in human capital or occupational specialization. In other words, we can imagine that investing in places can be a way for some families to compensate for less economic or educational opportunities. In this way, the spatial capital is really a capital that can be negotiated, inherited and, moreover, transformed into other resources.

Acknowledgments This work was supported by a grant from the French National Post Office (*La Poste*) and INRA. I would like to thank Béatrice Havet for her help in obtaining this funding. I am very grateful to Gilles Postel-Vinay for giving me the opportunity to work on the TRA project and for his continuous help and support. I also thank Jérôme Bourdieu and Muriel Roger for their comments on early versions of this chapter and two anonymous referees for their critical reading. Finally, I am indebted to Melinda Rice for her last review of the chapter. Funding and support was provided by IUSSP, INED, and EHESS.

References

Adams, J.W., A.B. Kasakoff, and J. Kok. 2002. Migration over the life course in XIXth century Netherlands and the American North: A comparative analysis based on genealogies and population registers. *Annales de Démographie Historique* 2: 5–28.

Bonvalet, C., A. Gotman, and Y. Grafmeyer (eds.). 1999. *La famille et ses proches. L'aménagement des territoires*. INED/PUF, Paris.

Bourdieu, J., G. Postel-Vinay, P-A. Rosental, and A. Suwa-Eisenmann. 2000. Migrations et transmissions inter-générationnelles dans la France du XIXe et du début du XXe siècle. *Annales Histoire, Sciences Sociales* 55(4): 749–90.

Bourdieu, J., G. Postel-Vinay, and A. Suwa-Eisenmann. 2004. Défense et illustration de l'enquête 3000 familles. *Annales de Démographie Historique* 1: 19–52.

Bourdieu, J. and L. Kesztenbaum. 2004. Vieux, riches et bien portants. Une application de la base 'TRA' aux liens entre mortalité et richesse. *Annales de Démographie Historique* 1: 79–105.

Chatelain, A. 1976. *Les migrants temporaires en France de 1800 à 1914*. Publications de l'université de Lille III, Lille.

Code-manuel (1873) *du recrutement de l'armée. Loi du 27 juillet 1872… Appel de classes. Engagements et réengagements. Opération du conseil de révision. Examen médical des jeunes gens. Textes officiels annotés avec table méthodique*. Librairie militaire J. Dumaine, Paris.

Courgeau, D. 1984. Relations entre cycle de vie et migrations. *Population* 39(3): 483–514.

Courgeau, D. 1993. Changements selon l'âge des flux de migration interne: La France du début du siècle, in J-P. Bardet, F. Lebrun, and R. Le Mée (eds.), *Mesurer et comprendre: Mélanges offerts à Jacques Dupâquier*, PUF, Paris, pp. 107–24.

Courgeau, D. and B. Baccaïni. 1989. Migrations et distance. *Population* 44(3): 659–63.

Courgeau, D. and E. Lelièvre. 2003. Les motifs individuels et sociaux des migrations, in G. Caselli, J. Vallin, and G. Wunsch (eds.), *Démographie: Analyse et Synthèse, vol. IV: Les déterminants de la migration*, INED/PUF, Paris, pp. 147–69.

Dupâquier, J. (eds.). 1988. *Histoire de la population française, tome 3—De 1789 à 1914*. PUF, Paris.

Dupâquier, J. and D. Kessler. 1992. *La société française au XIXe siècle. Tradition, transition, transformations*. Fayard, Paris.

Durlauf, S. and M. Fafchamps. 2005. Social capital, in S. Durlauf and P. Aghion (eds.), *Handbook of economic growth*, 1st edition, Elsevier, Amsterdam, Vol. 1B, pp. 1639–99.

Farcy, J-C. and A. Faure. 2003. *Une génération de Français à l'épreuve de la mobilité. Vers et dans Paris: recherche sur la mobilité des individus à la fin du XIXe siècle.* INED, Paris.

Fontaine, L. 1992. Droit et stratégies: La reproduction des systèmes familiaux dans le Haut-Dauphiné (XVIIe-XVIIIe siècles). *Annales E.S.C.* 47(6): 1259–77.

Greenwood, M. 1997. Internal migration in developed countries, in M. Rosenzweig and O. Stark (eds.), *Handbook of population and family economics*, Elsevier, Amsterdam, Vol. 1B, pp. 647–720.

Gribaudi, M. 1987. *Itinéraires ouvriers. Espace et groupes sociaux à Turin au début du XXème siècle.* EHESS, Paris.

Hontebeyrie, Y. and P-A. Rosental. 1998. Ségrégation sociale de l'espace et dynamiques longues de peuplement: La rue Wacquez-Lalo à Loos-lès-Lille (1866–1954), in Y. Grafmeyer and F. Dansereau (eds.), *Trajectoires familiales et espaces de vie en milieu urbain*, Presses Universitaires de Lyon, Lyon, pp. 73–100.

Kalbfleisch, J.D. and R.L. Prentice. 1980. *The Statistical Analysis of Failure Time Data.* Wiley, New York.

Kesztenbaum, L. 2006. *Une histoire d'espace et de patrimoine. Familles et migration dans la France de la Troisième République, 1800–1940.* Unpublished Doctoral Dissertation.

Lambert, S. 1994. La migration comme instrument de diversification intrafamiliale des risques: une application au cas de la Côte d'Ivoire. *Revue d'Économie du développement* 2: 3–38.

Lepetit, B. 1988. *Les villes dans la France moderne (1740–1840).* Albin Michel, Paris.

Lesger, C., L. Lucassen, and M. Schrover. 2002. Is there life outside the migrant network? German immigrants in XIXth century Netherlands and the need for a more balanced migration topology. *Annales de Démographie Historique* 2: 29–50.

Levy, J. 2003. Capital spatial, in J. Levy and J. Lussault (eds.), *Dictionnaire de la géographie et de l'espace des sociétés*, Belin, Paris, pp. 124–6.

Lin, N. 2001. Building a theory of social capital, in R.S. Burt, K.S. Cook, and N. Lin (eds.), *Social capital: Theory and research*, Aldine de Gruyter, New York, pp. 3–31.

Moch, L.P. 1992. *Moving Europeans. Migrations in Western Europe since 1650.* Indiana University Press, Indianapolis.

Motte, C., I. Seguy, and C. There. 2003. *Communes d'hier, communes d'aujourd'hui. Les communes de la France métropolitaine, 1801–2001. Dictionnaire d'histoire administrative.* INED, Paris.

Ogden, P.E. and P.E. White. (eds.) 1989. *Migrants in Modern France. Population Mobility in the Late 19th and 20th Centuries.* Unwin Hyman, London.

Rosental, P-A. 1999. *Les sentiers invisibles. Espace, familles et migrations dans la France du 19ème siècle.* Éditions de l'École des hautes études en sciences sociales, Paris.

Rosental, P-A. 2002. Pour une analyse mésoscopique des migrations. *Annales de Démographie Historique* 2: 145–60.

Roynette, O. 2000. *Bon pour le service. L'expérience de la caserne en France à la fin du XIXe siècle.* Belin, Paris.

Sandefur, G.D. and W.J. Scott. 1981. A dynamic analysis of migration: An assessment of the effects of age, family and career variables. *Demography* 18(3): 355–68.

Chapter 7
Inheritance, Environment, and Mortality in Older Ages, Southern Sweden, 1813–1894

Tommy Bengtsson[1] and Göran Broström[2]

Abstract This essay explores the role played by inheritance on human longevity. We estimate a model of overall mortality among married persons aged 50 years and above taking genetic as well as socioeconomic and environmental factors into account. We consider whether these factors have temporary or long-lasting effects on health. The demographic and economic individual level data come from the Scanian Demographic Database. These data cover five rural parishes in the southernmost part of Sweden for the period 1813–1894. To these, local grain prices, as an indicator of food costs, and the local infant mortality rate, as an indicator of the disease load, have been added. We find that age of death of the mother and the father have persistent impacts on their adult children's overall mortality regardless of sex, even after controlling for socioeconomic and environmental factors throughout the life course. In addition, we find strong birth cohort effects and effects of the disease load in the first year of life on male offspring. We are, however, unable to find any effects of socioeconomic status, neither at the time of birth or achieved later in life, a result consistent with earlier findings.

Keywords Sweden, mortality, historical demography, individual level, Cox regression, frailty, genetic factors, longevity, proportional hazards, socioeconomic and environmental factors

1 Introduction

There has been a growing interest in aging over the last years in parallel with improvements in survivorship to older ages and an increase in the proportion of the elderly.[1] We will here focus on survivorship, and more specifically on the role of

---

[1] Centre for Economic Demography and Department of Economic History, Lund University, Sweden

[2] Department of Statistics, Umeå University, Sweden

[1] The two phenomena are, however, not as closely related as one might believe since the increase in the proportion of the elderly has more than anything else been the result of declining fertility so far (Coale 1957; Bengtsson and Scott 2005).

T. Bengtsson and G.P. Mineau (eds.), *Kinship and Demographic Behavior in the Past.* 185
© Springer Science+Business Media B.V. 2009

inherited factors as the source of differences between individuals. The idea that inheritance played a part in human longevity dates back at least to the mid-nineteenth century (Smith and Griscom 1869; see Cohen 1964). Since then, scientists have tried to disentangle to what extent longevity is transferred from one generation to the next and, more distinctly, the role of genetic factors (Pearl 1931; Cohen 1964; Finch and Tanzi 1997).

While genes have successfully been linked to a variety of specific diseases, finding a link to overall longevity has proven to be problematic, and for two reasons. First, it is difficult to identify genes that give its bearers long life. Second, children share not only genes but also at least some environmental factors with their parents. We therefore expect the length of life of family members to be more strongly correlated than if genes were the only common factor. The general finding is that the correlation is weak (Pearl 1931; Cohen 1964; Wyshak 1978; Finch and Tanzi 1997) although examples can be found where the link is somewhat stronger (Wyshak 1978)—more so as regards the maternal link (Abbott et al. 1974).

The correlation of longevity between siblings is somewhat stronger than between parents and offspring (Cohen 1964; Wyshak 1978). Twin studies, based on Nordic registers, have estimated the genetic component separately, isolated from shared as well as nonshared environmental components, and show that up to one third of the variation in life span is caused by shared factors and 25 percent by genetic factors alone (Ljungquist, Berg, and Steen 1995; Christensen 2007). These studies are, however, restricted to married persons and to a certain period of life, most frequently older ages, which means that they do not answer the question of how important genetic factors are for the total life span, only for a certain part thereof.

The methodological approach usually applied to disentangle genetic from other factors has been to compare age at death between parents and their offspring, and between siblings and twins. Few methods allow for differentiation between monozygotic (genetically identical) and dizygotic twins. The basic assumption is that children, in comparisons with parents or with each other, are exposed to different environmental factors (see Wyshak 1978, 319–20). The correlation in length of life can therefore be interpreted as an outcome of genetic factors. The question is of course whether this assumption holds true—whether family members share no other factors that influence length of life but genes.

Siblings apparently share the household environment during childhood with each other as well as with their adult parents. Factors at household level that influence health, include food, clothing, housing, access to safe water, sanitation, etc. While some of these differences are due to economic resources that differ between socioeconomic groups, a certain variation (which we do not have information on) is likely to exist within these groups. Even in a society with a considerable degree of social mobility, family members nevertheless experience, if not the same, at least a similar household environment during periods of their lives, possibly throughout their lives. For example, in a rural area such as the one under study here, more than 80 percent of the sons of the landless groups remained landless throughout their lives (Lundh 1998). Furthermore, they share the local environment not only with each other but with their neighbors as well.

The assumption that environmental factors to a large extent can be controlled for by comparing family members is often an adaptation to the data. Few datasets on multiple generations contain information about occupation, landholding, or other indicators of income and wealth. Comparisons of generations without controlling for these shared factors will likely create a bias as the influence of genetic factors will be overstated. Whether this bias is large or not is difficult to assess if we do not have access to information on shared environmental factors, but it will obviously lead to an overestimation of the influence of genetic factors on length of life. The degree of bias depends on the environmental variation between parents and their offspring and between siblings during their life courses.

In a society with a low degree of social mobility, where future life to a great extent is determined by inherited, rather than achieved, socioeconomic status, it is difficult to distinguish between genetic and environmental factors in determining longevity. The reason is that there is simply too little environmental variation over the life course among family members. In such a case, correlation within the family might largely depend on socioeconomic factors, possibly also on environmental factors shared with neighbors, rather than on genetic factors.

In a society with a high degree of social mobility, not only in general but with large differences in social mobility between family members, it is easier to identify the role of inherited factors. It is likely that the achievements of individuals in that society are, relatively speaking, more important for longevity than in a setting where social mobility is low and where family-shared factors consequently are less important. Thus, the differences in results between various studies may be a result of differences in social mobility.

Environmental factors, whether shared with other family members or not, influence the health of a person from the fetal stage throughout life. Factors that affect the development of cells and organs may have a permanent influence on health although they are not manifested as illness until much later in life. We call them early-life factors since the speed of cellular development is high during gestation, infancy, and early childhood and then gradually declines between ages 20 and 30 when it almost comes to a halt. Later-life factors, by definition, affect us after our cells and organs are fully developed. Some factors, whether experienced early or late in life, cause only temporary health setbacks, while others cause lifelong health problems regardless of whether they manifest themselves immediately or not. It is therefore useful to distinguish between family factors shared early in life and those possibly shared later in life.

Epidemiologists and demographers showed interest in early-life factors, *cohort factors*, already in the 1920s and 1930s, when trying to explain the great mortality decline (Kermack, McKendrick, and McKinley 1934). While *period factors* came into focus from the 1950s onwards (UN 1953, 1973), cohort factors have in recent years gained renewed interest (Barker 1994; Bygren, Edvinsson, and Broström 2000; Elo and Preston 1992; Finch and Crimmins 2004; Fogel 1994; Fridlizius 1989; Kuh and Ben-Schlomo 1997; Preston, Hill, and Drevenstedt 1998). Fogel (1994) has proposed several plausible causal mechanisms that connect malnutrition *in utero* and during early life to chronic diseases in later life. These propositions have also been supported by the work of Barker (1994, 1995), who suggested that the preconditions for coronary heart disease, hypertension, stroke, diabetes, and chronic thyroiditis are initiated *in utero* without becoming clinically manifest until much later in life. Bygren et al. (2000) found that changes in food availability for mothers during pregnancy affected sudden death from cerebro- and cardiovascular disease in adult offspring.

The first years after birth are also important for mortality in later life. In two recent essays, based on the same geographical areas as we are analyzing, Bengtsson and Lindström (2000, 2003) show that the disease load experienced during the birth year, measured as the infant mortality rate in the local area, had a significant influence on old-age mortality, particularly with regard to airborne infectious diseases. Years with very high infant mortality, due to outbreaks of smallpox or whooping cough, had a strong impact, while modest changes had almost no impact at all. The causal relationship between cellular development during early childhood and mortality in old age has been supported by medical research (Liuba 2003; see Bengtsson and Lindström 2003 for further references).

Later-life factors, such as diet and working conditions, and in particular life style factors (smoking, etc.), have a strong impact on the life span. One such factor, short-term periods of stress caused by variations in consumption due to changes in food prices, had a strong impact on mortality in preindustrial populations both in Sweden (Bengtsson and Ohlsson 1985) and elsewhere (Bengtsson, Campbell, Lee et al. 2004), and also in the area that is under study here (Bengtsson 2004).

Family-shared factors that influence the development of the child during the fetal stage and early in life, in other words as long as organs and cells are developing rapidly, are of particular interest to us for two reasons. First, they have a strong impact on health in ages 50 years and above. Second, we know that the offspring share these conditions. Due to servant migration, which was common in all social groups, most children experienced different household environments starting in their early teens. Still, local environmental factors were shared by all children and youth.

The aim of this study is to establish whether the rather weak connection that has been found between length of life of parents and their offspring prevails after taking into consideration factors shared with the family and other members of the local community. We therefore estimate a model of old-age mortality for married adults taking into account not only genetic and other family-shared factors but also socioeconomic achievement and external environmental factors shared with all community members.

2   Data, Context, and Models

We analyze the mortality among all presently or previously married persons at the age of 50 years or above, and for whom we have information on age at death of both parents, in a rural area in southern Sweden between 1813 and 1895. Longitudinal demographic data on individuals and household socioeconomic data for parents and their offspring have been combined with community data on food costs and disease load. The data used come from the Scanian Demographic

Database, which covers nine rural parishes and one town situated in Scania in the southernmost part of Sweden. Five of the rural parishes are included in this study: Hög, Kävlinge, Halmstad, Sireköpinge, and Kågeröd. The material for two of the parishes dates back to 1646 and for the others to the 1680s. The publicly available records end in 1895, which is why our analyses end in this year. Our interest in life course effects on later-life mortality further limits our dataset. We need information about socioeconomic conditions at birth not only for those born in the parish but also for in-migrants. In order to gain such information, we need to know the birth parish of in-migrants, and that information is available only after 1813, hence the start-date of our analyses.[2]

The parish register material is of high quality and shows no gaps for births, deaths, or marriages. Migration records are less plentiful, but a continuous series exists from the latter part of the eighteenth century. Information concerning farm size and property rights, in addition to various sorts of information from poll tax records, land registers, and household examination records, are linked to family reconstitutions based on the parish records of marriages, births, and deaths. Taken together, we have very rich information on the household size and structure as well as socioeconomic conditions. In addition, we have good information on local food prices and the disease load, measured as the infant mortality rate.

The sampled parishes are compact in their geographical location, showing the variations that could occur in peasant society with regard to size, topography, and socioeconomic conditions, and they offer good source material. The entire area was open farmland, except for northern Halmstad and parts of Kågeröd, which were more wooded. Halmstad, Sireköpinge, and Kågeröd were predominantly noble parishes, while freehold and crown land dominated in Kävlinge and Hög. The parishes each had between 400 and 1,700 inhabitants in the latter half of the nineteenth century. The agricultural sector in Sweden, and Scania, became increasingly commercialized during the early nineteenth century. New crops and techniques were introduced. Enclosure reforms and other reforms in the agricultural sector influenced population growth, particularly in Sireköpinge which experienced fast population growth. In Kävlinge, the establishment of several factories and railroad communications led to rapid expansion from the 1870s onwards.

Land was the most important source of wealth in these societies. The social structure of the agricultural sector is often difficult to analyze since differences in wealth between the various categories of farmers and occupations are unclear and subject to change with the passage of time. Data from land registers on different types of tenure must be combined with information from poll tax records concerning farm size in order to arrive at a better understanding of each household's access to land. We here differentiate between two social groups: those with enough land to feed a family and those who needed to work for someone else to be able to support a family. The dividing line is set to 1/16 *mantal* based on well-founded arguments from numerous

---

[2] We have this information from 1813 in Kågeröd, from 1821 in Hög and Kävlinge, and from 1829 in Halmstad and Sireköpinge. The starting date consequently differs for the five parishes.

studies in this field of research, stating that peasants with smaller farms were not self-supporting (for an overview, see Bengtsson 2004; Bengtsson and Dribe 2005).

The nineteenth century was a period of considerable social change in the countryside. It has been described as a period of proletarization and pauperization. The share of landless increased (Carlsson 1968). Downward mobility was significant since many children of farmers were unable to obtain a farm themselves. This was true both for Sweden in general and for the area we study (Lundh 1998). Not only did the share of the lower strata increase, but their economic situation worsened as well. They became, for example, more vulnerable to short-term economic stress than before, as shown by their mortality and fertility response to food prices (Bengtsson and Dribe 2005).

Table 7.1 shows the socioeconomic position at birth (i.e., the parent's position) in relation to the achieved socioeconomic position at the age of 50 years for individuals still living in the parish at that age. The data includes all persons for whom we also have information on both parents' age at death. Upward mobility was modest but downward mobility strong. While only 13 percent of the sons and 10 percent of the daughters of landless couples were able to acquire access to land, 47 percent of the sons and 35 percent of the daughters of farmers and tenants could not maintain the socioeconomic position of their parents but became landless.

Downward mobility was also common among the elderly since many either sold their farms or gave them to their children. Those who transferred or sold their farms could, however, still be rather well-off as the new owner of the farm, whether a close relative or not, often had to provide for them in accordance with special contracts (Dribe and Lundh 2005; Lundh and Olsson 2002). Accordingly, it is important to consider not solely current socioeconomic status for the elderly, but also their status before they transferred their land.

The nineteenth century was also a period of rapidly expanding population in Scania as well as in the rest of Sweden. Fertility rates were rather stable and the mortality fell, initially among infants and children, later among adults and the elderly. Figure 7.1 shows the crude death rate for ages 50–100 years from 1813 to 1894.[3] The death rates of the elderly fell during this period, as in Sweden in general,

Table 7.1 Socioeconomic status at birth and at age 50 years for married persons

	SES at age 50 years			
SES at birth	Landless	Landed	Downward mobility	Upward mobility
Females				
Landless	279	32		10%
Landed	182	100	35%	
Males				
Landless	261	38		13%
Landed	135	121	47%	

This table includes all married persons whose parents died in the study area during the period 1813–1894.

[3] The higher variation up to 1829 is partly due to the fact that the population is smaller as all five parishes are not included before this year (see note 2).

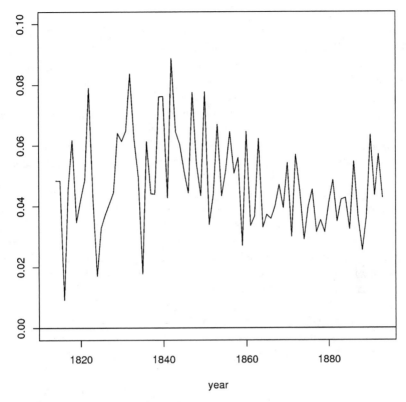

Figure 7.1 Crude death rate (CDR) in ages 50–100 years, 1813–1894

which is why we include the year at birth into our models. Life expectancy at birth for Swedish women was about 45 years in the 1840s, which was the highest recorded in the world (Oeppen and Vaupel 2002). The figures for men were a few years lower. Life expectancy in the area we are analyzing was much the same as for Sweden whereas the differences between the sexes were slightly smaller (Bengtsson and Dribe 1997, 8).

In order to separate the effects of family-shared environmental factors, community-shared environmental factors, and achieved factors from effects of genetic factors, we apply models that include a number of variables. While most factors are fixed, like sex, birth year, place of birth, the disease load at birth, socioeconomic status at birth and at age 50 years, some are time-variant, such as current socioeconomic status and current food prices.

Year at birth is the variable that captures the general improvement in health caused by factors shared by the members of all five communities, such as improved health care and better knowledge about disease control. We assume a log-linear influence over time, but test for curvilinear effects.

Individual life course factors that influence conditions in later life include one fixed variable, i.e., socioeconomic status at age 50, and two time-varying variables, namely present socioeconomic status and present price of food. There is reason for caution since socioeconomic status at age 50 years or later might partly be the result of inheritance. However, the substantial extent of social mobility, in part upward but mainly downward, indicates that this problem should not be overemphasized.

About 80 percent of the income of ordinary people was spent on food, the main share of which was grain products (Bengtsson 1993). We use the deviation from the log trend in annual rye prices, shown in Figure 7.2, as an indicator of short-term economic stress based on the fact that rye was the most common grain in this area (Bengtsson and Dribe 1997). The trend has been estimated using the Hodrick–Prescott filter with a smoothing parameter of 100. The aggregated economic information is used as a time-varying covariate common to all individuals in the risk set at each point in calendar time (Bengtsson 1993).

The disease load in the first year of life, a community variable measured as the infant mortality rate shown in Figure 7.3, is included since previous studies show a strong impact of this variable on later-life mortality, as discussed above. While this variable is time-varying, we assume that the effect of the disease load at year of birth is fixed and stays permanent throughout life. We have removed the trend using the same filter as used for food prices, in order to avoid the influence of other factors that are correlated and change slowly with time. Hence, we are estimating the influence of short-term variations in the disease load on mortality later in life. In particular, we are interested in years with outbreaks of highly virulent diseases, such as smallpox and whooping cough. We have therefore estimated the effects of

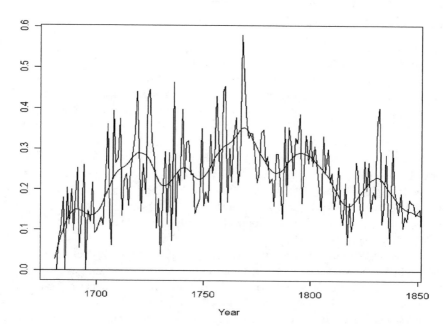

Figure 7.2 Local rye prices. Observed values and trend

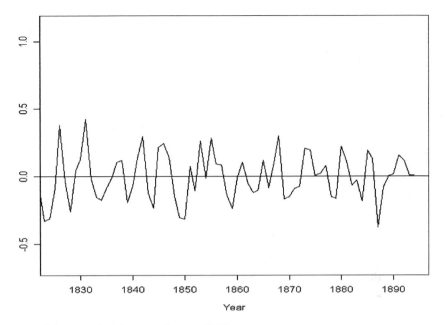

Figure 7.3 Cycles in infant mortality rate (IMR)

being born in a year in which the detrended infant mortality rate is 10 percent above the mean comparative to being born in other years. While this value is chosen arbitrarily, experiments show that the result is not sensitive to moderate changes.

Environmental factors transferred from parents are included both as an observable variable and as a nonobserved frailty component, which will be further discussed below. The observed factor is the socioeconomic situation of the family at the time of birth of the index person. Thus, we assume that the inherited environmental effects that influence health in childhood exert permanent influences throughout the life course. Since we are unable to differentiate between the effects of inherited and acquired land, our approach is likely to overestimate the effects of other environmental factors compared to those stemming from the family of birth. The bias should, however, not be large since there is a considerable amount of upward and, in particular, downward mobility throughout the life course.

The genetic factor included is parent's age at death. Here we encounter another problem since the mere presence of an elderly parent may be beneficial to the adult child as he or she grows older, e.g., by transfers of goods and services. But the presence of elderly parents might also generate costs. They need care and other resources, and elderly parents are assumed to be net consumers and thus, in economic terms, a burden to their offspring.

The cumulative hazard rates for married men and women of ages 50–100 years are shown in Figure 7.4. The gender deviation is minor and the developments of the two curves are smooth up to age 85 years. The number of individuals above that age is very small, in particular for males, which is why the curves jump around.

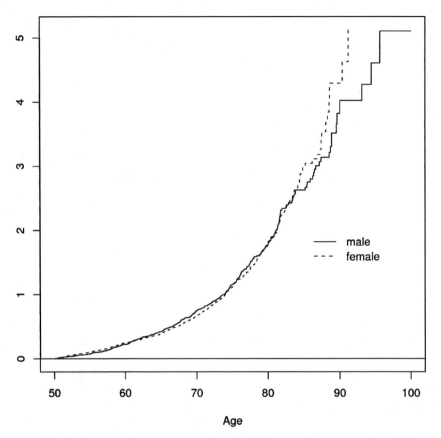

Figure 7.4 Cumulative hazard rate for males and females in ages 50–100 years, 1813–1894

We are assuming proportional hazards models (Cox 1972) which implies that a relative effect on mortality of any covariate is constant over age. The models also allow for time-varying covariates. It is very important to check the assumptions underlying this kind of model, especially the proportionality assumption. We have routinely tested all models for deviations from the proportionality assumption.[4] The test used is based on the correlation between log(t) and the Schoenfeld residuals for each covariate. A large correlation indicates that the corresponding coefficient varies with time; in other words, the hazards are not proportional. We found no signs of nonproportionality, neither on any of the covariates, nor globally.[5]

To control for possible effects of unobserved heterogeneity, which in our case means that we explore the possibilities of clustering effects of birth family on old-age mortality, we have estimated a model in which we assume that the frailty effect has a normal distribution. We find no significant effects of the frailty factor,

---

[4] The estimations are done in R using package *eha*, see Broström (2007).

[5] For a more detailed description of the proportionality test, see Therneau and Grambsch (2000, 127–152).

and the parameter estimates of the observed factors change only slightly. We have also estimated a model with lagged effects of current food prices to account for the possibility of delayed effects of food prices. Unlike our earlier findings for the period 1766–1865 (Bengtsson 2004), we find no delayed effects of food prices for this period. Finally, to control for factors related to area of residence, a model which includes parish of residence has been tested. We here find differences between the five parishes, but they only slightly alter the parameter estimates for other factors. In conclusion, of the three models that were used to check for alternative specifications of the model, none alter the results of the final model and therefore are not shown here.

3 Results

We start by displaying the raw correlation coefficients for age at death of offspring and parents (Table 7.2). The left column shows the figures for the entire sample and the right column for those whose parents were alive at age 50 years, just like the married persons included in the sample. The coefficients are stronger between mothers and sons and fathers and daughters than between individuals of the same sex. More important, the coefficients are overall low, whether due to lack of shared factors other than genetic ones or due to disturbing factors.

Table 7.2 Correlation between length of life of parents and offspring

	All	Those whose parents survived until 50 years of age
Daughters		
Father	0.092	0.099
Mother	0.075	0.039
Sons		
Father	0.105	0.079
Mother	0.147	0.127

All ever-married persons dying at ages 50 years and above with known age at death of parents are included.

Turning to the regression results, we find, as displayed in Tables 7.3a, b that mortality is declining by birth cohort. Persons being born 1 year later have a 1 percent lower mortality in ages 50 years and above, which is similar to what we have found in other studies covering this period (Bengtsson and Lindström 2000, 2003). We also find that boys, but not girls, who have been exposed to a heavy disease load in the birth year, face much higher mortality in later life than those who were not exposed. High infant mortality rates are typically due to outbreaks of either smallpox or whooping cough (Bengtsson and Lindström 2000). The effects were rather strong; boys born in a year with very high infant mortality rates showed mortality rates as adults that were about 70 percent higher than those born in years with a low disease load. While this phenomenon has been verified for several populations, this is the first time we have specifically investigated and identified sex differences.

Table 7.3a Estimation of female mortality

Covariate	Mean	Coeff.	Rel. risk	Wald p
Birthdate	1797.8	−0.010	0.990	0.000
IMR cycle at birth				
Low–high (ref.)	0.948	0	1	
Very high	0.052	−0.269	0.764	0.226
Food prices at birth	−0.006	−0.341	0.711	0.249
SES at birth				
Landless (ref.)	0.509	0	1	
Landed	0.491	0.037	1.038	0.712
SES at age of 50 years				
Landless (ref.)	0.739	0	1	
Landed	0.207	0.186	1.204	0.160
Food prices	0.001	0.479	1.614	0.133
SES current				
Landless (ref.)	0.877	0	1	
Landed	0.123	−0.180	0.835	0.401
Mother's age at death	66.2	−0.009	0.991	0.015
Father's age at death	67.6	−0.007	0.993	0.086
INTERACTIONS:				
Food prices at birth × SES at birth				
Landed		0.208	1.231	0.652
Food prices × SES at age of 50 years				
Landed		0.825	0.0283	0.245
Food prices × SES current				
Landed		−0.055	0.947	0.961
Events	434			
Overall *p*-value	0.0008			
	Df	AIC	LRT	Pr (Chi)
Single term deletions:				
None		4556.4		
Birth date	1	4571.6	17.1	0.00003****
IMR cycle at birth	1	4556.0	1.6	0.21175
Mother's death	1	4560.3	5.8	0.01585**
Father's death	1	4557.4	2.9	0.08829*
Food prices at birth × SES at birth	1	4554.7	0.2	0.65172
Food prices × SES at age of 50 years	1	4555.8	1.3	0.24569
Food prices × SES current	1	4554.4	0.00239	0.96097

*Significant at $p < 0.1$; **significant at $p < 0.05$; ***significant at $p < 0.01$; ****significant at $p < 0.001$.

Furthermore, and contrary to what we have found for earlier periods (Bengtsson 2004), elderly married persons did not suffer from high food prices. Over time, their situation thus improved.

Regarding socioeconomic status, we find no evidence that it has any impact on mortality level in older ages, neither at birth or at the peak of working life, nor at the time of observation. This evidence might seem peculiar since we are used to finding large socioeconomic differences in health and mortality today (Valkonen 1993). This link is, however, likely to be a rather modern phenomenon. Some socioeconomic

Table 7.3b Estimation of male mortality

Covariate	Mean	Coeff.	Rel. risk	Wald p
Birthdate	1797.1	−0.009	0.991	0.000
IMR cycle at birth				
Low–high (ref.)	0.964	0	1	
Very high	0.036	0.554	1.741	0.020
Food prices at birth	−0.006	0.472	1.603	0.119
SES at birth				
Landless (ref.)	0.505	0	1	
Landed	0.495	0.030	1.031	0.786
SES at age of 50 years				
Landless (ref.)	0.701	0	1	
Landed	0.299	−0.076	0.927	0.576
Food prices	0.001	−0.102	0.903	0.733
SES current				
Landless (ref.)	0.812	0	1	
Landed	0.188	−0.040	0.961	0.831
Mother's age at death	66.8	−0.008	0.992	0.040
Father's age at death	67.8	−0.012	0.989	0.005
INTERACTIONS:				
Food prices at birth × SES at birth				
Landed		−0.436	0.647	0.370
Food prices × SES at age of 50 years				
Landed		0.218	1.244	0.747
Food prices × SES current				
Landed		1.123	3.073	0.237
Events	396			
Overall *p*-value	0.0028			
	Df	AIC	LRT	Pr (Chi)
Single term deletions:				
None		4098.7		
Birth date	1	4109.2	12.4	0.00424****
IMR cycle at birth	1	4101.5	4.7	0.02976**
Mother's death	1	4100.9	4.1	0.04201**
Father's death	1	4104.5	7.8	0.00528***
Food prices at birth × SES at birth	1	4097.5	0.8	0.36958
Food prices × SES at age of 50 years	1	4096.8	0.1	0.74664
Food prices × SES current	1	4098.1	1.4	0.23798

*Significant at $p < 0.1$; **significant at $p < 0.05$; ***significant at $p < 0.01$; ****significant at $p < 0.001$.

differences in mortality first started to develop during the course of the nineteenth century, at about the same time as the sex differences in mortality appeared (Smith 1983). In the local area of this analysis, we find that socioeconomic differences among children emerged in the mid-nineteenth century (Bengtsson and Dribe 2007).

Finally, turning to the issue of the connection between length of life of parents and their offspring, we find persistent effects of parents' longevity on the mortality of their adult married children. The effects are the same for both daughters and sons. Children of both sexes gained from having long-lived mothers and fathers.

A person having a mother or father who lived 1 year longer meant 1 percent lower adult mortality for him-/herself. The effects are of the same magnitude as being born 1 year later. In both cases, the effects are quite strong: being born 10 years later, or having a parent who died at an age 10 years above average, lowers the mortality risk among married adults aged 50 years and over by 10 percent.

4   Summary and Discussion

For a long time, the idea that inheritance played a part in human longevity has been puzzling. Scientists have tried to disentangle to what extent longevity is transferred from one generation to the next and, more specifically, to understand the role of genetic factors. While genes have successfully been linked to a variety of specific diseases, it has proven to be problematic to find a link to overall longevity, the reasons being that it is difficult to identify genes that give its bearers long life, and that children share not only genes but also environmental conditions with their parents.

For a nineteenth-century rural population in southern Sweden, we find that the correspondence between length of life of parents and of their offspring is rather weak, as has been shown in many other similar studies. The question is whether this is due to strong influences of other than inherited factors, such as local environmental factors and social mobility, or simply that length of life of parents does not provide us with information about inherited factors of importance to length of life. Since the dataset we are using is very rich in terms of details about occupation and landholding, as well as local conditions such as food prices and mortality outbreaks, we have estimated a model taking a number of factors—shown to be important in other studies—into account by using a Cox regression framework. We are not only considering observed factors but also unobserved factors at family level shared by siblings.

After controlling for socioeconomic status at birth, at age 50 years and current status, the disease load in the first year of life, current food prices and food prices at year of birth, and birth year, as well as unobserved factors at birth family level, we find a persistent influence of parents' longevity on their children's mortality at older ages. If either of the parents lived 1 year longer, both sons and daughters experience 1 percent lower mortality in ages 50 years and above. The effect is the same as being born 1 year later. Another important factor for men's mortality in older ages was the exposure to diseases in first year of life. Men born in years of outbreaks of epidemic diseases, such as smallpox and whooping cough, have much higher mortality in older ages. Thus, the scarring effect is dominating over the selection effect. But throughout, we find no effects of socioeconomic status. The lack of a socioeconomic divergence may seem odd, but it is in fact consistent with most historical studies, which show that the social gradient in mortality is a rather modern phenomenon. Accordingly, in the rural nineteenth-century population that we analyze, in which all are equally exposed to communicable infectious diseases for which no medication was available, access to resources could not improve survival.

The most difficult, and controversial, question is whether the length of life of parents is genetically transferred to their children. Most previous studies, if not all, showing a correlation between length of life of parents and children have not been able to include other shared factors that might contribute to such a relationship. An important strength of this study is that we have included various factors shared with relatives or members of the local community, as well as achieved socioeconomic status. We have also included a frailty factor to account for unobserved factors at birth family level. After controlling for these factors, length of life of parents has a significant and strong impact on the mortality of their children at an older age. Still, we cannot conclude that this is entirely a genetic effect, only that genetics may well play an important role in determining length of life.

It is essential to bear in mind that these results should not be interpreted as if inherited environmental factors, like the socioeconomic situation of the family, are never important. Our findings should not be extrapolated into the twentieth century, perhaps not even to other nineteenth-century populations, particularly not urban ones. Our results instead refer to a certain context in which the socioeconomic differences in mortality were modest, although emerging, which most likely was the case in most of nineteenth-century rural Europe. This means that the methodological issues that we brought into our analysis may be far more important elsewhere than they were here.

Acknowledgments This work has been done within three projects: Early-Life Conditions, Social Mobility, and Longevity: Social Differences and Trends in Adult Mortality in Sweden, 1650–1900, financed by the Swedish Council for Working Life and Social Research; Early-Life Conditions, Social Mobility, and Health in Later Life, financed by the Bank of Sweden Tercentenary Foundation; and Early-Life Conditions, Social Mobility, and Longevity, financed by the National Institute of Aging, USA. The data come from the Scanian Demographic Database, which is a collaborative project between the Regional Archives in Lund and the Centre for Economic Demography at Lund University. We gratefully acknowledge comments on an earlier version of this paper from Kaare Christensen and Martin Lindström.

References

Abbott, M., E. Murphy, D. Bolling, and H. Abbey. 1974. The familial component in longevity. A study of offspring of nonagenarians. II. Preliminary analysis of the completed study. *Johns Hopkins Medical Journal* 134(1): 1–16.

Barker, D. 1994. *Mothers, Babies, and Disease in Later Life*. British Medical Journal Publishing Group, London.

Barker, D. 1995. Fetal origins of coronary heart disease. *British Medical Journal* 1: 171–4.

Bengtsson, T. 1993. Combined time-series and life event analysis: The impact of economic fluctuations and air temperature on adult mortality by sex and occupation in a Swedish mining parish, in D.S. Reher and R. Schofield (eds.), *Old and new methods in historical demography*, Clarendon/Oxford University Press, Oxford, England/New York, pp. 239–58.

Bengtsson, T. 2004. Mortality and social class in four Scanian parishes, 1766–1865, in T. Bengtsson, C. Campbell, J.Z. Lee et al. (eds.), *Life under pressure. Mortality and living standards in Europe and Asia 1700–1900*, MIT, Cambridge, MA, pp.135–72.

Bengtsson, T., C. Campbell, J.Z. Lee et al. (eds.). 2004. *Life under Pressure. Mortality and Living Standards in Europe and Asia 1700–1900*, MIT, Cambridge, MA.

Bengtsson, T. and M. Dribe. 1997. Economy and demography in Western Scania, Sweden, 1650–1900. Working Paper Series No. 10. International Research Center for Japanese Studies, Kyoto.

Bengtsson, T. and M. Dribe. 2005. New evidence on the standard of living in Sweden during the eighteenth and nineteenth centuries: Long-term development of the demographic response to short-term economic stress, in R.C. Allen, T. Bengtsson, and M. Dribe (eds.), *Living standards in the past. New perspectives on well-being in Asia and Europe*, Oxford University Press, Oxford, pp. 341–72.

Bengtsson, T. and M. Dribe. 2007. Socioeconomic differences and family clustering of infant and child mortality: A multilevel analysis of rural southern Sweden, 1766–1895. Conference paper for the PAA Annual Meeting, Session 110: Long-run trends and differentials in mortality, New York, NY.

Bengtsson, T. and M. Lindström. 2000. Childhood misery and disease in later life: The effects on mortality in old age of hazards experienced in early life, southern Sweden, 1760–1894. *Population Studies* 52: 263–77.

Bengtsson, T. and M. Lindström. 2003. Airborne infectious diseases during infancy and mortality in later life, southern Sweden, 1766–1894. *International Journal of Epidemiology* 32: 286–94.

Bengtsson, T. and R. Ohlsson. 1985. Age-specific mortality and short-term changes in the standard of living: Sweden, 1751–1859. *European Journal of Population* 1(4): 309–26.

Bengtsson, T. and K. Scott. 2005. Varför Sveriges befolkning åldras. Vad vi kan och inte kan göra åt det. *Sociologisk Forskning* 3: 3–12.

Broström, G. 2007. *eha: Event History Analysis*, R package version 0.97-6. http://www.stat.umu.se/personal/goran.brostrom/eha/

Bygren, L-O., S. Edvinsson, and G. Broström. 2000. Change in food availability during pregnancy: Is it related to adult sudden death from cerebro- and cardiovascular disease in offspring? *American Journal of Human Biology* 12: 447–53.

Carlsson, S. 1968. *Yrken och samhällsgrupper: Den sociala omgrupperingen i Sverige efter 1866*. Almqvist & Wiksell, Stockholm.

Christensen, K. 2007. Early life events and later life health: Twin and famine studies, in T. Bengtsson (ed.), *Perspectives on mortality forecasting. V. Cohort models*. Swedish National Insurance Board, Stockholm.

Coale, A.J. 1957. How the age distribution of a human population is determined. *Cold Spring Harbor Symposia on Quantitative Biology* 22: 83–9.

Cohen, B. 1964. Family pattern of mortality and life-span. *Quarterly Review of Biology* 39: 130–81.

Cox, D. 1972. Regression models and life-tables (with discussion). *Journal of the Royal Statistical Society* Series B 34: 187–220.

Dribe, M. and C. Lundh. 2005. Retirement as a strategy for land transmission: A micro study of pre-industrial rural Sweden. *Continuity and Change* 20(2): 165–91.

Elo, I. and S. Preston. 1992. Effects of early-life conditions on adult mortality: A review. *Population Index* 58(2): 86–212.

Finch, C.E. and R.E. Tanzi. 1997. Genetics of aging. *Science* 278(17): 407–11.

Finch, C.E. and E.M. Crimmins. 2004. Inflammatory exposure and historical changes in human life-spans. *Science* 305: 1736–9.

Fogel, R. 1994. The relevance of Malthus for the study of mortality today: Long-run influences on health, mortality, labour-force participation and population growth, in K. Lindvall and H. Landberg (eds.), *Population, economic development, and the environment: The making of our common future*, Oxford University Press, Oxford/New York, pp. 231–84.

Fridlizius, G. 1989. The deformation of cohorts: Nineteenth-century mortality in a generational perspective. *Scandinavian Economic History Review* 37: 3–17.

Kermack, W.O., A.G. McKendrick, and P.L. McKinley. 1934. Death rates in Great Britain and Sweden: Some regularities and their significance. *Lancet* 226: 698–703.

Kuh, D. and Y. Ben-Schlomo. 1997. *A life course approach to chronic disease epidemiology.* Oxford University Press, Oxford.

Liuba, P. 2003. *Arterial injury due to infections in early life: A possible link in coronary heart disease.* Lund University Hospital, Lund.

Ljungquist, E., S. Berg, and B. Steen. 1995. Prediction of survival in 70-year olds. *Archives of Geronotology and Geriatrics* 20(3): 295–307.

Lundh, C. 1998. The social mobility of servants in rural Sweden, 1740–1894. *Continuity and Change* 1(14): 57–89.

Lundh, C. and M. Olsson. 2002. The institution of retirement on Scanian estates in the nineteenth century. *Continuity and Change* 17(3): 373–403.

Oeppen, J. and J.W. Vaupel. 2002. Broken limits to life expectancy. *Science* 296(5570): 1029–31.

Pearl, R. 1931. Studies on human longevity. IV: The inheritance of longevity. *Human Biology* 3: 245–69.

Preston, S., M. Hill, and G. Drevenstedt. 1998. Childhood conditions that predict survival to advanced ages among African-Americans. *Social Science and Medicine* 47: 1231–46.

Smith, D.S. 1983. Differential mortality in the United States before 1900. *Journal of Interdisciplinary History* 13(4): 735–59.

Smith, J.V.C. and J.H. Griscom. 1869. *The Two Price ($500 each) Essays on the Physical Indications of Longevity Written for the American Popular Life Insurance Co.* William Wood & Co., New York.

Therneau, T. and P. Grambsch. 2000. *Modeling Survival Data: Extending the Cox Model.* Springer, New York.

United Nations. 1953. The determinants and consequences of population trends. *Population studies No. 17.* United Nations, New York.

United Nations. 1973. The determinants and causes of population trends. *Population studies No. 50.* United Nations, New York.

Valkonen, T. 1993. *Socio-economic mortality differences in Europe.* NIDI, The Hague.

Wyshak, G. 1978. Fertility and longevity in twins, sibs, and parents of twins. *Social Biology* 25(4): 315–30.

Chapter 8
The Influence of Consanguineous Marriage on Reproductive Behavior and Early Mortality in Northern Coastal Sweden, 1780–1899

Inez Egerbladh[1] and Alan Bittles[2]

Abstract Remarkably few studies have been conducted into the prevalence and possible influence of close kin marriage on fertility and mortality in northern European populations. The Demographic DataBase at Umeå University offers a unique opportunity to correct this situation, with data on births, deaths, and marriages in the Skellefteå region of Sweden for the period 1720–1899 collected by the State Lutheran Church. The data are made more interesting by the fact that until 1680 first cousin unions were prohibited in Sweden; and from 1680 until 1844 a royal dispensation was needed before such unions could proceed. Of the 14,639 marriages initially studied, 20.8 percent were between couples related as sixth cousins or closer, with a significant increase in first cousin marriages post-1844. Using logistic regression, two subsets of marriages contracted from 1780 to 1899 were investigated with respect to fertility and mortality. First cousin marriages were strongly favored by freeholders and peasant landowning families; and in some families they had been preferentially contracted across successive generations. Consanguinity appeared to exert no influence on fertility. However, first cousin couples had higher rates of stillbirths and more deaths in infancy and early childhood among their progeny. This excess mortality was probably associated with the expression of detrimental recessive genes, although nongenetic factors may also have been involved. There was evidence of the clustering of multiple deaths within first cousin families, which likewise would be consistent with a genetic aetiology. Overall, the data confirm the significance of close consanguinity as an important demographic variable in this European population.

Keywords Consanguineous marriage, fertility, mortality, Sweden, 19th century

[1] Centre for Population Studies, Demographic DataBase, Umeå University, Sweden

[2] Centre for Human Genetics, Edith Cowan University, Perth, Australia

T. Bengtsson and G.P. Mineau (eds.), *Kinship and Demographic Behavior in the Past.*
© Springer Science+Business Media B.V. 2009

1 Introduction

1.1 Consanguineous Marriage: A Historical Background

Marriages between close biological relatives are strongly favored in many human populations (Bittles et al. 1991; Bittles 1998; http://www.consang.net). However, historical sources suggest a longstanding prejudice against consanguineous unions in most European populations (Bittles 2003a), as evidenced by the prohibition of first cousin marriages introduced by the Emperor Theodosius the Great (ca.384). Although the ban was revoked by his son Arcadius in 400, and the validity of first cousin marriages was also confirmed in the Institutes of Justinian in 533, by 692 first cousin marriages had been proscribed by the Orthodox Christian Churches (Knight 2003), with the continuing exception of the Coptic Church.

According to the Venerable Bede, in 597 Pope Gregory I advised Augustine, the first Archbishop of Canterbury, that "sacred law forbad a man to uncover the nakedness of his near kin", and in addition, that "unions between consanguineous spouses did not result in children" (Bede ca.731). Subsequently this opinion was formally endorsed by the Latin Church; and by the Fourth Lateran Council in 1215 Diocesan fee-based dispensation was required for marriages up to and including third cousins ($F \geq 0.0039$) (Goody 1983). These regulations were approved by the post-Reformation Council of Trent in 1563. They remained in force within the Roman Catholic Church until 1917, when the requirement for dispensation was initially reduced to marriages between couples who were related as second cousins or closer, and then to first cousins or closer ($F \geq 0.0625$) (Cavalli-Sforza, Moroni, and Zei 2004).

Demands for the cessation of obligatory dispensation payments for consanguineous marriages were an important feature of the Reformation movement. As a result, in the post-Reformation era the various Protestant denominations treated the consanguinity regulations imposed by the Pope as prohibitions additional to the rules of marriage ordained by God (Goody 1983). For this reason, the Protestant Churches in general reverted to the guidelines on consanguinity established in Leviticus 18: 7–18, with first cousin marriages freely permissible.

1.2 Consanguineous Marriage in Sweden

Among the Protestant denominations, the Lutheran State Church of Sweden was an important exception in its attitude towards consanguineous marriage, and until 1680 first cousin unions were proscribed by the Church. From 1680, a dispensation to permit first cousin marriage could be granted by the King in Council. This was an expensive process as it involved the payment of fees both to the Crown and to the Commissioners who acted as intermediaries in the dispensation process. Therefore, during this period first cousin marriages were principally contracted among the nobility, bourgeoisie, and peasantry (Alström 1958; Gaunt 1983; Göransson 1990). After unsuccessful attempts to dismiss the requirement for first cousin marriage dispensation in 1809 and 1823, the compulsory fee for consanguinity dispensation was removed by the *Riksdag* (Parliament) in 1829. Then in 1844, the *Riksdag* formally revoked the requirement for royal dispensation leaving first cousins of any social background free to marry should they so desire.

1.3 Consanguinity and Reproductive Behavior

As previously indicated, consanguinity-associated infertility was one of the early reasons cited by the Latin Church for the restriction on first cousin unions. Unfortunately, information on the relationship between consanguinity and fertility is limited; and where empirical information has been collected in human populations the studies have often relied on very small sample numbers, which makes the results difficult to assess. Various biological factors have been suggested for reduced fertility in consanguineous matings. Some studies, based on female olefactory responses to male body odors, have claimed a significant role for major histocompatibility complex (MHC) haplotypes in sexual attractiveness, with a marked preference for MHC-dissimilar partners and hence inbreeding avoidance (Wedekind et al. 1995). Other authors, however, either failed to confirm nonrandom mating at human leucocyte antigen (HLA) loci, or even indicated a greater likelihood of HLA-sharing between couples, suggesting increased attractiveness between biological relatives (reviewed in Bittles et al. 2002).

A lower than expected incidence of HLA haplotype matches was observed in the S-leut Hutterites, a highly endogamous Anabaptist sect resident in South Dakota, USA, which once again was interpreted as evidence of inbreeding avoidance (Ober et al. 1997). However, in their series of investigations over some 16 years, the authors had accepted the Hutterites as a natural fertility population, an assumption which was later recognized as incorrect (Ober, Hyslop, and Hauck 1999). Information on the various contraceptive practices favored by the Hutterites, including abstinence or infrequent intercourse, prolonged breast-feeding, and various methods of barrier, hormonal, and surgical birth control, was subsequently provided by a detailed study conducted in a Dariusleut Hutterite Colony (Curtis White 2002). In fact, even if the results of Ober et al. had been confirmed, their general relevance would be difficult to gauge, particularly in the many populations where consanguineous unions are strongly preferential and marriage partner choice is largely governed by parental decision (Bittles et al. 2002).

Similar conflicting opinions have arisen with respect to the effect of consanguinity on fertility. Some reports have indicated that antigenic disparity between the mother and fetus is beneficial to fetal development (Clarke and Kirby 1966; Adinolfi 1986; Ober 1998). The alternative view is that the enhanced genetic compatibility between mother and fetus in consanguineous unions, because of the increased proportion of shared genes between the parents, results in lower rates of intrauterine mortality and hence greater overall fertility (Philippe 1974). This opinion was supported by evidence indicating that both maternal-fetal Rhesus incompatibility and pre-eclamptic toxaemia were lower in consanguineous pregnancies (Stern and Charles 1945; Stevenson et al. 1971, 1976), which would favor fetal survival.

Appropriate caution is needed in the interpretation of retrospective data on pregnancies and prenatal losses, which are known to be unreliable and subject to major recall problems (Wilcox and Horney 1984; Wilcox et al. 1988), and so often lead to low levels of prenatal losses being cited. By comparison, when assays based on a systematic assessment of human chorionic gonadotrophin (hcG) levels were used, postimplantation losses of 48–92 percent were reported, dependent on maternal age (O'Connor, Holman, and Wood 1998).

1.4   Consanguinity and Mortality

While genetic similarity between mother and fetus may be beneficial in terms of prenatal survival, consanguinity can exert an adverse effect on health due to the expression of specific disease mutations inherited via both parents from a common ancestor (Bittles 2001). On average, couples related as first cousins have 1/8 of their genes in common, which means that their offspring would be expected to inherit identical genes at 1/16 (6.25%) of all gene loci. By convention, the level of inbreeding in an individual is expressed as the coefficient of inbreeding (F), which theoretically can range from 0 in an individual with nonidentical alleles from both parents at all gene loci to 1 in a person who has inherited identical alleles from each parent at all loci. For first cousin progeny $F = 0.0625$; while for second and third cousin offspring, who predictably inherit identical genes at 1/64 and 1/256 of loci, the comparable figures are $F = 0.0156$ and 0.0039 respectively. In populations where consanguineous unions have been sequentially contracted across several generations, the cumulative level of inbreeding may exceed these values. When a detailed pedigree is available, a correction can be applied to account for ancestral inbreeding using the formula:

$$F = \Sigma \, (1/2)_n \, (1 + F_A)$$

where F_A is the ancestor's inbreeding coefficient, n is the number of individuals in the path connecting the parents of the individual, and the summation (Σ) is taken over each path in the pedigree that goes through a common ancestor.

In general, estimates of the detrimental effects of consanguinity have declined through time, mainly reflecting less-biased sampling strategies (Bittles and Makov 1988). Unfortunately, many studies into the biological effects of inbreeding still lack adequate control for major sociodemographic variables. This is especially important in low income countries where factors associated with increased infant and childhood mortality, including maternal illiteracy, young maternal age, short birth intervals, and high parity are more common in consanguineous unions

(Bittles, Grant, and Shami 1993; Bittles 1994; Grant and Bittles 1997; Hussain and Bittles 1998, 2000).

1.5 Subjects and Methods

According to the Swedish Ecclesiastical Law of 1686, ministers of the State Lutheran Church were required to record all births, marriages, and deaths within their parish (O'Brien et al. 1989). The present investigation initially focused on the period 1720–1899 and was based on the population of the rural Skellefteå region of northern Sweden, located on the western coast of the Gulf of Bothnia. The information was derived from individuals listed in the catechetical registers of the Lutheran Church, with the data entries digitized by the Demographic DataBase at Umeå University (www.ddb.umu.se/ddnmaterial/kb_eng.htm). The study data were compiled from five complementary sources: (i) the examination registers for 1720–1899, which are similar in structure to censuses but with current recording for time periods[1]; (ii) birth registers for 1699–1899; (iii) death registers for 1815–1901; (iv) marriage registers for 1801–1895; and (v) migration registers for 1831–1895.

Records for each individual were linked into biographies; and the individuals were initially linked to first-degree relatives, i.e., parents, spouses, and children, with both biological and nonbiological relationships then added. Subsequent steps involved the generation of more distant kin links from these family data. Both the birth registers dating from 1699 and the catechetical registers that commenced in 1720 largely contained information on explicit parent–offspring relationships. Therefore, more distant biological relationships are probably underestimated for the population resident in the region during the early eighteenth century.

A total of 14,639 marriages contracted in Skellefteå between 1720 and 1899 were examined, with details of all consanguineous unions collected from the extended pedigrees constructed. The information analyzed included data on marriages ranging from first cousin ($F = 0.0625$) to sixth cousin ($F = 0.00006$) and beyond (Bittles and Egerbladh 2005). Mean coefficients of inbreeding (α) were calculated for the population at differing time intervals according to the formula:

$$\alpha = \Sigma p_i F_i$$

where Σ is the sum of the proportion of couples (p_i) in each consanguinity category (F_i), e.g., from first to beyond third cousins. Across the entire time period (1720–1899), the mean coefficient of inbreeding for the study population was $\alpha = 0.00204$.

---

[1] Date of birth, death, marriage, and other events also exist in the examination registers, but the specific event registers have more detailed information about such events. Hence, a shorter time span for a specific event register entry than the examination register does not necessarily denote missing information about events, for instance, spouses and dates of marriage.

Very few consanguineous marriages occurred during the eighteenth century ($\alpha = 0.00041$); and marriages between couples related as third cousins or closer ($F \geq 0.0039$) accounted for 95% of the cumulative coefficient of inbreeding (Bittles and Egerbladh 2005). For these reasons, only marriages contracted from 1780 to 1899 were included for detailed study. The analysis was further limited to unions between spouses related as first, second, or third cousins, and to nonconsanguineous controls with no records of consanguineous marriages among their ancestors. The final requirement imposed for mortality studies was a minimum observation period of more than 1 year. Subject to these restrictions, the impact of consanguinity on mortality was examined in a total of 6,017 marriages.

The influence of consanguinity on fertility was separately investigated by logistic regression analysis (SPSS 12.0) in high and low fertility families. In both cases, women aged <35 years at marriage were observed for 10+ years. Women in the high fertility families had borne 8+ children, whereas women in the low fertility families had 0–4 children, with a total of 4,301 families investigated. Controls for age at marriage, observation time, and husband's occupation were incorporated in the regression analyses of fertility.

Logistic regression analysis (SPSS 12.0) of mortality in terms of stillbirths, infant deaths, and deaths at ages 1–4 years old was performed, using data on multiple births, birth date, mother's age at delivery, birth interval, sex of the progeny, and father's occupation to control for the effects of possible confounding of sociodemographic and economic variables on survival. Parity was excluded due to its correlation with mother's age at delivery and to the quite wide range in the age at marriage of fecund females (age range 15–47 years). To examine possible family dependency with respect to mortality, covariates referring to the survival of previously born siblings were additionally included.

2 Results

2.1 Basic Demographic Profile

During the eighteenth and nineteenth centuries, there was an increase in the population density of Skellefteå from 1.3 to 9.7 inhabitants per km^2, with a growth in population from 3,650 inhabitants in 1749 to 26,100 in 1890. This increase in population density was principally driven by high marital fertility and low mortality, with only a low level of recorded illegitimacy (Sundbärg 1910; Alm-Stenflo 1994). Approximately 12.0 percent of all individuals recorded in the parish record books were migrants into the region, but only half of these individuals became permanent residents. Over the same time period, 12.4 percent of the population is known to have migrated from Skellefteå. Following the Great Nordic War at the beginning of the eighteenth century, and after the war between Sweden and Russia at the start of the nineteenth century, there was an excess of females in Skellefteå that remained until 1870–1880. Administrative changes introduced in the early nineteenth century resulted in a reduction in the population of Skellefteå of about 11 percent, and in its total area by approximately 50 percent to 2,700 km².

Skellefteå followed the general demographic pattern of northern Sweden with high marital fertility, low illegitimacy, and low mortality. The total fertility rate remained relatively high during the nineteenth century with about five children per woman, although somewhat fewer children were born during the first decade. The crude mortality rate decreased from around 20 per thousand in the late eighteenth century to 15 per thousand at the turn of the twentieth century. However, death rates fluctuated over time and, for example, they were lower from 1830–1840 but with peaks of mortality due to war in the early nineteenth century and following severe crop failures in the 1860s. Infant mortality decreased from around 200 per thousand in risk years to approximately half that level by the 1840s and for the remainder of the century. No specific trend was observed in child mortality because of temporal fluctuations (Alm-Stenflo 1994; Edvinsson 2004).

2.2 Prevalence and Patterns of Consanguineous Marriage Through Time

The numbers of marriages contracted in Skellefteå from 1780 to 1899 are listed by decade in Table 8.1, subdivided into first, second, and third cousin unions, and nonconsanguineous marriages. Contrary to theoretical expectation (Hajnal 1963), the increasing total number of marriages in the region was accompanied by a marked positive trend in the numbers and percentages of consanguineous unions, suggesting their greater social acceptability through time (Bittles and Egerbladh 2005). Thus, during the last 20-year period examined in Skellefteå (1880–1899), 8.8 percent of marriages were between couples related as third cousins or closer, and a further 29.3 percent of marriages were between more remote biological relatives, equivalent to an α value of 0.00273 for the population as a whole.

The increased popularity of first cousin unions was especially apparent after 1844 when royal dispensation ceased to be a prerequisite to marriage. First cousin unions increased from 1.5% during 1820–1839, to 2.6%, 2.7%, and 2.9% in the three following 20-year periods (Table 8.1). There also was convincing evidence that close kin marriages were favored by landowning families in particular, with 86.2% of first cousin marriages involving landowning parents of both the groom and bride, and 82.8% of women in a first cousin union marrying a spouse who was a peasant (Table 8.2).

2.3 Consanguinity and Fertility

As in other, non-European populations (Bittles et al. 1993; Bittles 1994), mean male and female ages were lower at marriage and the mean spousal age differences between the main consanguineous and nonconsanguineous categories were smaller (Table 8.3). Some of the observed difference in these mean values was, however, accounted for by a small number of unions in the nonconsanguineous group where either the husband or wife was much older than their spouse.

When all marriages that met the requisite preconditions were considered ($n = 6,350$), only minor differences were observed in the numbers of total births, livebirths, and children surviving to 5 years in the different consanguinity categories (Table 8.4). As indicated in Tables 8.5 and 8.6, regression analyses on women aged <35 years at marriage and observed for 10+ years confirmed that consanguinity had no significant effect on fertility either in high fertility or low fertility families. However, in both cases, female age at marriage and the time period under observation after marriage exerted a significant impact. Economic conditions also affected fertility, since landowning peasants had higher fertility whereas both unskilled laborers and husbands with an unknown occupation had lower fertility.

Table 8.1 Consanguineous marriages by degree of relationship, Skellefteå 1780–1899

Marriage types	1780–1799	1800–1819	1820–1839	1840–1859	1860–1879	1880–1899	Total numbers
First cousin	5	17	24	59	80	111	296
Second cousin	17	23	34	79	76	95	324
Third cousin	1	9	61	96	130	129	426
Beyond third cousin	4	27	44	310	582	1,122	1,989
Nonconsanguineous	950	1,200	1,492	1,786	2,137	2,369	9,934
All marriages	979	1,276	1,655	2,230	3,005	3,826	12,969

Table 8.2 Consanguinity and parental landownership (%), and husband's occupation as landowner (%), Skellefteå 1780–1899

Marriage type	Husband's father	Wife's father	Both fathers	Neither father	Husband
First cousin	5.2	6.6	86.2	2.1	82.8
Second cousin	6.4	12.5	79.5	1.7	82.4
Third cousin	5.9	8.6	83.6	1.8	77.7
Nonconsanguineous	12.9	27.6	48.3	11.2	72.1
All marriages	11.7	24.5	53.7	9.7	73.5

Table 8.3 Consanguinity and mean age at marriage (with SD) in years, all marriages, Skellefteå 1780–1899

Type of marriage	Husband		Wife		Age difference	
	Mean	SD	Mean	SD	Mean	SD
First cousin	27.9	6.2	25.7	5.7	4.9	3.5
Second cousin	27.0	5.1	25.0	4.7	4.7	3.7
Third cousin	27.1	5.3	25.3	5.3	4.7	3.4
Nonconsanguineous	29.6	8.8	27.4	7.4	5.9	4.9

Table 8.4 Consanguinity and mean fertility (with SD), all marriages, Skellefteå 1780–1899

	All births		Livebirths		Surviving to age 5 years	
Type of marriage	Mean	SD	Mean	SD	Mean	SD
First cousin	4.8	3.2	4.7	3.4	3.8	2.7
Second cousin	5.1	3.3	5.0	3.2	4.2	2.8
Third cousin	5.1	3.3	5.0	3.3	4.2	2.8
Nonconsanguineous	5.0	3.4	4.9	3.4	4.0	2.9

Table 8.5 Binary logistic regression analysis of high fertility families with 8+ children, Skellefteå 1780–1899. (From Demographic DataBase, Umeå University.)

Covariate	B	S.E	Wald	Sign. level	Exp(B)
Kin					
Reference: nonconsanguinity			2.623	0.453	
First cousins	0.041	0.176	0.053	0.818	1.041
Second cousins	−0.198	0.160	1.533	0.216	0.821
Third cousins	−0.147	0.138	1.132	0.287	0.863
Wife's age at marriage					
Reference: <25 years old			413.205	0.000**	
Age 25–29	−1.089	0.075	210.973	0.000**	0.336
Age 30–34	−2.902	0.177	268.717	0.000**	0.055
Observed time after marriage					
Reference: 10–14 year			214.864	0.000**	
15–19 year	1.868	0.178	109.901	0.000**	6.474
20+ year	2.286	0.159	207.782	0.000**	9.835
Husband's occupation					
Reference: unknown			24.139	0.000**	
Peasants	1.231	0.468	6.932	0.008**	3.426
Officials and skilled labor	0.939	0.490	3.669	0.055	2.557
Unskilled labor and crofters	0.796	0.477	2.785	0.095	2.217
Constant	−3.031	0.488	38.557	0.000**	0.048

*Significant at $p < 0.05$; **significant at $p < 0.01$.

2.4 Consanguinity and Mortality

The mean levels of stillbirths, infant deaths, and deaths between years 1–4 are summarized in Table 8.7 for the progeny of first, second, and third cousins, and nonconsanguineous couples. There was a positive relationship between mortality and increasing level of inbreeding and, comparing first cousin and nonconsanguineous progeny, the total excess mortality from stillbirths to 5 years of age was 3.2%. This compares with an estimated 3.5% excess mortality reported for first cousin progeny in Italy during the early to mid-twentieth century (Cavalli-Sforza et al. 2004); and a mean 4.4% excess first cousin deaths from late pregnancy to approximately age 10 years in a meta-analysis conducted on 38 mid- to late twentieth-century populations (Bittles and Neel 1994).

In general, infant mortality in Skellefteå was significantly less common among the children of peasants (Edvinsson 2004), and, as shown in Table 8.2, landowners

Table 8.6 Binary logistic regression analysis of low fertility families with 0–4 children, Skellefteå 1780–1899. (From Demographic DataBase, Umeå University.)

Covariate	B	S.E	Wald	Sign. level	Exp(B)
Kin					
Reference: nonconsanguinity			1.963	0.580	
First cousins	0.100	0.186	0.289	0.591	1.105
Second cousins	−0.128	0.178	0.522	0.470	0.880
Third cousins	−0.168	0.159	1.121	0.290	0.845
Wife's age at marriage					
Reference: <25 years old			291.789	0.000**	
Age 25–29	0.595	0.084	50.345	0.000**	1.814
Age 30–34	1.727	0.101	291.789	0.000**	5.626
Observed time after marriage					
Reference: 10–14 year			56.844	0.000**	
15–19 year	−0.703	0.134	27.699	0.000**	0.495
20+ year	−0.731	0.098	55.358	0.000**	0.481
Husband's occupation					
Reference: unknown			18.624	0.000**	
Peasants	0.210	0.155	1.834	0.176	1.234
Officials and skilled labor	0.287	0.103	7.775	0.005*	1.333
Unskilled labor and crofters	1.026	0.309	11.056	0.001**	2.791
Constant	−1.106	0.103	115.093	0.000**	0.331

*Significant at $p < 0.05$; **significant at $p < 0.01$.

Table 8.7 Consanguinity and mean mortality (%), Skellefteå 1780–1899

	First cousin progeny ($F = 0.0625$)	Second cousin progeny ($F = 0.0156$)	Third cousin progeny ($F = 0.0039$)	Nonconsanguineous progeny
Stillbirths	2.7	2.4	2.0	1.6
Infant deaths	13.2	10.2	10.2	12.2
Deaths 1–4 years	8.3	7.9	7.5	6.9
Total mortality	23.6	23.2	19.3	20.4
Total numbers of progeny	1,404	1,624	2,096	25,796

were more likely to contract consanguineous marriages. Thus, the lower-bound level of excess consanguinity-associated mortality (3.2%) indicated in Table 8.7 may be explained by the high rate of infant mortality observed among nonconsanguineous progeny whose parents had less adequate access to economic resources.

The influence of consanguinity and of possible confounding sociodemographic variables on stillbirths, infant deaths, and deaths between 1–4 years of age were determined by logistic regressions (Tables 8.8–8.10). Among first cousin progeny, consanguinity had a major negative impact on survival during all three time periods, with a particularly adverse outcome in terms of infant mortality (p < 0.01), whereas the comparable data for second and third cousin progeny were statistically nonsignificant.

Negative influences on survival were also observed at varying levels of statistical significance for multiple births, earlier year of birth (prior to 1840), short birth

Table 8.8 Binary logistic regression analysis of stillbirths, Skellefteå, 1780–1899. (From Demographic DataBase, Umeå University.)

Covariate	B	S.E	Wald	Sign. level	Exp(B)
Kin					
Reference: nonconsanguinity			11.512	0.023*	
First cousins	0.534	0.188	11.108	0.005**	1.706
Second cousins	0.173	0.202	0.650	0.393	1.188
Third cousins	0.267	0.176	0.877	0.128	1.306
Multiple birth					
Reference: not	1.292	0.181	64.286	0.000**	3.639
Birth date					
Reference: 1880+			88.071	0.000**	
1860–1879	−0.031	0.125	0.941	0.805	0.970
1840–1859	−1.339	0.198	58.524	0.000**	0.262
1820–1839	−0.391	0.151	3.693	0.010**	0.676
<1820	−1.753	0.245	36.227	0.000**	0.173
Mother's age					
Reference: 25–29 years old			23.473	0.371	
Age <20	−0.134	0.600	0.002	0.823	0.874
Age 20–24	−0.176	0.209	0.927	0.400	0.839
Age 30–34	0.110	0.154	1.409	0.476	1.117
Age 35–39	0.141	0.158	6.694	0.374	1.151
Age 40+	0.324	0.178	16.302	0.068	1.382
Birth interval					
Reference: child 1			17.795	0.001**	
Interval <18 months	−0.191	0.190	0.567	0.316	0.826
Interval 18–35 months	−0.594	0.173	5.402	0.001**	0.552
Interval 36+ months	−0.364	0.206	0.762	0.077	0.695
Sex					
Reference: son			442.995	0.000**	
Daughter	−0.216	0.104	5.632	0.038*	0.806
Unknown sex	6.756	0.276	420.666	0.000**	859.484
Father's occupation					
Reference: peasants			0.722	0.401	
Entrepreneurs, officials, and skilled labor	−0.238	0.271	0.345	0.380	0.788
Crofters and unskilled labor	−0.013	0.144	0.005	0.930	0.987
Unknown occupation	−1.054	0.709	0.371	0.137	0.349
Stillborn siblings					
Reference: 0 previous siblings			426.830	0.000**	
1 sibling	1.724	0.151	142.861	0.000**	5.607
2+ siblings	2.892	0.203	369.349	0.000**	18.030
Infant deaths siblings					
Reference: 0 previous siblings			0.001	0.005**	
1 sibling	0.397	0.125	0.000	0.001**	1.488
2 siblings	0.121	0.198	0.000	0.541	1.129
3+ siblings	0.852	0.409	0.000	0.037*	2.345
Siblings dead 1–4 years					
Reference: 0 previous siblings			0.075	0.969	
1 sibling	0.044	0.139	0.005	0.751	1.045
2 siblings	−0.100	0.293	0.005	0.733	0.905
3+ siblings	0.016	0.618	0.063	0.979	1.016
Constant	−3.978	0.195	432.298	0.000**	0.019

*Significant at $p < 0.05$; **significant at $p < 0.01$.

Table 8.9 Binary logistic regression analysis of infant mortality, Skellefteå, 1780–1899. (From Demographic DataBase, Umeå University.)

Covariate	B	S.E	Wald	Sign. level	Exp(B)
Kin					
Reference: nonconsanguinity			19.007	0.000**	
First cousins	0.346	0.084	17.082	0.000**	1.413
Second cousins	−0.082	0.086	0.903	0.342	0.921
Third cousins	0.071	0.078	0.837	0.360	1.074
Multiple birth	1.322	0.078	286.564	0.000**	3.752
Reference: not					
Birth date					
Reference: 1880+			279.338	0.000**	
1860–1879	0.115	0.060	3.646	0.056	1.122
1840–1859	−0.003	0.064	0.003	0.960	0.997
1820–1839	0.391	0.061	41.208	0.000**	1.479
<1820	0.770	0.057	179.588	0.000**	2.159
Mother's age					
Reference: 25–29 years old			21.072	0.001**	
Age <20	0.489	0.159	9.397	0.002**	1.630
Age 20–24	0.084	0.064	1.715	0.190	1.087
Age 30–34	−0.065	0.052	1.589	0.207	0.937
Age 35–39	0.019	0.055	0.115	0.735	1.019
Age 40+	0.128	0.065	3.836	0.050*	1.136
Birth interval					
Reference: child 1			61.966	0.000**	
Interval <18 months	0.213	0.064	11.156	0.001**	1.237
Interval 18–35 months	−0.148	0.058	6.465	0.011*	0.862
Interval 36+ months	−0.160	0.074	4.741	0.029*	0.852
Sex					
Reference: son	−0.273	0.036	57.642	0.000**	0.761
Father's occupation					
Reference: peasants			11.778	0.008**	
Entrepreneurs, officials, and skilled labor	0.092	0.092	0.993	0.319	1.096
Crofters and unskilled labor	0.123	0.051	5.757	0.016*	1.130
Unknown occupation	0.316	0.127	6.208	0.013*	1.372
Stillborn siblings					
Reference: 0 previous siblings			10.596	0.005**	
1 sibling	0.322	0.101	10.081	0.001**	1.380
2+ siblings	0.195	0.240	0.658	0.417	1.215
Infant deaths siblings					
Reference: 0 previous siblings			145.639	0.000**	
1 sibling	0.267	0.047	32.597	0.000**	1.306
2 siblings	0.540	0.064	71.768	0.000**	1.717
3+ siblings	1.216	0.131	86.630	0.000**	3.374
Siblings dead 1–4 years					
Reference: 0 previous siblings			22.572	0.000**	
1 sibling	0.096	0.051	3.518	0.061	1.100
2 siblings	0.345	0.095	13.347	0.000**	1.412
3+ siblings	0.608	0.206	8.721	0.003**	1.837
Constant	−2.389	0.074	1040.353	0.000**	0.092

*Significant at $p < 0.05$; **significant at $p < 0.01$.

Table 8.10 Binary logistic regression analysis of child mortality, Skellefteå, 1780–1899. (From Demographic DataBase, Umeå University.)

Covariate	B	S.E	Wald	Sign. level	Exp(B)
Kin					
Reference: nonconsanguinity			12.475	0.006**	
First cousins	0.300	0.103	8.541	0.003**	1.350
Second cousins	0.169	0.097	3.028	0.082	1.184
Third cousins	0.154	0.089	2.969	0.085	1.166
Multiple birth					
Reference: not	0.621	0.125	24.726	0.000**	1.862
Birth date					
Reference: 1880+			70.290	0.000**	
1860–1879	0.514	0.071	53.080	0.000**	1.672
1840–1859	0.393	0.074	28.040	0.000**	1.481
1820–1839	0.165	0.081	4.107	0.043*	1.179
<1820	0.467	0.076	37.598	0.000**	1.596
Mother's age					
Reference: 25–29 years old			9.277	0.099	
Age <20	0.476	0.210	5.120	0.024*	1.609
Age 20–24	−0.026	0.084	0.094	0.760	0.975
Age 30–34	0.040	0.065	0.392	0.531	1.041
Age 35–39	0.087	0.069	1.572	0.210	1.090
Age 40+	0.146	0.082	3.153	0.076	1.158
Birth interval					
Reference: child 1			11.633	0.009**	
Interval <18 months	0.191	0.084	5.140	0.023*	1.210
Interval 18–35 months	−0.024	0.073	0.111	0.739	0.976
Interval 36+ months	0.042	0.090	0.218	0.641	1.043
Sex					
Reference: son	−0.089	0.045	3.949	0.047*	0.915
Father's occupation					
Reference: peasants			12.508	0.006**	
Entrepreneurs, officials and skilled labor	0.121	0.113	1.151	0.283	1.128
Crofters and unskilled labor	0.187	0.063	8.919	0.003**	1.206
Unknown occupation	0.331	0.172	3.710	0.054	1.393
Stillborn siblings					
Reference: 0 previous sibling			1.475	0.478	
1 sibling	−0.100	0.144	0.482	0.487	0.905
2+ siblings	−0.374	0.370	1.020	0.312	0.688
Infant deaths siblings					
Reference: 0 previous siblings			19.925	0.000**	
1 sibling	0.059	0.061	0.941	0.332	1.061
2 siblings	0.143	0.091	2.492	0.114	1.154
3+ siblings	0.837	0.194	18.573	0.000**	2.310
Siblings dead 1–4 years					
Reference: 0 previous siblings			28.035	0.000**	
1 sibling	0.298	0.061	24.320	0.000**	1.348
2 siblings	0.311	0.124	6.309	0.012*	1.365
3+ siblings	−0.101	0.352	0.083	0.773	0.904
Constant	−2.977	0.094	1001.851	0.000**	0.051

*Significant at $p < 0.05$; **significant at $p < 0.01$.

intervals (< 18 months), and male sex. Lower paternal socioeconomic status/occupation (crofters, i.e., tenant smallholders, and unskilled) and younger maternal age showed significantly higher risks for infant and child deaths, but the impact of the other covariates differed with type of mortality, e.g., with advanced maternal age (40+ years) impacting mainly on infant deaths.

There was evidence of mortality clustering within certain families, which is in keeping with research reported from other populations (Das Gupta 1990, 1997; Guo 1993; Lynch and Greenhouse 1994; Edvinsson et al. 2005). To further assess this phenomenon, the risk of death was examined where a previously born sibling had been stillborn, or had died in infancy or early childhood. This analysis showed that: (i) stillbirths were associated with previous siblings being stillborn or having died in infancy; (ii) the risk of infant death increased when stillbirths or infant or childhood deaths had been reported for previous siblings; and (iii) both infant and childhood deaths among previous siblings had a significant positive impact on childhood deaths.

These findings are in keeping with the concept of specific high-risk families and could represent the expression of detrimental genes or unfavorable socioeconomic conditions (Stoltenberg et al. 1999). Given the generally more privileged socioeconomic position of first cousin spouses in terms of land ownership (Table 8.2), and hence better access to food and other material resources, a genetic aetiology would seem to be a probable explanation for the increased occurrence of multiple deaths in close kin families. Support for this hypothesis is provided by examination of the pedigrees of single gene disorders reported in the present-day population of Skellefteå and neighboring areas (Bittles and Egerbladh 2005).

3 Discussion

Prior to the introduction of the royal dispensation in 1680, first cousin marriages were extremely rare in Sweden; but thereafter their prevalence increased nationally to an estimated 0.2% in 1750, 1.0% in 1800, and 1.5% by the mid-nineteenth century (Alström 1958). This study also reported a distinct north-south cline in consanguineous marriage, with the highest rates of consanguinity in the more sparsely populated northern regions abutting Finland that are home to most of the Swedish Sami (Lapp) community. Reports on cousin marriage conducted in neighboring Norway (Saugstad 1977) and Finland (Jorde and Pitkanen 1991) also suggest that consanguinity may be higher in Sami communities, possibly reflecting either preferred marriage patterns or restrictions on marriage partner choice. Among non-Sami settlers, kinship groups preferentially lived in close proximity and at a distance from other settlers, which through time resulted in the establishment of kin-based freeholder settlements (Bylund 1960).

It is generally believed that first cousin marriages are chosen for economic reasons and to strengthen family ties whereas more remote levels of kin marriage primarily reflect spouse availability. According to the Hajnal (1963) model, which assumes random inbreeding, the expected ratio of first cousin to second cousin marriage in an isolated population is 1:4 (0.25). A ratio greater than 0.25 would suggest possible preference for first cousin marriage whereas a ratio ≤ 0.25 would indicate either a preponderance of marriages between more remote relatives, effectively contracted on a random basis, or avoidance of close kin unions. In both cases, however, the observed ratio could have been significantly influenced by partner availability, social or religious norms which favored or prohibited certain forms of consanguineous unions, and by socially acceptable age differentials between marriage partners (Barrai, Cavalli-Sforza, and Moroni 1962; Bittles 1994; Cavalli-Sforza et al. 2004).

There was steady growth in the total population of Skellefteå during the eighteenth century and more especially the nineteenth century. As shown in Table 8.1, across the study period 1780–1899 the numbers of first cousin ($n = 296$) and second cousin marriages ($n = 324$) were quite similar, with a high overall ratio of 0.91. However, when the ratios of first to second cousin marriages were compared across time, they had increased from 0.29 during 1780–1799 to 1.17 in 1880–1899, suggesting greatly increased acceptance of first cousin marriages in Skellefteå once the economic disincentives associated with compulsory royal dispensation had been removed (Bittles and Egerbladh 2005).

Within Scandinavia, the requirement for dispensation to marry a first or second cousin was rescinded by the Danish-Norwegian king in 1800 (Saugstad and Ødegård 1977), and a first cousin–second cousin marriage ratio of 1.0 was reported in Norway during the early twentieth century (Gedde-Dahl 1973). The situation was quite different in Finland where studies based on royal dispensation records and national population statistics showed a very low level of first cousin marriage during the nineteenth century, although with Sami communities a possible exception. Avoidance of first cousin marriage in Finland appears to have resulted both from the requirement for royal dispensation payments which continued until 1872 and a cultural prohibition in parts of eastern Finland against paternal parallel cousin marriages (Jorde and Pitkänen 1991). This latter prohibition may have stemmed from the restrictions on first and second cousin marriages applied by the Orthodox Church which would have been quite influential in regions of the country bordering on Russia (Ignatius 1994–1995). But even among the Swedish Lutheran population of the western Åland Islands in the Gulf of Bothnia, there was general avoidance of first, second, and third cousin marriages throughout the eighteenth, nineteenth, and early twentieth centuries (O'Brien et al. 1989).

The data on attitudes towards consanguineous marriage in nineteenth-century Skellefteå are therefore at marked variance with neighboring Finland, but they are in close accord with reports from populations resident in many other parts of the world. Besides the perceived benefits of consanguinity in terms of enhanced family solidarity, there is a particular preference for first cousin unions among landowning groups, indicative of their desire to maintain the integrity of their landholdings (Bittles 1994; Hussain 1999). In Skellefteå, infant and childhood mortality, and multiple deaths within specific families, were higher among first cousin progeny which is consistent with the expression of detrimental recessive gene(s) inherited from a common ancestor. In particular, the much higher rate of infant mortality is in keeping with the results of previous studies into the effects of consanguinity on early postnatal mortality (Dorsten, Hotchkiss, and King 1999; Bittles 2001, 2003b).

Despite the higher levels of early postnatal mortality among first cousin couples, there was no indication of any differences in fertility among the different consanguinity groups. Therefore, the present study does not provide support for reproductive compensation, i.e., the rapid replacement of an infant dying at an early age which has been reported in other populations (Schull et al. 1970; Rukanuddin 1982; Bittles et al. 1991) and may involve a conscious decision by parents to achieve their desired family size (Scrimshaw 1978; Gyimah and Fernando 2002). It has been suggested that reproductive compensation could be difficult to demonstrate when women are reproducing at or close to their maximum biological and social potential (Ober et al. 1999), and in this respect the relatively late mean ages at marriage in Skellefteå during the late eighteenth and nineteenth centuries may have acted as a practical constraint to replacement. In the present instance, however, the failure to demonstrate any obvious difference between the effects of consanguinity in both high and low fertility families effectively negates this possibility.

Childhood deaths tend to cluster in certain families (Zenger 1993; Ronsmans 1995; Sastry 1997; Stoltenberg et al. 1999). Although the precise mechanisms remain poorly understood, and may vary across and within high-risk families and communities, the predisposing factors for death clustering appear to be both familial and environmental, acting independently or in a synergistic manner. As has been widely reported, consanguinity usually is positively associated with increased postnatal mortality (Bittles and Neel 1994), described in the biological literature in terms of "inbreeding depression". The strength of inbreeding depression is dependent on the percentage and types of genes shared by a couple and, as previously indicated, multiple deaths may be observed in a proportion of families (Bittles et al. 1991; Stoltenberg et al. 1999). In the present study, marriages beyond first cousins ($F \leq 0.0625$) did not appear to be adversely affected in terms of stillbirths, infant deaths, or mortality in years 1–4. However, this conclusion, and the possible influence of more remote levels of consanguinity on survival in the age group 1–4 years, may require revision when an assessment of multiple consanguineous relationships across generations has been conducted. Data on stillbirths also may be incomplete prior to 1820. By comparison, post-1820, the clergy had to report annually the numbers of stillbirths in their parish to the Commission of the Tabellverket (the State Organization responsible for gathering demographic statistics).

The Skellefteå mortality data presented in Tables 8.8–8.10 suggest that increasing consanguinity during the nineteenth century could have significantly influenced the subsequent prevalence and patterns of inherited disease genes in the region and thus morbidity and early deaths. The switch from nonconsanguineous to consanguineous marriage during the study period would in itself have been significant since it made the expression of otherwise rare recessive genes more probable, particularly in first cousin unions where the partners would have inherited identical genes from each parent at 6.25 percent of their gene loci.

It is also probable that the population gene pool would have been subject to the underlying influences of founder effect and genetic drift, which can cause variation in disease gene frequencies in an essentially random manner. The effect of genetic drift would have been reinforced by imbalanced tertiary sex ratios, by familial clustering with respect to consanguineous marriages in the majority farming community (Table 8.2), and by village endogamy (Bittles and Egerbladh 2005). The net effect of both preferential consanguinity and endogamy-associated genetic drift is that specific inherited diseases would be confined to particular pedigrees or sub-communities (Bittles 2002, 2005). In support of this hypothesis, there have been well-documented reports of a high prevalence of genetic disorders in particular northern Swedish communities (Backman and Holmgren 1988; Holmgren 2000) some of which can be traced back over multiple generations (Sjögren and Larsson 1957; Nordström and Thorburn 1980).

From a more general social perspective, the increasing prevalence of first cousin marriage during the course of the nineteenth century illustrates the quite rapid change in community marital preferences that followed the revised civil legislation on consanguineous marriage. This emphasizes the potential role of consanguinity as a significant demographic variable in the many other populations where cousin marriage has yet to be investigated. It also suggests the possibility of an effective trade-off between the perceived social and economic benefits of close kin marriage and the greater probability of premature deaths among consanguineous progeny. The higher prevalence of deaths among first cousin progeny may have become increasingly obvious with declining overall local mortality rates during the course of the nineteenth century (Alm-Stenflo 1994; Edvinsson 2004). This could in part explain the subsequent decline in the popularity of consanguineous unions during the first half of the twentieth century—a trend that was reinforced by modernization leading to greater spatial mobility and declining fertility, both of which in turn would have restricted the numbers of first cousins available within the marriage pool.

Acknowledgments Funding provided by IUSSP, Demographic DataBase, Umeå University, and Edith Cowan University.

References

Adinolfi, M. 1986. Recurrent abortion, HLA sharing and deliberate immunization with partner's cells: A controversial topic. *Human Reproduction* 1: 45–8.

Alm-Stenflo, G. 1994. *Demographic Descriptions of the Skellefteå and Sundsvall Regions During the 19th Century*. Demographic DataBase, Umeå University, Umeå.

Alström, C.H. 1958. First-cousin marriages in Sweden 1750–1844 and a study of the population movement in some Swedish subpopulations from the genetic-statistical viewpoint. *Acta Genetica* 8: 295–369.

Backman, B. and G. Holmgren. 1988. Amelogenesis imperfecta: A genetic study. *Human Heredity* 38: 189–206.

Barrai, I., L.L. Cavalli-Sforza, and A. Moroni. 1962. Frequencies of pedigrees of consanguineous marriages and mating structure of the population. *Annals of Human Genetics* 25: 347–76.

Bede. *The Ecclesiastical History of the English People, ca.731*. Revised edition 1990. Penguin, London.

222

I. Egerbladh and A. Bittles

Bittles, A.H. 1994. The role and significance of consanguinity as a demographic variable. *Population and Development Review* 20: 561–84.

Bittles, A.H. 1998. Empirical estimates of the global prevalence of consanguineous marriage in contemporary societies. Morrison Institute for Population and Resource Studies, Working Paper 0074. Stanford University, Stanford.

Bittles, A.H. 2001. Consanguinity and its relevance to clinical genetics. *Clinical Genetics* 60: 89–98.

Bittles, A.H. 2002. Endogamy, consanguinity and community genetics. *Journal of Genetics* 81: 91–8.

Bittles, A.H. 2003a. The bases of Western attitudes to consanguineous marriage. *Developmental Medicine and Child Neurology* 45: 135–8.

Bittles, A.H. 2003b. Consanguineous marriage and childhood health. *Developmental Medicine and Child Neurology* 45: 571–6.

Bittles, A.H. 2005. Consanguinity, endogamy and community health. *Community Genetics* 8: 17–20.

Bittles, A.H. and I. Egerbladh. 2005. The influence of past endogamy and consanguinity on genetic disorders in northern Sweden. *Annals of Human Genetics* 69: 1–10.

Bittles, A.H., J.C. Grant, and S.A. Shami. 1993. Consanguinity as a determinant of reproductive behaviour and mortality in Pakistan. *International Journal of Epidemiology* 22: 463–7.

Bittles, A.H., J.C. Grant, S.G. Sullivan, and R. Hussain. 2002. Does inbreeding lead to decreased human fertility? *Annals of Human Biology* 29: 111–30.

Bittles, A.H. and U. Makov. 1988. Inbreeding in human populations: Assessment of the costs, in C.G.N. Mascie-Taylor and A.J. Boyce (eds.), *Mating patterns*, Cambridge University Press, Cambridge, pp. 153–64.

Bittles, A.H., W.H. Mason, J. Greene, and N. Appaji Rao. 1991. Reproductive behavior and health in consanguineous marriages. *Science* 252: 789–94.

Bittles, A.H. and J.V. Neel. 1994. The costs of human inbreeding and their implications for variations at the DNA level. *Nature Genetics* 8: 117–21.

Bylund, E. 1960. Theoretical considerations regarding the distribution of settlement in inner North Sweden. *Geografiska Annaler* 42: 225–31.

Cavalli-Sforza, L.L., A. Moroni, and G. Zei. 2004. *Consanguinity, Inbreeding and Genetic Drift in Italy*. Princeton University Press, Princeton, NJ.

Clarke, B. and D.R.S. Kirby. 1966. Maintenance of histocompatibility polymorphisms. *Nature* 211: 999–1000.

Curtis White, K.J. 2002. Declining fertility among North American Hutterites: The use of birth control within a Dariusleut colony. *Social Biology* 49: 58–73.

Das Gupta, M. 1990. Death clustering, mother's education and determinants of child mortality in rural Punjab, India. *Population Studies* 44: 489–505.

Das Gupta, M. 1997. Socio-economic status and clustering of child deaths in rural Punjab. *Population Studies* 51: 191–202.

Dorsten, L.E., L. Hotchkiss, and T.M. King. 1999. The effect of inbreeding on early childhood mortality: Twelve generations of an Amish settlement. *Demography* 36: 263–71.

Edvinsson, S. 2004. Social differences in infant and child mortality in nineteenth century Sweden, in M. Breschi and L. Pozzi (eds.), *The determinants of infant and child mortality in past European populations*, Forum, Editrice Universitaria Udinese, Udine, pp. 67–87.

Edvinsson, S., A. Brändström, J. Rogers, and G. Broström. 2005. High-risk families: The unequal distribution of infant mortality in nineteenth-century Sweden. *Population Studies* 59: 321–37.

Gaunt, D. 1983. *Familjeliv i Norden*. Gidlunds, Malmö.

Gedde-Dahl, T. 1973. Population structure in Norway. *Hereditas* 73: 211–32.

Goody, J. 1983. *The Development of the Family and Marriage in Europe*. Cambridge University Press, Cambridge.

Göransson, A. 1990. Kön, släkt och ägande. Borgerliga maktstrategier 1800–1850. *Historisk Tidskrift* 4: 525–44.

Guo, G. 1993. Use of sibling data to estimate family mortality effects in Guatemala. *Demography* 30: 15–32.

Grant, J.C. and A.H. Bittles. 1997. The comparative role of consanguinity in infant and child mortality in Pakistan. *Annals of Human Genetics* 61: 143–9.

Gyimah, S.O. and R. Fernando. 2002. The effects of infant deaths on the risk of subsequent births: A comparative analysis of DHS data from Ghana and Kenya. *Social Biology* 49: 44–57.

Hajnal, J. 1963. Concept of random mating and the frequency of consanguineous marriage. *Proceedings of the Royal Society* Series B 159: 125–77.

Holmgren, G. 2000. Det norrländska ärftliga sjukdomspanoramat. Arkiven, genetiken och sjukdomen. *Arkiv i Norrland* 17: 104–17.

Hussain, R. 1999. Community perceptions of reasons for preference for consanguineous marriages in Pakistan. *Journal of Biosocial Science* 31: 449–61.

Hussain, R. and A.H. Bittles. 1998. The prevalence and demographic characteristics of consanguineous marriages in Pakistan. *Journal of Biosocial Science* 30: 261–79.

Hussain, R. and A.H. Bittles. 2000. Sociodemographic correlates of consanguineous marriage in the Muslim population of India. *Journal of Biosocial Science* 32: 433–42.

Ignatius, J. 1994–1995. Consanguineous marriages in Finland and their implications for genetic disease. *Yearbook of Population Research in Finland* 32: 45–53.

Jorde, L. and K.J. Pitkänen. 1991. Inbreeding in Finland. *American Journal of Physical Anthropology* 84: 127–39.

Knight, K. 2003. Consanguinity (in Canon Law), in *The Catholic Encyclopedia*, Online edition, Vol. IV. http://www.knight.org.advent/cathen/

Lynch, K.A and J. Greenhouse. 1994. Risk factors for infant mortality in nineteenth-century Sweden. *Population Studies* 48: 117–33.

Nordström, S. and W. Thorburn. 1980. Dominantly inherited macular degeneration (Best's disease) in a homozygous father with 11 children. *Clinical Genetics* 18: 211–6.

Ober, C. 1998. HLA and pregnancy: The paradox of the fetal allograft. *American Journal of Human Genetics* 62: 1–5.

Ober, C., T. Hyslop, and W.W. Hauck. 1999. Inbreeding effects on fertility in humans: Evidence for reproductive compensation. *American Journal of Human Genetics* 64: 225–31.

Ober, C., L.R. Weitkamp, N. Cox, H. Dytch, D. Kostyu, and S. Elias. 1997. HLA and mate choice in humans. *American Journal of Human Genetics* 16: 497–504.

O'Brien, E., L.B. Jorde, B. Rönnlof, J.O. Fellman, and A.W. Eriksson. 1989. Consanguinity avoidance and mate choice in Sottunga, Finland. *American Journal of Physical Anthropology* 79: 235–46.

O'Connor, K.A., D.J. Holman, and J.W. Wood. 1998. Declining fecundity and ovarian ageing in natural fertility populations. *Maturitas* 30: 127–36.

Philippe, P. 1974. Amenorrhea, intrauterine mortality and parental consanguinity in an isolated French Canadian population. *Human Biology* 46: 405–24.

Ronsmans, C. 1995. Patterns of clustering of child mortality in a rural area in Senegal. *Population Studies* 49: 443–61.

Rukanuddin, A.R. 1982. Infant-child mortality and son preference as factors influencing fertility in Pakistan. *Population and Development Review* 21: 297–328.

Sastry, N. 1997. Family-level clustering of childhood mortality risk in Northeast Brazil. *Population Studies* 51: 245–61.

Saugstad, L.F. 1977. The relationship between inbreeding, migration and population density in Norway. *Annals of Human Genetics* 40: 331–41.

Saugstad, L.F. and Ø. Ødegård. 1977. Predominance of extreme geographical proximity of the spouses of heirs to independent farms in a mountain valley in Norway between 1600 and 1850. *Annals of Human Genetics* 40: 419–30.

Schull, W.J., T. Furusho, M. Yamamoto, H. Nagano, and I. Komatsu. 1970. The effect of parental consanguinity and inbreeding in Hirado, Japan. IV. Fertility and reproductive compensation. *Humangenetik* 9: 294–315.

Scrimshaw, S.C.M. 1978. Infant mortality and behavior in the regulation of family size. *Population and Development Review* 4: 383–404.

Sjögren, T. and T. Larsson. 1957. Oligophrenia in combination with congenital ichthyosis and spastic disorders: A clinical and genetic study. *Acta Psychiatrica et Neurologica Scandinavica* 32 (Suppl. 113): 1–112.

Stern, C. and D.R. Charles. 1945. The Rhesus gene and the effect of consanguinity. *Science* 101: 305–7.

Stevenson, A.C., B.C.C. Davison, B. Say, S. Ustuoglu, D. Liya, M. Abul-Einem, and H.K. Toppozada. 1971. Contribution of feto-maternal incompatibility to aetiology of pre-eclamptic toxaemia. *Lancet* 298: 1286–9.

Stevenson, A.C., B. Say, S. Ustaoglu, and Z. Durmas. 1976. Aspects of pre-eclamptic toxaemia of pregnancy, consanguinity, and twinning in Ankara. *Journal of Medical Genetics* 13: 1–8.

Stoltenberg, C., P. Magnus, A. Skrondal, and R.T. Lie. 1999. Consanguinity and recurrence risk of stillbirth and infant death. *American Journal of Public Health* 89: 517–23.

Sundbärg, G. 1910. Ekonomisk-statistisk beskrifning öfver Sveriges olika landsdelar, in *Emigrationsutredningen, Bilaga V. Bygdestatistik*. Stockholm.

Wedekind, C., T. Seebeck, F. Bettens, and A.J. Paepke. 1995. MHC-dependent mate preference in humans. *Proceedings of the Royal Society of London* Series B 260: 245–9.

Wilcox, A.J and L.F. Horney. 1984. Accuracy of spontaneous abortion recall. *American Journal of Epidemiology* 120: 727–33.

Wilcox, A.J., C.R. Weinberg, J.F. O'Connor, D.D. Baird, J.P. Schlatterer, R.E. Canfield, E.G. Armstrong, and B.C. Nisula. 1988. Incidence of early loss of pregnancy. *New England Journal of Medicine* 319: 189–94.

Zenger, E. 1993. Siblings neonatal mortality risks and birth spacing in Bangladesh. *Demography* 30: 477–88.

Website: International Consortium on Consanguinity: http://www.consang.net

Chapter 9
Postreproductive Longevity in a Natural Fertility Population

Alain Gagnon[1], Ryan Mazan[1], Bertrand Desjardins[2], and Ken R. Smith[3]

Abstract Fertility patterns may be useful markers for rates of biological aging. From historical data for the population of Quebec (taken in the "Registre de population du Québec ancien", at the University of Montreal), we examine the effects of reproduction on longevity from evolutionary and sociodemographic perspectives. Using Cox hazard models on 1,923 women and 1,926 men married in the colony before 1740, we show that women bearing their last child late in life had longer postreproductive lives, suggesting that late menopause is associated with an overall slower rate of aging. Increased parity had an opposite, detrimental effect on women's postreproductive survival. On the other hand, husbands' longevity was less sensitive to parity and reproductive history. For husbands, increased effective family size (EFS), i.e., the number of children who survived up to age 18 in a "compressed" reproductive time span meant higher chances for survival past age 60. Children may serve as valuable economic assets on farmsteads during colonization, which would mostly benefit fathers. In a collaborative effort to unveil postreproductive aging patterns in historical populations, the results are compared to previous analyses conducted on the Utah Population Database and evolutionary and sociodemographic theories are addressed in light of these results.

Keywords menopause, longevity, fertility, effective family size

1 Introduction

It is well-established that childbirth has significant health effects on mothers during child-bearing years. Far less is known about the influences of fertility patterns on longevity of both men and women. Following Smith and colleagues (2002), we address this question

---

[1] Population Studies Center, Department of Sociology, University of Western Ontario, Canada

[2] Programme de recherches en démographie historique, Département de Démographie, Université de Montréal, Canada

[3] Department of Family and Consumer Studies and Huntsman Cancer Institute, University of Utah, Salt Lake City, USA

T. Bengtsson and G.P. Mineau (eds.), *Kinship and Demographic Behavior in the Past.*
© Springer Science+Business Media B.V. 2009

from biological and social perspectives. We briefly review the theories on both subjects and, using historical data from Quebec, attempt to replicate the original study based on the Utah population and compare the results obtained from the two populations.

Demography has traditionally addressed the interplay between aging and fertility in terms of population dynamics and structure. Lower infant mortality mechanically increases life expectancy, and reduced fertility leads to an increased proportion of the population at older ages. Based on the theory of natural selection, biodemographers propose additional theoretical connections between the two phenomena. Natural selection has no direct role in longevity but indirectly molds it through differential reproductive success (Charlesworth 1994; Hamilton 1966), which depends on parents' survival (Kirkwood 1997; Smith, Mineau, and Bean 2002; Vaupel et al. 1998; Wachter et al. 1997; Westendorp and Kirkwood 1998). This molding of aging and senescence could be achieved through three evolutionary mechanisms, which form the basis of the current main three evolutionary theories of longevity.

The first affirms that aging is an inevitable result of the decline of the force of natural selection with age. Any mutation having a lethal effect prior to the reproductive period cannot not be transmitted and will thus be quickly eliminated from a population. On the other hand, harmful mutations expressed only later in life are relatively neutral to selection because their bearers have already passed on their genes to the next generation. Over time, all deleterious mutations having a late age of onset will then freely accumulate. This theory, referred to as the "mutation accumulation theory", is believed to have originated in a discussion between Medawar and Haldane on Huntington's disease in the 1940s.

The second, related theory confers a more active role to natural selection. Instead of supposing the passive accumulation of detrimental mutations after reproductive age, it posits the antagonistic action of so-called pleiotropic genes that would favor vigor and reproduction at younger ages at the expense of vitality at older ages. A recurrent hypothesis in the literature (but not demonstrated so far) is a mutation that increases the fixation of calcium in bones. Such a mutation would have a positive effect early in life and indirectly help reproduction by reducing the risk of bone fracture. The negative counterpart would be an increase in the risk of osteoarthritis later in life due to excessive calcification (Gavrilov and Gavrilova 2002). Put forward by Williams (1957), the theory predicts that early and higher levels of fertility should correlate with reduced life span (Le Bourg et al. 1988; Le Bourg et al. 1993).

A third mechanism, proposed by Kirkwood (1977), could also link the age at first birth to senescence and aging. Each organism makes trade-offs between investing resources into somatic growth or maintenance and into reproduction (Kirkwood 1977; Kirkwood and Holliday 1979; Lycett, Dunbar, and Voland 2000). It is selectively advantageous to adopt an energy-saving strategy of reduced accuracy in somatic cells to accelerate development and reproduction. This would mean, however, faster postreproductive deterioration and death. This "disposable soma theory" represents a special variant of the antagonistic pleiotropy theory and leads to similar predictions: young ages at first birth and high parities would entail high somatic costs, with the consequence of a shorter postreproductive life span. In this scenario, the hypothesized antagonistic mutations save energy for reproduction by partially disabling molecular accuracy for somatic maintenance (Gavrilov and Gavrilova 2002; Kirkwood and Holliday 1979; Reznick et al. 2001).

Despite notable differences and subtleties, the three theories somewhat fit into each other and lead to the general prediction that the forces postponing the period of female reproduction will postpone aging and increase female longevity. Empirically, provided that sufficient polymorphism is maintained in populations (Houle et al. 1994), later ages at last birth among females (a proxy for late menopause) should be associated with greater postreproductive longevity. Additionally, Kirkwood's disposable soma theory provides more specific perspectives on the effects of age at first birth and parity on longevity (i.e., a shorter life for women with high parities and early ages at first birth).

These arguments do not seem to apply to males to the same extent as they do for females. Men invest much less in their progeny than their female counterparts, and this may explain why, in comparison, their reproductive success does not critically depend on their survival. Consequently, very few biologists have addressed the effects of reproduction on men's longevity in an evolutionary perspective. While they propose appealing biological arguments, evolutionists generally fail to account for social factors, subsuming these factors into the environmental component—a residual or nuisance category that further complicates an already complex model. Sociologists and demographers, on the other hand, may be able to offer some clues and, at the same time, furnish ways of reinterpreting women's reproductive life history traits.

It is well known that access to social and family support leads to better health and lower levels of mortality (Connidis 2001; House, Landis, and Umberson 1988). After the spouse or marriage partner, children are generally regarded as the most important component of an adult's social and family network (Lye 1996). In agricultural and preindustrial societies, children may also serve as important assets, particularly during the first phases of the colonization of a new territory. They may represent a valuable addition to the workforce in the fields when young and, as adults, may provide health-enhancing social and economic support to their elderly parents. On the pioneer front, the crude number of family members may determine which kin group will take over the best available resources, which family will have access to the most fertile lands, etc. (Bouchard 1996; Bouchard and De Braekeleer 1991; Gagnon and Heyer 2001a, b).

It has been found that the upward flow of resources (social support, workforce, income) from children to parents was small in other preindustrial families (Lee 1997) as well as in contemporary families (Hogan 1993). Moreover, upward genealogical transfer may be limited by the fact that adult children are themselves rearing offspring of their own. Given that fertility patterns are transmitted across generations (Anderton et al. 1987; Gagnon and Heyer 2001b), the capacity for children to provide assistance to their parents may be further reduced in lineages with high parities. This argument suggests that, in natural fertility populations, parents with many children could be adversely rather than beneficially affected since the children will devote resources to their own children (Smith et al. 2002).

As high parities do not necessarily lead to high numbers of children who survive (high parity often comes with high infant mortality), Smith et al. (2002) introduced "number of children who died before age 18" as a control in various models. In the present chapter, we used the effective family size, or EFS (Gagnon and Heyer 2001b), defined as the number of children who reach adulthood. Parity alone would capture the physiological and biological processes affecting women's reproductive health and longevity, while EFS would capture the socioeconomic benefits or costs of having many or few children, for both women and men. As explained above, large EFS may favor a family's ability to take over freely available resources in a colonization context. We propose that females' longevity will be more influenced by figures pertaining to total parity than to EFS, while the converse would be true for males.

Concerning the interplay between the timing of fertility and the flow of resources in families, parents bearing their first children at younger ages will be more likely to invest their limited resources into the children rather than into their own personal health and development (Hofferth 1984; Waldron, Weiss, and Hughes 1998). In historical times, the production of children too early in life may have impeached or slowed the accumulation of critical resources for later days. On the other hand, women bearing children at very old age could have experienced adverse health consequences because of an extended period of childrearing during years in which an individuals' frailty increases dramatically.

The evolutionary theories and social support theories linking reproduction with longevity lead to the formulation of several hypotheses to explain preindustrial mortality patterns (Table 9.1). Scenarios with effects pointing towards opposite directions are more amenable to the formulation of tests that could delineate the action of social and evolutionary forces. For example, a positive association between age at first birth and age at death could be indicative of either evolutionary or social support influences. On the other hand, positive association between age at last birth and age at death would clearly offer support to the evolutionary perspective. Note, however, that in many cases, evolutionary forces themselves are hard to distinguish from more proximal determinants. Under a natural fertility regime, a considerable amount of women's energy is spent on gestation and lactation, rather than on somatic maintenance (Doblhammer and Oeppen 2003). Premature and compressed fertility schedules can create adverse health conditions lasting to late adulthood. We show in the discussion how some researchers have overlooked this aspect.

Table 9.1 Hypothesized effect of reproductive variables on longevity from Evolutionary biology and Social Support theories[a]

Theoretical perspective	Age at first birth	Age at last birth	Parity (and EFS)
Evolutionary/biology	(H1) *Positive*	(H2) *Positive*	(H3) *Negative*
Social Support	(H4) *Positive*	(H5) *Negative*	Either (H6A) *positive* (greater access to social support from children) or (H6B) *negative* (greater wealth flows from parents to children)

[a]Taken from Smith et al. (2002).

2 Data and Methods

2.1 Data and Selection of Cases

The data used here originate from the *Registre de population du Québec ancien*, compiled by the *Programme de recherche en démographie historique* (PRDH) at the University of Montreal (Desjardins 1998; Légaré 1988). For individuals that lived in the Saint Lawrence Valley in the seventeenth and eighteenth centuries, the database contains date and place of birth, death and marriage(s), names of parents and spouse(s) and secondary information on occupation (if available), and places of residence and of origin. The population remained quasi-closed until the nineteenth century because of particular historical and geographical circumstances, and thus the usual problem of missing observations because of migration was greatly reduced (Charbonneau et al. 1993; Desjardins 1999). The database covered information on the entire period of French rule. Births were matched with individuals up to the year 1770 and deaths up to around 1830 (relating to people born before 1730). All the ancestors of every individual who married before 1800 were traced back to the founders of the population. Previous studies have shown that the population of that period lived under "natural fertility" conditions, as defined by Henry (1972), in that it was free of deliberate fertility control (Charbonneau et al. 1993; Desjardins, Bideau, and Brunet 1994; Desjardins et al. 1991).

The database contains more than 712,000 vital rate certificates spanning more than two centuries. However, the highly constraining selection criteria pertaining to longevity studies, as well as the necessity of a complete knowledge of couples' reproductive histories, resulted in final samples of 1,923 women and 1,926 men in this study. Families with no birth certificate for the first- and last-born child were removed from the analysis. For comparability purposes, we used the same criteria as employed by the Utah study, except that we made two separate samples, one for each sex, in order to preserve a reasonable sample size. For simplicity and homogeneity, only first marriages were considered. Given the current advancement of the record linkages at the PRDH, this criterion led us to retrieve all couples who married before 1740, thus enabling both husbands and wives to complete reproductive life and survival to age 100 within the database limits. Husbands were no more than 10 years younger or 15 years older than their wives, which reduced large differences in age and cohort experiences. Wives were required to have married no later than their 35th birthday in order to ensure that they had a clear opportunity to bear children. All the selected women lived to at least age 60 to assure that they would all have completed childbearing and childrearing. Bias-free analysis also required couples with husbands fathering past age 60 to be removed because they would have, by definition, lived over the "time origin" of our study. Finally, individuals who were widowed before their 60th birthday were also removed because of the critical lack of resources and social support they endured.

2.1.1   Variables

The main variables of interest in this study are (1) age at first birth, (2) age at last birth, (3) parity, and (4) effective family size (EFS). Each was first entered as a continuous variable (Table 9.3) and then with categorical specifications (Table 9.4). Although the focus was on reproductive history, we examined the possibilities of coincidental associations by including a set of control variables such as the year of marriage, the number of children who died before age 18, residential status (urban or rural), and geographic location (eastern or western part of the colony).

Tables 9.2a, and b present the descriptive statistics concerning our variables of interest and controls as well for the response variable, i.e., age at death or, more appropriately, the number of years lived past age 60. Age at death was approximately

Table 9.2 Descriptive statistics for (a) women and (b) men

(a) women (N = 1,923)

Variables	Min	Max	Mean	Std. Dev.
Age at death	60.0	99.6	74.1	7.98
Husband's age at death	48.0	99.8	73.1	8.11
Year of marriage	1632	1739	1716	17.94
Immigrant to New France (=1)			0.02	0.15
Husband immigrant to New France (=1)			0.17	0.37
Residence in the eastern part of the colony (=1)			0.43	0.50
Lived in an urban area (=1)			0.21	0.41
Age difference between spouses (husband – wife)	–9.3	15	4.7	4.91
Age at first birth	14.6	45.2	22.9	4.19
Age at last birth	18.1	50	40.9	4.34
Mean age at childbearing	18.1	45.2	31.5	2.98
Total number of children born (parity)	1	23	10.3	3.66
Fraction of children who survived to age 18 and/or married			0.62	0.22
Total number of children who survive to age 18 and/or married	0	17	6.3	2.88

(b) men (N = 1,926)

Variables	Min	Max	Mean	Std. Dev.
Age at death	60.0	94.7	73.2	7.61
Wife's age at death	42.0	97.5	71.0	10.29
Year of marriage	1639	1739	1716	18.73
Immigrant to New France (=1)			0.10	0.29
Wife is immigrant to New France (=1)			0.05	0.21
Residence in the eastern part of the colony (=1)			0.47	0.50
Lived in an urban area (=1)			0.20	0.40
Age difference between spouses (husband – wife)	–9.5	15.0	5.1	4.53
Age at first birth	18.5	44.4	27.5	4.04
Age at last birth	20.8	57.9	45.9	5.95
Mean age at childbearing	20.8	48.2	36.2	4.12
Total number of children born (parity)	1	23	10.4	3.60
Fraction of children who survived to age 18 and/or married			0.62	0.22
Total number of children who survive to age 18 and/or married	0	17	6.4	2.86

74 years on average and did not differ appreciably between the sexes. Both males and females survived an average of 14 years after the cut-off point of age 60. One woman was very close to giving the colony its first centenarian. Marguerite St-Julien Daragon was born January 28, 1714, and died almost 100 years later, on August 28, 1813. In her death certificate, the priest declared that she was 106 years old. This demonstrates why investigators of longevity should be extremely careful with declared ages. The latter were shown to be consistently exaggerated, especially for older people (Desjardins 1999).

The figures and numbers pertaining to fertility are quite high, although not uncommonly so for natural fertility populations. Families averaged 10.3 children, of whom about 6.3 could survive up to age 18 or marry in the colony. Mean age at first birth was 22.9 years for wives and 27.5 years for husbands. Women gave birth to their last child at a mean age of 41, while men on average had their last child 5 years later. About 20 percent of the selected individuals lived in Quebec City, Montreal, or Trois-Rivières (urban areas).

2.1.2   Survival Models

A series of Cox regression models were fitted to the data in order to test whether the predictors had any influence on survival times. The Cox regression model expresses a transformation of the hazard as a linear function of the predictors. A continuous hazard function is a rate with no upper bound and thus the logarithm of the hazard is treated as the outcome variable:

$$\log h(t_i) = \log h_\circ(t) + [\,\beta_1 X_1 + \beta_2 X_2 + \dots + \beta_i X_i\,].$$

The log hazard $\log h(t_i)$ equals the baseline function $\log h(t_i)$ plus a weighted linear combination of predictors β that measure the effect of the covariates on $\log h(t_i)$. There are two main assumptions involved in the Cox regression model: first, that there is a log-linear relationship between the covariates and the underlying hazard function; and second, that there is a multiplicative relationship between the underlying hazard function and the log-linear function of the covariates. This is also known as the proportionality assumption. It is assumed that the hazard function of any two individuals with different values of the covariates have parallel age patterns (Elandt-Johnson and Johnson 1980).

Potential violations of the proportionality assumption were checked with $\log S(t)$ plots of the categorical variables and with Schoenfeld residual plots of all covariates. For women, the main variables of interest showed no deviation from the time invariance assumption. Additionally, there were no significant correlations between the residuals and the time variable (years lived over age 60) for each of the covariates. Some of the control variables (for instance, urban/rural), however, had a significant interaction with time. Consequently, we introduced additional cross-product terms with the time variable for any of these variables when necessary. For men, the picture was much less clear and one must exercise caution when interpreting the

Table 9.3 Hazard rate models for survival past age 60 in early Quebec (entries are Cox hazard regression coefficients multiplied by 10^3)

	MODEL							
	1	2	3	4	5	6	7	8
Women								
Age at first birth	−6.4				1.7	1.4		
Age at last birth		−18.1****			−23.9****	−23.7***		
Parity			−1.1		18.6*			
EFS[a]				−7.4		14.8		
Model-2LL vs Null-2LL	45.46	57.03	48.67	48.58	58.93	58.67		
Model df vs Null df	12	12	12	12	14	14		
Men								
Age at first birth	−4.9				−9.2	−9.7	−13.1	16.2
Age at last birth		−2.0			2.3	2.7	3.2	3.6
Parity			−0.4		−6.5	−6.7		
EFS[a]				−3.5	−11.0			−15.0
Age at first birth × Parity						−2.2		
Age at first birth × EFS								−3.5**
Model-2LL vs Null-2LL	58.62	56.91	56.16	56.52	57.19	58.0	59.69	60.83
Model df vs Null df	9	9	9	9	11	11	12	12

Adjusted for marriage year, immigration status, age difference between the spouses, age at death of spouse, and fraction of children who died before age 18; standard errors were estimated using the "robust" command in STATA.

*$p<0.10$; **$p<0.05$; ***$p<0.01$; ****$p < 0.001$.

[a]EFS: Effective Family Size.

corresponding coefficients. Since we observed several crossings of the hazard functions for the categorical variable on age at first birth, we introduced a term for interaction with time for this variable in the continuous models (Table 9.3). This interaction term proved to be significant at the 0.056 level. There was some evidence that this variable interacted with the EFS. The variables age at last birth, parity, and effective family size, however, appeared to meet the proportionality assumption after visual inspection of Schoenfeld residual plots and more formal tests. All Cox models were run in STATA, using "sandwich" robust estimators of variances. Shared frailty models and parametric models including unobserved heterogeneity were also briefly tested for women, with no important variations in the parameter estimates and their significance from the results obtained from the Cox models (not shown here).

3   Results

Table 9.3 lists results for several Cox proportional hazard models for females (upper panel) and males (lower panel). All variables were measured as continuous variables (except for eastern/western part of the colony and urban/rural setting, which are categorical by nature). When each of the reproductive history variables were introduced separately (Models 1–4), only age at last birth was found to affect female postreproductive survival. However, the simultaneous inclusion of all three fertility measures appeared to remove the suppressor effect on parity, that is, it becomes significant at the 0.1 level. Notice also the increase (in absolute terms) of the parameter estimate for age at last birth from Model 2 to Model 4 (from −0.018 to −0.024). Women who had few (relatively!) children and who bore their last child at a late age would have had lower risks of mortality past age 60. For example, a delivery of one more child would have increased the postreproductive hazard rate by about 1.9 percent ($e^{0.0186} = 1.0188$); while a decrease of 1 year in the age at last birth would have increased this rate by 2.4 percent ($e^{0.0239} = 1.0242$). A woman terminating reproduction 5 years earlier with five more children would have faced a hazard about 24 percent greater ($e^{5(0.0186 + 0.0239)} = 1.237$). Age at first birth and EFS had no significant effects. The best model simultaneously included age at last birth and parity (Model 5). These results largely agree with those reported by Smith et al. (2002) for the nineteenth- to twentieth-centuries Utah population. There are only two slight differences. First, in the Utah population, the variable that stood alone with a significant effect was *parity*, not *age at last birth* as in Quebec. Second, we found no significant interaction between age at last birth and parity. The effect sizes of most variables, however, were surprisingly close in both populations (between 0.010 and 0.025); a striking result considering that they refer to different populations during different epochs.

Table 9.3 also shows that none of the reproductive history variables, when measured as main effects on a continuous scale, significantly affected male survival. When only one of the reproductive history variables was entered, the overall fit was slightly better for men than for women, but this was because of a stronger implication of the (not listed) control variables in the case of men. For instance, wife's age at death strongly influenced husband's age at death, while the converse was not true. Adding more variables did not seem to improve the fit, suggesting that factors pertaining to the intensity and the timing of reproduction did not have much effect on males' survival. Nevertheless, a significant interaction between age at first birth and EFS was detected (Model 8). As the parameter is negative, increasing both variables multiplicatively increases males' longevity, meaning that, typically, men who started reproducing later but still had many children *who survived*, had the best prospects of reaching older ages. For example, an individual who would have begun reproduction 10 years later than the average age and who still ended up with five more children than average would have faced a hazard that was 84 percent of the hazard faced by individuals with the average for these two variables ($e^{-0.0035 \times 10 \times 5}$) $= 0.839$, $p < 0.05$.

In principle, nothing "forces" the relationship between survival and reproductive history to be strictly linear. To further explore the relationship, Cox models were re-estimated with the fertility indicators included as categorical variables (Table 9.4). To facilitate the comparison with the Utah study, we now present hazard ratios instead of parameter estimates. Categorized hazard ratios largely confirmed previous results. Again, when entered alone, the most important variable for women was

Table 9.4 Hazard rate models for survival past age 60 in early Quebec (entries are hazard ratios based on Cox proportional hazard coefficients)[a]

	MODEL					
	1	2	3	4	5	6
Women						
Age at first birth						
<19	0.92				0.89*	0.91
19–26	Ref.				Ref.	Ref
27+	0.80***				0.80***	0.81***
Age at last birth						
<38		1.26****			1.25***	1.27***
38–43		Ref.			Ref.	Ref.
44+		0.90**			0.88**	0.89**
Parity						
<7			1.09		1.02	
7–13			Ref.		Ref	
14+			1.16**		1.22***	
EFS[b]						
<4				1.07		1.01
4–9				Ref.		Ref.
10+				1.06		1.12
Model-2LL vs Null-2LL	60.6	63.4	54.6	49.8	83.5	78.8
Model df vs Null df	13	13	13	13	17	17
Men						
Age at first birth						
<24	1.09				1.11	1.13*
24–30	Ref.				Ref.	Ref.
31+	1.04				1.05	1.01
Age at last birth						
<40		1.15*			0.87**	0.82***
40–51		Ref.			Ref.	Ref.
52+		1.06			0.94	0.96
Parity						
<7			0.89*		0.95	
7–13			Ref.		Ref.	
14+			0.89*		0.89*	
EFS[b]						
<4					0.98	1.08
4–9				Ref.		Ref
10+				0.89*		0.86**
Model-2LL vs Null-2LL	58.5	62.6	60.3	62.14	68.4	71.7
Model df vs Null df	10	10	10	11	14	14

"Ref." equals reference category.
*$p < 0.10$; **$p < 0.05$; ***$p < 0.01$; ****$p < 0.001$.
[a]Adjusted for marriage year, immigration status, age difference between spouses, spousal age at death, and fraction of children who died before age 18; standard errors were estimated using the "robust" command in STATA.
[b]EFS: Effective Family Size.

the age at which they terminated reproduction (Model 2). Having a child late appeared to be a sign of a slower rate of aging, with a reduction of about 10 percent in the postreproductive hazard ($p < 0.05$) for women who bore their last child after age 44, relative to modal women who bore their last child between ages 38 and 43. In comparison to women having their last child before age 38, these "late-fertile" women could expect to be submitted to hazard rates about 29 percent lower ($0.90/1.26 = 0.71$) in the postreproductive period.

This time, when parity was entered alone, it proved to be significant, at least at the extreme of the distribution. After age 60, women who previously gave birth to 14 children or more had hazard rates that were about 16 percent higher than those of women who had fewer children ($e^{0.1464} = 1.16$, $p < 0.01$). Introducing the two other reproductive history variables, the parameter estimate for this group of women increased from 0.1464 ($p = 0.015$) to 0.1982 ($p = 0.002$), which demonstrates how a suppressor effect can be removed with the adjunction of controls. Here, we categorized the variable in order to have approximately 15 percent of the women at each extreme of the distribution, with the remaining 70 percent in the modal size family groups. When we categorized the variable as binary, with families comprising more than 13 children in the large parity category, the parameter estimate slightly decreased to 0.183 ($p = 0.002$). Using family sizes of 12 and then 11 as the cut-off points defining large families resulted in important decreases of the parameter estimates and in loss of significance; for example, with 11 or more births as the demarcation point, the parameter fell to 0.052 ($p = 0.302$). Hence, there could be a threshold after which adding more children would result in decreased longevity. However, postreproductive survival under this threshold (of about 12–13 births) was relatively unaffected. Note that this conclusion applies to fertility alone, and not to effective family size. Comparing Model 6 to Model 5 (highlighted here because it provided the strongest measure of good fit), we observed that the influence of net EFS was, as predicted, less strong, if not negligible, than that of crude parity among women.

The effect of age at first birth was more mitigated and difficult to interpret than those of age at last birth and parity. It appeared to be u-shaped, as both *younger* and *older* primiparous women enjoyed higher chances for survival than most women, although the significance was not strong for younger primiparous mothers. These results were exclusively based on the almost complete reproductive history of the selected families. All dates of birth and death for husbands, wives, first born and last born children were precisely known because they were directly taken from the parish registers. With the technique of family reconstitution, researchers at the PRDH were able to link many children for whom the birth certificate was not found in the registers, but for whom we have a declared age. When these families with incomplete history (admittedly far less reliable than those with all vital statistics confirmed) were added to the sample, the apparent beneficial effect of early age at first birth completely disappeared (not shown here). In this new sample comprising 2,280 families (instead of 1,923), all other measures remained consistent, including those pertaining to parity and age at last birth. We also ran several models using age 50 and age 55 as the starting point of postreproductive survival, with no appreciable changes in the parameter estimates. The significance of the parameters even increased due to larger sample sizes.

The picture appeared diametrically inverted among men, for whom Model 6 (and not Model 5) offered the best fit. As predicted, EFS was positively related to males' reproductive survival, while parity in itself had no clear effect: the hazard ratio of men who had 10 or more *surviving children* to those with 9 or less was 0.86 (p < 0.05). As hypothesized by Smith et al. (2002), early age at first child can be detrimental to men, although the effect was less significant (p < 0.1) in the Quebec data. We were surprised to find a strong, positive influence of early age at last child for men. In light of previous results, the best scenario for men was to have a maximum number of surviving children in the shortest time! This result is truly intriguing considering what it meant for their wives (a highly intensive and compressed reproductive period). Although all parameters remained relatively stable in the enlarged sample (N = 2,280) for men (while the one pertaining to age at first birth lost significance in the case of women), caution and deeper analyses are warranted.

4   Discussion

Replication is not a road often taken by social scientists. It is largely believed that human behaviors are too complex and particular to be repeated and tracked more than once. Many interesting theoretical issues remain irresolvable and subject to debate, definitively because of variations in data sources and methods. As shown in this chapter, the field of biodemography may offer opportunity to prove the contrary. Isolating the hypothesized association between longevity, timing, and intensity of reproduction in a natural fertility population is complicated by the fact that women bearing children during a longer reproductive period usually have higher parity. Nevertheless, adjusting for coincidental associations, lower parity, and late age at last birth were clearly associated with greater postreproductive longevity among women of both populations. As noted above, the parameter estimates were even surprisingly close in the two populations. However, the results on age at first birth were less consistent. We first discuss this variable.

In contrast with what was found in the Utah population, there is some evidence that late age at first birth enhanced female longevity in the early French Canadian population (providing support for both hypotheses H1 and H4). This evidence is inconclusive, however, as early age at first birth also appeared favorable (Table 9.4). We would thus recommend further analysis of this variable. Westendorp and Kirkwood (1998) also reported a longer life for British aristocratic women who started reproduction later, and they directly interpreted this evidence as strong support for the disposable soma theory. Following Gavrilova et al. (2004), we would argue that this conclusion was premature because in most human populations, the age at which women bear their first child depends primarily on the age at which they marry. Across societies and throughout history, kinship systems, inheritance rules, or demographic pressure determine the variations on the timing of marriage and reproduction (Laslett and Wall 1972; Wall, Robin, and Laslett 1983), not genes. Polymorphism on some fertility loci may well account for a certain part of the variation in age at menarche. This variation, however, seems to have no direct effect on the timing of nuptiality.

An alternative explanation for Westendorp and Kirkwood's results is that women who started reproduction too early dipped into essential somatic resources. Without the opportunity to fully recover after each successive birth (because of maternal depletion), they would have exhausted their potential for a healthy long life. In other words, they would simply have acquired that frailty over an exhausting reproductive life. Although this alternative explanation is phrased in terms of energy costs for the organisms (biological constraints), it rather refers to the action of social forces that account for variations on nuptiality and fertility schedules. The results for Quebec are, however, quite different. There is some evidence that early fertility is associated with longer postreproductive survival in this population. As noted by Van de Putte et al. for the Belgian case (Chapter 2 in this volume), good health may be associated with early marriage, and thus with early fertility. Early fertility and longevity could thus be positively associated because of their joint association with health. This selection effect may blur the reversed association that is expected from the consideration of evolutionary mechanisms.

Using French Canadian data (the same as those used in this article but at an earlier stage of completion of the database), Le Bourg et al. (1993) failed to find support for a trade-off between early fecundity and later-age survival. The measure they used as a proxy for early fecundity, i.e., age at first birth, was ill-chosen for the reason given above: the strongest determinant of age at first birth is age at marriage, and there is no reason to believe that this age would be under the influence of pleiotropic genes having a simultaneous effect on fecundity and longevity. The best measure would be the protogenesic interval (the interval between marriage and first birth) as a proxy for fecundability. After several tests in our data, we found that very short intervals were in fact associated with longer life, although the association was not significant. If pleiotropic genes with antagonistic effects on reproduction and survival really exist, their effect is probably too mild to be detected, at least in historical data. Strong selective pressures would likely oppose these rare variants. The critical advantage of prolonged parental investment offers a good example.

A similar argument could be put forward in the case of parity. The association between high parity and higher hazard rates at older ages disclosed here is consistent with the predictions based on the disposable soma theory (H3, Table 9.1): mutations increasing fecundity with adverse side effects on soma maintenance could have segregated in the seventeenth- and eighteenth-centuries' Quebec gene pool, and produced the expected results that surface today in our data. We gain additional support on the fact that for this variable, the same relationship with longevity was found in the Utah population. One must be cautious, however, before discarding a more proximal explanation. Again, frailty may simply be acquired during life through excessive energy expenditure in reproduction. There is no critical necessity to call upon the presence of heritable genetic variants that would simultaneously affect women's fertility and longevity.

Using the same database as we do, other researchers came to the counterintuitive view that higher parity was linked to an increased rather than decreased postreproductive survival (Muller et al. 2002). They wrote: "highly fertile women will tend to have small children at age 50, and their increased longevity is likely to improve the chances of survival for their offspring" (ibid., p. B204). This conclusion is not supported by the French Canadian data, let alone the Utah data. In some of our bivariate analyses, we also noticed negative and significant relationships between parity and postreproductive death rates (not shown here; but notice the negative coefficient in Table 9.3). However, when other controls were taken into consideration, large family size was systematically associated with high hazard rates. In Utah, low parity was beneficial to survival throughout the models (Smith et al. 2002). We believe that Muller and his associates simply confused the effect of parity with that of age at last birth. Conceptually, it is easy to figure how a slow rate of aging could simultaneously delay menopause and senescence. How biological pathways would affect both fecundity and longevity is less obvious.

We feel that the close association between age at last birth and age at death (highly significant and stable in both Quebec and Utah) can be taken as a more reliable support for an underlying evolutionary mechanism in natural fertility populations. Several genes affecting the rate of senescence could segregate into the populations. Delineating evolutionary forces and social forces is here easier to achieve because their respective effects lean towards opposing directions (i.e., H2 and H5, Table 9.1). The cost and the risks associated with reproduction sharply increase with age and, in this respect, one should expect better survival prospects for women who have their last child at an early age. The fact that the data tell the contrary strongly favors the claim for a slower rate of aging in women with a late fertility schedule. Whether the association ultimately rests on genetic factors cannot be definitively proven. Varying environmental conditions could still lead to varying rates of aging. But other (unpublished) results support the genetics/evolutionary view; among persons with a long-lived opposite sex sibling in Utah, those with a late fertile sister enjoyed a significantly higher probability of reaching older ages than those whose sisters completed their childbearing earlier (Smith et al. 2005).

Since women's reproductive life rests on a set of strong biological constraints, their reproductive (and, presumably, longevity) outcomes will tend to be stable from one population to another. Provided that researchers use similar sampling procedures and methods, the results should be replicable. In comparison, men's reproductive prospects appear to depend more on social factors. It is thus expected that these patterns will vary from one population to another, as seen for Quebec and Utah. In Utah, the direction of the effects was consistent for the two sexes, although compared to their wives, husbands experienced weaker longevity benefits of low parity and late fertility (Smith et al. 2002). As seen in Tables 9.3 and 9.4, in Quebec an earlier age at last birth may have been detrimental for men while the contrary was true for women. Delayed fertility may be associated with larger accumulation of resources and wealth, and hence reduce mortality for men (Smith et al. 2002). Reproductive success, as measured by the number of children who survived up to age 18 (i.e., EFS), also clearly advantaged men, but did not advantage women because it meant a higher parity for them. The most striking result was a positive influence on longevity of an early cessation of reproduction for men, contrary to what was observed for women. Pending further model testing, the relationships between fertility and survival among men in historical Quebec appears to match all the predictions originating from the social support theories (H4, H5, and H6A). This was not the case for the Utah study.

Particular incentives associated with the peopling of a new territory might have pushed the reproductive capacity of the female inhabitants of the early French Canadian colony to the limits. Ironically, such strong incentives for reproduction seem to have benefited their husbands, for whom a large effective family was probably a key to old age survival. We could portray these early Quebec male settlers as "using" their wife's reproductive capacity to their benefit, i.e., to facilitate their takeover of largely free lands by increasing their family size. The economic benefits of large families, and perhaps the associated stronger access to social support provided by adult children, may have translated into longevity gains for postreproductive males, in agreement with social support theories.

Acknowledgments We thank Benjamin Beall and Andrea Flynn for helpful suggestions, as well as Lee Bean for his review of an earlier version of this manuscript.

References

Anderton, D.L., N.O. Tsyua, L.L. Bean, and G.P. Minaeu. 1987. Intergenerational transmission of relative fertility and life course patterns. *Demography* 24: 467–80.

Bouchard, G. 1996. *Quelques arpents d'Amerique: Population, économie, famille au Saguenay, 1838–1971*. Boréal, Montreal.

Bouchard, G. and M. De Braekeleer. 1991. *Histoire d'un génome: Population et génétique dans l'est du Québec*. Presses de l'Université du Québec, Sillery.

Charbonneau, H., B. Dejardins, A. Guillemette, Y. Landry, J. Légaré, and F. Nault. 1993. *The First French Canadians: Pioneers in the St. Lawrence Valley*. University of Delaware/Associated University Presses, Newark/London/Toronto.

Charlesworth, B. 1994. *Evolution in Age-Structured Populations*. Cambridge University Press, Cambridge/New York.

Connidis, I.A. 2001. *Family Ties and Aging*. Sage Publications, Thousands Oaks, California/London.

Desjardins, B. 1998. Le Registre de population du Québec ancien. *Annales de démographie historique* 2: 215–26.

Desjardins, B. 1999. Validation of extreme longevity cases in the past: The French-Canadian experiences, in B. Jeune and J.W. Vaupel (eds.), *Validation of exceptional longevity*, Odense Monographs on Population Aging Vol. 6, Odense University Press, Odense, pp. 65–73.

Desjardins, B., A. Bideau, and G. Brunet. 1994. Age of mother at last birth in two historical populations. *Journal of Biosocial Science* 26: 509–16.

Desjardins, B., A, Bideau, E. Heyer, and G. Brunet. 1991. Intervals between marriage and first birth in mothers and daughters. *Journal of Biosocial Science* 23: 49–54.

Doblhammer, G. and J. Oeppen. 2003. Reproduction and longevity among British peerage: The effect of frailty and health selection. *Proceedings Biological Sciences* 270: 1541–7.

Elandt-Johnson, R.C. and N.L. Johnson. 1980. *Survival Models and Data Analysis*. Wiley, New York.

Gagnon, A. and E. Heyer. 2001a. Fragmentation of the Québec population genetic pool (Canada): Evidence from the genetic contribution of founders per region in the 17th and 18th centuries. *American Journal of Physical Anthropology* 114: 30–41.

Gagnon, A. and E. Heyer. 2001b. Intergenerational correlation of effective family size in early Québec (Canada). *American Journal of Human Biology* 13: 645–59.

Gavrilov, L.A., and N.S. Gavrilova. 2002. Evolutionary theories of aging and longevity. *The Scientific World Journal* 2: 339–56.

Gavrilova, N.S., V.G. Semyonova, G.N. Evdokushikina, and L.A. Gavrilov. 2004. Does exceptional human longevity come with a high cost of infertility? *Annals of the New York Academy of Science* 1019: 513–7.

Hamilton, W.D. 1966. The moulding of senescence by natural selection. *Journal of Theoretical Biology* 12(1): 12–45.

Henry, L. 1972. *On the Measurement of Human Fertility; Selected Writings.* Translated by M.C.S. a. E. Lapierre-Adamcyk. Elsevier, Amsterdam.

Hofferth, S.L. 1984. Long-term economic consequences for women of delayed childbearing and reduced family size. *Demography* 21: 141–55.

Hogan, D.P. 1993. The structure of intergenerational exchanges in American Families. *American Journal of Sociology* 98: 1428–68.

Houle, D., K.A. Huges, D.K. Hoffmaster, J. Ihara, S. Assimacopoulos, D. Canada, and B. Charlesworth 1994. The effects of spontaneous mutation on quantitative traits. I. variances and covariances of life history traits. *Genetics* 138: 773–85.

House, J.S., K.R. Landis, and D. Umberson. 1988. Social relationships and health. *Science* 241: 540–5.

Kirkwood, T.B. 1977. Evolution of ageing. *Nature* 270: 301–4.

Kirkwood, T.B. 1997. Genetics and the future of human longevity. *Journal of the Royal College of Physicians of London* 31(6): 669–73.

Kirkwood, T.B. and R. Holliday. 1979. The evolution of ageing and longevity. *Proceedings of the Royal Society of London* Series B. *Biological Sciences* 205(1161): 531–46.

Laslett, P. and R. Wall. 1972. *Household and Family in Past Time.* Cambridge University Press, Cambridge.

Le Bourg, E., F.A. Lints, J. Declince, and C.V. Lints. 1988. Reproductive fitness and longevity in Drosophila melanogaster. *Experimental Gerontology* 23: 491–500.

Le Bourg, E., B. Thon, J. Légaré, B. Desjardins, and H. Charbonneau. 1993. Reproductive life of French-Canadians in the 17th–18th centuries: A search for a trade-off between early fecundity and longevity. *Experimental Gerontology* 28: 217–32.

Lee, R.D. 1997. Intergenerational relations and the elderly, in K. Wachter, A.C. Finch, and National Research Council (US) Committee on Population (eds.), *Between Zeus and the salmon: The biodemography of longevity*, National Academy Press, Washington, DC, pp. 212–33.

Légaré, J. 1988. A population register for Canada under the French regime: Context, scope, content, and applications. *Canadian Studies in Population* 15: 1–16.

Lycett, J.E., R.I. Dunbar, and E. Voland. 2000. Longevity and the costs of reproduction in a historical human population. *Proceedings Biological Sciences* 267(1438): 31–5.

Lye, D.N. 1996. Adult child parent relationships. *Annual Review of Sociology* 22: 79–102.

Muller, H.G., J.M. Chiou, J.R. Carey, and J.L. Wang. 2002. Fertility and life span: Late children enhance female longevity. *The Journals of Gerontology Series A: Biological Sciences and Medical Sciences* 57: B202–6.

Reznick, D., G. Buckwalter, J. Groff, and D. Elder. 2001. The evolution of senescence in natural populations of guppies (Poecilia reticulata): A comparative approach. *Experimental Gerontology* 36: 791–812.

Smith, K.R., G.P. Mineau, and L.L. Bean. 2002. Fertility and post-reproductive longevity. *Social Biology* 49: 185–205.

Smith, K.R., G.P. Mineau, R. Kerber, E. O'Brien, and R.M. Cawthon. 2005. Increased longevity in the siblings of late fertile women, in Inherited dimensions of human populations in the past: Exploring intergenerational dimensions of human behaviour. Conference arranged by GEPS (Grupo de Estudios Población y Sociedad) at Mahón, Spain.

Vaupel, J.W., J.R. Carey, K. Christensen, T.E. Johnson, A.I. Yashin, N.V. Holm, I.A. Iachine, V. Kannisto, A.A. Khazaeli, P. Liedo, V.D. Longo, Y. Zeng, K.G. Manton, and J.W. Curtsinger. 1998. Biodemographic trajectories of longevity. *Science* 280: 855–60.

Wachter, K.W. and C.E. Finch (eds.) 1997. *Between Zeus and the Salmon: The Biodemography of Longevity*. National Academy Press, Washington, DC.

Waldron, I., C.C. Weiss, and M.E. Hughes. 1998. Interacting effects of multiple roles on women's health. *Journal of Health and Social Behavior* 39(3): 216–36.

Wall, R., J. Robin, and P. Laslett. 1983. *Family Forms in Historic Europe*. Cambridge University Press, Cambridge.

Westendorp, R.G. and T.B. Kirkwood. 1998. Human longevity at the cost of reproductive success. *Nature* 396: 743–6.

Williams, G.C. 1957. Pleiotropy, natural selection, and the evolution of senescence. *Evolution* 11: 398–411.

Chapter 10
Familial Aggregation of Elderly Cause-Specific Mortality: Analysis of Extended Pedigrees in Utah, 1904–2002

Richard Kerber[1], Elizabeth O'Brien[2], Ken R. Smith[3], and Geraldine P. Mineau[1]

Abstract This study addresses the impact of family history of disease and family history of longevity on cause-specific mortality in a large population-based cohort. We identified a cohort of 464,494 people born between 1830 and 1984 from the Utah Population Database, a resource of linked genealogy, vital statistics, and disease data. To be eligible, a cohort member must have lived at least 65 years and died between 1904 and 2002. We measured familial disease risks using the familial standardized mortality ratio (FSMR), and familial longevity using familial excess longevity (FEL). For each of the leading causes of death in the U.S., we constructed a nested case-control study using cohort members dying of a specific cause (cases) and individually matched cohort members who remained at risk at the time of the cases' deaths (controls). Our results indicate that family histories of cause-specific mortality greatly affect risk of death from the same cause, especially for heart disease, cancer, and diabetes. However, familial excess longevity is associated with decreased risks of almost all causes of death, suggesting that whatever factors link kin survival, an important component is the familiality of longevity within their extended family. The one major disease for which familial longevity confers no substantial protection is cancer, suggesting that there may be some antagonism between genetic mechanisms that protect against aging and those that protect against cancer.

Keywords Mortality, longevity, kinship, cause of death, genealogy

1 Introduction

Scholars have long observed that life span is more positively correlated between close relatives than between unrelated individuals (e.g., Beeton and Pearson 1899). Numerous studies have demonstrated a substantial familial component to human

[1] Department of Oncological Sciences and Huntsman Cancer Institute, University of Utah, USA

[2] Huntsman Cancer Institute, University of Utah, USA

[3] Department of Family and Consumer Studies and Huntsman Cancer Institute, University of Utah, USA

T. Bengtsson and G.P. Mineau (eds.), *Kinship and Demographic Behavior in the Past.*   243
© Springer Science+Business Media B.V. 2009

longevity (Carey and Tuljapurkar 2003; Carey 2003; Wachter and Finch 1997). While this body of work is impressive, much of it suffers from three general limitations. First, many analyses have relied on restricted sampling schemes where the family is defined by dyads, typically parent-child and sibling pairs. Information about other kin is not considered, largely due to data limitations. Second, much of this work has relied on data pertaining to small geographic areas where continual migration processes introduce considerable data censoring. Third, little attention has been given to familial aggregation of mortality due to shared risks of specific causes of death. More frequently familial mortality risks have been evaluated based on all-cause mortality. The limited attention given to familial aggregation of cause-specific mortality is largely attributable to a lack of suitable mortality data linked to large pedigrees.

With the increasing availability of large, high-quality human genealogies linked to vital records, including death certificates (Smith and Mineau 2003; Gavrilov et al. 2002), it is possible to consider how individuals' ages at death due to specific causes may be related among close and distant relatives, irrespective of their geographic proximity (Gudmundsson et al. 2000; Kerber et al. 2001). The reason that relatives share a propensity for premature death or long life may be due to shared genetic, social, or environmental factors that predispose them to specific causes of death. Alternatively, familial aggregation of mortality and longevity may result from inherited variation among individuals in the rate at which they age.

In this study we analyze the familial aggregation of cause of death for persons surviving to age 65 using the linked records of the Utah Population Database (UPDB). Of particular interest is the relationship between overall familial mortality and familial longevity with respect to specific causes of death. If familial longevity is simply a function of variability in genetic predisposition to the major diseases of old age (e.g., heart disease, cancer, and cerebrovascular disease), we would not expect to find that overall familial longevity is especially associated with disease-specific mortality risk after adjusting for family history of the disease. On the other hand, if familial longevity is related to variation in rates of aging, we would expect to find an association between increased familial longevity and reduced mortality risks for the major diseases of old age. Finally, we also consider temporal changes in familial cause-specific mortality by analyzing the consistency with which family history predicts mortality for the same cause over different historical periods.

2   Study Population

The Church of Jesus Christ of Latter-day Saints (LDS Church or Mormons) was established in 1830 in the state of New York. In the years immediately following its establishment, church members migrated and created settlements in Ohio, Missouri, Illinois, and Iowa. The Mormons first entered the Salt Lake Valley in 1847 and this was the beginning of an organized migration. Between 1846 and 1870, over 60,000 pioneers and adherents of the LDS Church migrated from eastern and midwestern United States, as well as from Western Europe, into the U.S. intermountain west (Wahlquist 1974). In the 1880 census, 143,963 residents were enumerated in Utah Territory. The state of Utah was created in 1896, and in 1900 the census enumerated 276,749 residents. Since early in the *twentieth* century, about three fourths of Utah's population has professed church membership, and 9 out of 10 of these have been members of the Mormon Church (Allen 1989, 609). About two thirds of Utah's current 2.6 million residents are members of the LDS Church.

This analysis draws upon the UPDB for information as to the influences of a range of demographic and family characteristics on the risk of familial mortality from 1904 to 2002. The purpose of the UPDB is to represent genealogical, demographic, and health information about the settlers of Utah and their Utah descendants. Genealogical records originated as "Family Group Sheets" filled out by members of LDS Church. These records were selected from the Family History Library of the LDS Church in 1975–1976 and again in 1978–1979, under the criterion that one or more family members of a group sheet was born or died on the Mormon Pioneer Trail or in Utah (Bean, Mineau, and Anderton 1990). They have been updated and verified using the LDS Church's Ancestral File, as needed. Genealogical information for Utah's early migrants and their families represent birth cohorts that date back to about 1760. More than 185,000 family group sheets (and 1.6 million individuals) have been linked across generations and, in some instances, the genealogy records encompass as many as seven generations.

Over time, the utility of the UPDB as a research tool has been enhanced well beyond the information contained in the original core genealogy records. To improve the power of the UPDB, the genealogy records have been linked to other data sets, including Utah vital records, state-wide cancer records, driver license records, the 1880 manuscript census, records from Social Security Death Index, and other medical records. The UPDB is a dynamic database and receives annual electronic updates from data sources. This has increased the number of generations in families and some are now 10 generations deep. Extending the value of the UPDB depends on effective record linking capabilities (i.e., to matching person records from multiple datasets). Through record linking techniques, longitudinal person records are created which capture the many events associated with an individual over time. In addition, record linking activities impose important quality controls on the process of accumulating demographic and genealogical data, especially regarding the management of duplicate records. Containing almost 9 million records today, the UPDB stands as a unique population data resource in the U.S., and one of only a few in the world.

The Utah Resource for Genetic and Epidemiologic Research (RGE) at the University of Utah administers access to these data through a review process of the project proposal. The protection of privacy and confidentiality of individuals represented in these records has been negotiated with agreements between RGE and the data contributors. This project has received approval from the University of Utah's Institutional Review Board and RGE Review Committee (Wylie and Mineau 2003).

3   Previous Research Using UPDB

This population is biologically representative of a broad spectrum of the white U.S. population and is genetically similar to other Northern European-derived populations. The population has a low inbreeding rate that is very similar to that of the U.S. population due to a large founding population and high rates of immigration from a diverse group of outside populations (Jorde 1989, 2001). The representative nature of the genealogy file has been demonstrated in a variety of demographic studies on infant mortality (Lynch, Mineau, and Anderton 1985; Bean et al. 1990) and maternal mortality (Bardet et al. 1981) that have compared Utah rates and patterns to other populations. Other studies have analyzed fertility (Bean et al. 1990), birth spacing (Anderton and Bean 1985), widowhood (Mineau 1988; Mineau, Smith, and Bean 2002), familial excess longevity (Kerber et al. 2001), the relationship between reproductive behavior and adult longevity (Smith et al. 2002), and the effect of religious affiliation on adult mortality (Mineau et al. 2004).

Various studies have explored the relationship between familial effects and disease using UPDB data. O'Brien et al. (1994) examined the relationship of founder gene contributions to disease incidence from a theoretical perspective by simulating founder gene contributions in comparison to two other populations. An extensive evaluation of familial cancer risk in Utah reported on familial effects up to the fifth degree of relationship for 40 cancer sites (Kerber and O'Brien 2005). Other studies have drawn upon death certificates to study familial disease effects. A study of coronary heart disease (CHD) (Williams 1980; Hunt et al. 1986) in Utah identified a positive association between family history of CHD and an increased CHD mortality risk, and examined the reliability of death certificates listing myocardial infarction as the underlying cause of death (Williams et al. 1978). More recently, Cannon-Albright et al. (2003) conducted a genealogical assessment of the familial predisposition to aneurysms in an analysis of common ancestry among Utah patients who died of aneurysms.

4   Material and Methods

Using a combination of genealogy, birth certificates, driver license, Social Security death index (SSDI), and death certificate data, we identified a cohort of 2,195,808 people born between 1830 and 1984 for whom we had vital status follow-up in the form of either a Utah death record (from the genealogical data, death certificates, SSDI) or a current Utah driver license. A subset of 464,494 cohort members who met the above criteria also linked to at least one other family member in UPDB and survived to at least 65 years of age. The cohort is left-truncated in that individuals who died before age 65 or before the origin of death certification in 1904 are not part of the sample; it is right-censored in that individuals alive at the time of last

Table 10.1 Characteristics of cohort members by birth cohort

Birth cohort	Males	Females	Number of relatives			Generation depth (median)	Year of death[a]	
			Median	Min	Max		Min	Max
1830–1850	12,007	9,464	485	1	62,412	2	1904	1952
1851–1870	20,805	19,931	1,138	3	75,089	3	1917	1974
1871–1890	33,561	33,822	2,105	2	77,597	4	1937	1995
1891–1910	56,628	61,072	4,068	1	102,242	5	1957	2002
1911–1930	82,585	84,212	6,525	1	117,128	6	1977	2002
1931–1937	24,919	25,488	9,733	1	142,217	6	1997	2002
Total	230,505	233,989						

[a]Excludes those still living.

follow-up are censored thereafter. Table 10.1 provides basic characteristics of the cohort by year of birth. More males than females survived to age 65 and older in the early cohorts; this is likely the result of maternal mortality. Particularly noteworthy is the large number of relatives of each cohort member that are available for study. Cohort members in recent generations can trace ancestry to multiple founding ancestors, each of whom may have thousands of descendants. In contrast, the founding ancestors themselves are related only to their own descendants. Thus, the number of known relatives per cohort member tends to increase with increasing generation.

4.1 Death Information

Death certificate data for Utah are available in the UPDB with coded underlying causes of death for the years beginning in 1904 and include more than 708,000 deaths. In this study, we analyze death certificates from the years 1904–2002. Utah death records follow the coding conventions of the International Classification of Diseases (ICD). Multiple code revisions have been enacted since 1904 and all are represented over the long period of time covered by this study. Revision codes 6 to 10 were provided by the Utah Department of Health for certificates recorded 1957–2002: 1957 = ICD-6; 1958–1967 = ICD-7; 1968–1978 = ICD-8; 1979–1998 = ICD-9; and 1999–2002 = ICD-10. For deaths from 1904 to1956, about 80 percent of these records were coded to ICD-10 using World Health Organization software by a UPDB research project. The remaining 20 percent of certificates from this period were coded manually to ICD-10. The underlying cause of death was classified to 1 of the 10 leading causes of death in the U.S. in 2002 (Anderson and Smith 2005). Table 10.2 shows the codes included in each definition and the number of deaths from each cause.

Table 10.2 ICD Codes related to the 10 leading causes of death in 2002

Category		Cases	ICD-6	ICD-7	ICD-8	ICD-9	ICD-10
1	Cardiovascular (heart) disease	67,625	410–416, 420–422, 430–434, 440–443	410–416, 420–422, 430–434, 440–443	393–398, 400, 402, 404, 410–414	393–398, 402, 404, 410–414	I00–I09, I11, I13, I20–I51
2	Neoplasms	31,452	140–205	140–205	140–209	140–208	C00–C97
3	Cerebrovascular diseases	23,757	330–334	330–334	430–438	430–438	I60–I69
4	Chronic lower respiratory diseases	3,167	522	522	490–493	490–493	J40–J47
5	Accidents	4,346	E800–E936	E800–E936	E800–E949	E800–E949	V01–X59, Y85–Y86
6	Diabetes mellitus	6,163	260	260	250	250	E10–E14
7	Influenza and pneumonia	11,009	480–483, 490–493	480–483, 490–493	470–474, 480–486	480–487	J10–J18
8	Alzheimer's disease	1,216				331	G30
9	Nephritis, nephrotic syndrome, and nephrosis	3,569	590–594	590–594	580–584	580–589	N00–N07, N17–N19, N25–N27
10	Septicemia	1,030	53	53	38	38	A40–A41

4.2 Nested Case-Control Design

Since we are interested in repeatedly analyzing disease-specific subsets of the data, a nested case-control design was chosen for our study (Liddell, McDonald, and Thomas 1977; Langholz and Thomas 1991). This study design is an efficient alternative to survival analysis as a method of analyzing epidemiologic cohort data.

We constructed nested case-control datasets by identifying cases as individuals who died of one or more of the 10 leading causes of death categories selected. Controls were individually matched to cases on sex and year of birth, with the requirement that they be alive at the time of the cases' death or dead at the same age from another cause. Cases for a given cause of death were eligible as controls for the same cause of death prior to the date of their death. We selected one control per case. For a small number of cases, the desired number of controls could not be matched because the stratum of candidates was exhausted. Conditional logistic regression models were used to estimate odds ratios and confidence intervals for familial factors.

4.3 Historical Comparisons

Not all of the leading causes of death in the U.S. as of 2002 were recognized or diagnosed during the entire period of the study. As an example, Alzheimer's disease had no ICD code until the ninth revision and was not given as a cause of death in Utah until 1979. Although the ICD-10 codes were applied based on review of all text fields on death certificates from 1904 to1956, only two certificates mentioned Alzheimer's disease; thus, this diagnosis effectively does not exist in our data prior to 1979. Changes in nomenclature and medical science undoubtedly affect the classification of other diseases in more subtle ways as well (Anderton and Leonard 2004). To investigate this, we stratified our death certificate data into three historical periods, corresponding to changes in the ICD codes and the format of the death certificates themselves. Deaths from 1904 to 1956 were classified as "early." These were all coded to the ICD-10 revisions from the literal text fields on each death certificate. The "middle" period consists of death certificates coded to ICD revisions 6 (1957), 7 (1958–1967), and 8 (1968–1978). The "late" period consists of death certificates from 1979 to present, coded to either ICD-9 or ICD-10.

We anticipate several possible patterns of variation that may be indicative of the reliability of historic death records used for the purpose of developing indicators of familial disease predisposition. First, if the strength of the relationship between familial mortality and family history effects is stable over all time periods, then cause-of-death diagnoses are reasonably reliable and the pattern consistent with genetic predisposition. Alternatively, if the strength of the relationship between family history and mortality increases from the early to the late periods, then it may be difficult to distinguish whether the difference is due to changes in diagnostic assignments and coding, or to actual changes in shared (familial) environmental factors over time. Finally, if the strength of the relationship between family history and mortality declines over time, this would indicate a substantial redistribution of familial factors affecting risk, due to a decline in the relative importance of shared hereditary effects (genetic) compared to nonhereditary effects (environmental), or due to an overall decline in shared environmental factors.

4.4 Familial Standardized Mortality Ratio (FSMR)

The *familial standardized mortality ratio* (FSMR) measures mortality in terms of its familial expression (Kerber 1995). It is the ratio of observed to expected deaths from a particular cause summarized over all relatives of every class (i.e., first degree, second degree, etc.). The expression of each relative is weighted by the kinship coefficient (Malecot 1948) which is the probability that two individuals share a given gene identical by descent from a common ancestor. We use a further refinement of FSMR in this analysis, a simple logarithmic transformation that improves the behavior of FSMR as a covariate in a regression model: LFSMR = ln(FSMR+1). In this study, we use LFSMR as a covariate in conditional logistic regression models of cause-specific mortality in the cohort, adjusted for sex and year of birth.

4.5 Population Attributable Risk (PAR)

Population attributable risk (PAR) is used in epidemiology to estimate the fraction of reduction in a population outcome that would result if its cause was eliminated. Here we calculate PAR for the familial fraction of deaths due to each cause. The calculation assumes independence of each cause of death from all others. Using the effect estimates from the conditional logistic regression analysis of cause-specific mortality in relation to LFSMR, we calculated PARs according to the method of Bruzzi et al. (1985). Briefly, the PAR is the mean over all disease cases of

$$\frac{e^{x\beta}-1}{e^{x\beta}}$$

where x is the quantity of exposure of interest for each case, and β is the associated effect estimate from the conditional logistic regression model—thus $e^{x\beta}$ is the estimated odds ratio.

4.6 Familial Excess Longevity (FEL)

We are interested not only in the degree to which each cause of death has a familial component but also in the possibility that there is a familial predisposition to longevity which reduces the risk of death from multiple outcomes at advanced ages (and perhaps before). A familial predisposition to longevity might confound the analysis of familial predisposition to specific diseases and vice versa. To assess this possibility, we estimated familial excess longevity for all subjects. *Familial excess longevity* (FEL) measures the familial component of longevity just as we use FSMR to measure the familial component of mortality. With the two measures, we can address potential confounding between familial factors that condition longevity through adulthood as well as mortality risks associated with age-related common diseases. In addition, we note that there are numerous factors unrelated to genetic variation in longevity which nonetheless contribute to variation in individual lifespan, e.g., gender and year of birth; others have a substantial familial component as well, e.g., exposure to infectious disease, variability in social support, and behavioral factors such as smoking.

We begin by estimating individual *excess longevity*, defined as the difference between an individual's attained age and the age to which that individual was expected to live. To minimize the influence of some potential confounders, we incorporate gender and birth year in the model.

We estimate expected longevity ($\hat{y}$) from an accelerated failure time model in the following manner:

$$\hat{y} = e^{\alpha + \beta_1 \cdot gender + \beta_2 \cdot birthyear}$$

where α is the intercept, $\beta_1 \ldots \beta_n$ are slope coefficients, and the excess longevity (l) is simply $y-\hat{y}$, where y is the attained age in years. This approach to estimating excess longevity is similar to the method of Bocquet-Appel (1990) in estimating the heritability of longevity at Arthez d'Asson.

We estimate $\hat{y}$ and l using only individuals who survived at least to age 65 in order to reduce the impact on our analyses of familial mortality that presumably results from familial predisposition to diseases, such as heart disease, cancer, or diabetes, which commonly conclude in deaths attributed to those causes.

The concept of excess longevity can be extended to the family members of each subject, excluding those who did not live at least 65 years. Averaging the excess longevities of all of a subject's family members, with an appropriate weighting scheme, yields an estimate of the *familial excess longevity* (FEL). For the present analysis, we have chosen two primary weighting schemes, each corresponding to a different model of transmission of familial longevity. The kinship coefficient, the probability that an individual shares a single autosomal gene with another individual, is used as a weight in calculating FEL (Kerber et al. 2001):

$$\text{FEL}_i = \frac{\sum_{k \in K} f(i,k) \cdot l_k}{\sum_k f(i,k)}$$

where FEL_i is the familial excess longevity for subject i; K is the set of all relatives of subject i; l_k is the excess longevity of the kth member of K; and $f(i,k)$ is the kinship coefficient. Because of the large number of relatives available for study, ranging from a median of 485 for cohort members born 1830–1850, to a median of 9,733 for those born after 1930, the estimates of FEL that we can calculate for each cohort member are relatively stable. This is also true (but to a lesser degree) for our estimates of LFSMR, which are subject to additional variability introduced by changes in disease coding and the underlying variation among disease rates in the population.

5 Results

5.1 Familiality by Cause

Table 10.3 shows the relative risk associated with a 1 standard deviation change in LFSMR (s = 0.42) and FEL (s = 2.2 years), representing normal variation within the population, as well as the PAR for familial risk of each of the 10 leading broad causes of death. The estimated contribution to risk of specific familial factors, measured by the relative risk and population attributable risk estimates for LFSMR, varies widely by cause of death. PAR is calculated only for the cause-specific LFSMR values, as an estimate of the total fraction of deaths from each cause attributable to family histories of each disease. The PAR estimates range from nearly 0 for septicemia disease, to 40% for neoplasms (cancer), 41% for diabetes, and 57% for heart disease.

Table 10.3 Relative risk associated with a 1 standard deviation change in LFSMR (0.42) and FEL (2.2), and population attributable risk for familial risk of each of the 10 leading causes of death in the U.S. in 2002

| | | | Full data | | |
| | | | LFSMR[a] | | FEL[d] |
Code	Category	Cases	RR[b]	PAR[c]	RR
1	Cardiovascular (heart) disease	67,625	1.69*	0.57*	0.93*
2	Neoplasms (cancer)	31,452	1.47*	0.39*	1.00
3	Cerebrovascular diseases	23,757	1.27*	0.32*	0.91*
4	Chronic lower respiratory diseases	3,167	1.21*	0.19*	0.91*
5	Accidents	4,346	1.22*	0.24*	0.94*
6	Diabetes mellitus	6,163	1.47*	0.41*	0.87*
7	Influenza and pneumonia	11,009	1.18*	0.24*	0.95*
8	Alzheimer's disease	1,216	1.10*	0.10*	0.99
9	Nephritis, nephrotic syndrome, and nephrosis	3,569	1.04*	0.06*	0.96*
10	Septicemia	1,030	1.04	0.05	0.87*

*p-value < 0.05.
[a]LFSMR: (log 1+) familial standardized mortality ratio.
[b]RR: relative risk.
[c]PAR: population attributable risk.
[d]FEL: familial excess longevity.

In contrast to the LFSMR estimates, the estimated effects of a 2.2 year increase in FEL (1 standard deviation) are quite consistent across the various causes of death, with only cancer deaths failing to show an effect of familial longevity on reduced risk. The strongest protective effect for FEL is for diabetes (RR = 0.87) and septicemia, while the weakest effect (but still statistically significant) is for nephritis (RR = 0.96).

5.2 Historical Comparisons

Each historical comparison can be viewed as a three-by-three matrix of effect estimates. A potentially useful indicator of the importance of genetic factors in disease susceptibility is the relative strength of the main diagonal of the matrix (for which the family history and the risk period of the subject are contemporaneous) to its off-diagonal elements (where the family history and the risk period of the subject are separated in time).

Table 10.4 shows how family histories of death from varying causes in each of the three time periods affect risks of death from the same cause in each period. In general, relative risk estimates for LFSMR remain stable or increase with time, so that the effects are usually strongest for the recent family histories of the most recent deaths. This is particularly true for cardiovascular (heart) disease, neoplasms (cancer), cerebrovascular disease, diabetes, and influenza/pneumonia. With the exception of nephritis, septicemia, and accidents in the early period (period I), there are substantial off-diagonal effects, indicating that effects of family history in periods before or after the time an individual is at risk contribute to their risk of death in a manner most consistent with genetic causation. This also appears to be true for causes of death that are affected by immediate shared environments, such as accidents (e.g., a family history of accidental death after 1978 is a significant predictor of accidental death prior to 1956), or influenza and pneumonia (a family history of death from influenza or pneumonia in any period significantly increases the risk of death from the same cause in any period). Figures 10.1 through 10.3 show the pattern of changes in relative risk estimates for heart disease, cancer, and influenza/pneumonia described above.

6 Discussion

6.1 Family Histories and Cause-Specific Risk of Death

We have seen that family histories of cause-specific mortality greatly affect risk of death from the same cause. It is axiomatic that this familial aggregation results from some combination of genetic causes, the effects of shared environments, and

Table 10.4 Relative risks for a 1 standard deviation increase in LFSMR by time period: period I
(early) 1904–1956, period II (middle) 1957–1978, and period III (late) 1979–2002

Code	Category	Period	Cases	LFSMR[a] (by period)		
				I	II	III
1	Cardiovascular (heart) disease	I	19,141	1.17*	1.23*	1.24*
		II	23,074	1.26*	1.29*	1.30*
		III	25,410	1.27*	1.38*	1.46*
2	Neoplasms (cancer)	I	5,888	1.09*	1.15*	1.21*
		II	7,777	1.08*	1.16*	1.25*
		III	17,787	1.14*	1.20*	1.37*
3	Cerebrovascular diseases	I	5,935	1.11*	1.10*	1.13*
		II	8,040	1.10*	1.10*	1.09*
		III	9,782	1.10*	1.05*	1.22*
4	Chronic lower respiratory diseases	I	737	1.08*	1.02	1.09*
		II	598	1.08*	1.09*	1.25*
		III	1,832	1.07*	1.09*	1.19*
5	Accidents	I	463	1.08	1.07	1.13
		II	1,756	1.04	1.13*	1.11*
		III	2,127	1.06*	1.13*	1.21*
6	Diabetes mellitus	I	1,140	1.21*	1.21*	1.20*
		II	1,400	1.19*	1.21*	1.36*
		III	3,623	1.12*	1.14*	1.39*
7	Influenza and pneumonia	I	4,123	1.11*	1.05*	1.05*
		II	1,986	1.09*	1.05*	1.08*
		III	4,900	1.10*	1.04*	1.21*
9	Nephritis, nephrotic syndrome, and nephrosis	I	1,941	1.03	1.03	1.00
		II	304	1.04	1.09	1.04
		III	1,324	1.03	1.02	1.11*
10	Septicemia	I	96	1.03	0.95	0.98
		II	98	0.98	1.24	0.80
		III	836	1.08	0.97	1.06

*p-value < 0.05.
[a]LFSMR: (log 1+) familial standardized mortality ratio.

perhaps from biases present in data or analytic methods. Although a small number
of genes are known to affect the risk of death from major killers like heart disease,
stroke, and cancer, variability in these genes collectively accounts for little of the
observed familial clustering of these diseases; nor are genes known at present that
affect accident-proneness. In recent years, geneticists have become increasingly
aware of the complex nature of late-onset chronic disease etiology and have posited
models involving interactions among multiple genetic loci, with or without environmental modifiers of risk. Yet the pattern of inherited risk we have observed in
this study is relatively simple—LFSMR is optimized to detect autosomal dominant
genetic effects and recessive alleles or interactions across multiple loci rapidly disappear with increasing genealogical distance. So the large, outbred genealogical
dataset we have analyzed would show little familial aggregation of disease if the
genetics in question were complex. Complex etiologies do not automatically imply
complex genetics.

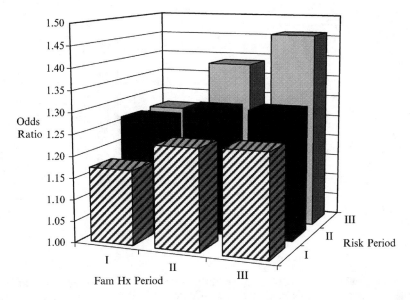

Figure 10.1 Heart disease: Relative risk of death from heart disease for a 1 standard deviation change in LFSMR in each of three historical periods, compared to family histories of heart disease accumulated in one of the same three periods

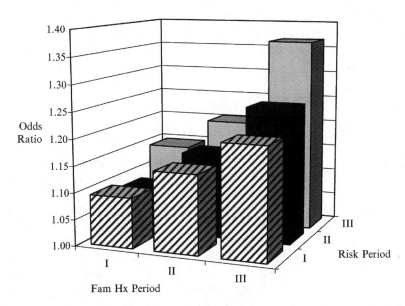

Figure 10.2 Cancer: Relative risks of death from cancer for a 1 standard deviation change in LFSMR in each of three historical periods, compared to family histories of cancer accumulated in one of the same three periods

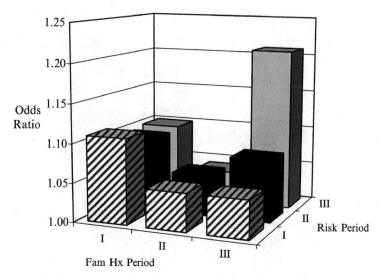

Figure 10.3 Influenza/Pneumonia: Relative risks of death from influenza/pneumonia for a 1 standard deviation change in LFSMR in each of three historical periods, compared to family histories of influenza/pneumonia accumulated in one of the same three periods

Shared environments account for an unknown proportion of the familial disease risk, but they too are unlikely to be replicated among the very many distant relatives (third- through tenth-degree relatives) that members of the cohort have. While a typical individual selected from UPDB may have 10 or more first-degree relatives, he or she will have several orders of magnitude more relatives separated by five or ten generations. It is the collective experience of these relatives that is summarized most effectively by LFSMR and FEL.

6.2   *Familial Excess Longevity*

We consider FEL to be a potentially important and observable indicator of frailty. We have observed that increased FEL is associated with decreased risks of almost all the 10 leading causes of death, and that the magnitude of reduction in risk is remarkably similar across very dissimilar causes. This observation is further supported by a comparison between Cox models that incorporate frailty but exclude FEL and models that incorporate frailty and include FEL. When FEL is excluded, we find significant effects of frailty (not shown) suggesting that there are shared factors among siblings that contribute to a common excess risk of mortality. When FEL is added to the model, FEL becomes the strongest predictor of mortality and frailty effects disappear. This finding suggests that whatever factors link kin survival, an important component is the familiality of longevity within their extended family, suggesting that they share alleles affecting survival. Genealogies may be helpful for demographers to get observable measures of frailty, and one way of procuring this information (in the absence of a UPDB resource) is to seek a family history of longevity from research subjects.

The results of this study provide additional support to the notion that familial longevity can result not only from an absence of genetic predisposition to specific diseases, but also from a genetic predisposition to be less susceptible, at any age, to the major chronic diseases that afflict, and ultimately kill, the elderly. In demographic terms, this indicates that people with strong family histories of longevity experience a reduced rate of aging. It remains to be seen in what manner, and to what degree, this reduction in the demographic rate of aging is observable in biological terms.

Acknowledgments We wish to thank the Pedigree and Population Resource of Huntsman Cancer Foundation, University of Utah, for providing the data and valuable computing support. This work was supported by NIH grants AG13748 (Kinship and Socio-Demographic Determinants of Mortality, Smith PI) and AG22095 (The Utah Study of Fertility, Longevity and Ageing, Smith PI). Funding and support provided by: IUSSP, INED, and EHESS.

References

Allen, R.D. 1989. Religion in twentieth-century Utah, in R.D. Poll, T.G. Alexander, E.E. Campbell, and D.E. Miller (eds.), *Utah's history*, Utah State University Press, Logan, pp. 609–27.

Anderson, R.N. and B.L. Smith. 2005. Deaths: Leading causes for 2002. *National Vital Statistics Reports* 53(17): 1–89.

Anderton, D.L. and L.L. Bean. 1985. Birth spacing and fertility limitation: A behavioral analysis of a nineteenth century frontier population. *Demography* 22: 169–83.

Anderton, D.L. and S.H. Leonard. 2004. Grammars of death: An analysis of nineteenth-century literal causes of death from age of miasmas to germ theory. *Social Science History* 28(1): 111–43.

Bardet, J.P., K.A. Lynch, G.P. Mineau, M. Hainsworth, and M. Skolnick. 1981. La mortalité maternelle autrefois: Une étude comparée. *Annales de Démographie Historique*: 31–49.

Bean, L.L., G.P. Mineau, and D.L. Anderton. 1990. *Fertility Change on the American Frontier, Adaptation and Innovation*. University of California Press, Berkeley.

Beeton, M. and K. Pearson. 1899. Data for the problem of evolution in man. II. A first study on the inheritance of longevity and the selective death rate in man. *Proceedings of the Royal Society London* 65: 290–305.

Bocquet-Appel, J.P. 1990. Familial transmission of longevity. *Annals of Human Biology* 17(2): 81–95.

Bruzzi, P., S.B. Green, D.P. Byar, L.A. Brinton, and C. Schairer. 1985. Estimating the population attributable risk for multiple risk factors using case-control data. *American Journal of Epidemiology* 122: 904–14.

Cannon-Albright, L.A., N. Camp, J.M. Farnham, J. MacDonald, K. Atbin, and K. Rowe. 2003. A genealogical assessment of heritable predisposition to aneurysms. *Journal of Neurosurgery* 99: 637–43.

Carey, J.R. 2003. *Longevity: The Biology and Demography of Life Span*. Princeton University Press, Princeton, NJ.

Carey, J.R. and S. Tuljapurkar (eds.). 2003. *Life Span: Evolutionary, Ecological, and Demographic Perspectives*. Population Council, New York.

Gavrilov, L.A., N.S. Gavrilova, S.J. Olshansky, and B.A. Carnes. 2002. Genealogical data and the biodemography of human longevity. *Social Biology* 49(3–4): 160–73.

Gudmundsson, H., D.F. Gudbjartsson, M. Frigge, J.R. Gulcher, and K. Stefansson. 2000. Inheritance of human longevity in Iceland. *European Journal of Human Genetics* 8(10): 743–9.

Hunt, S.C., K. Blickenstaff, P.N. Hopkins, and R.R. Williams. 1986. Coronary disease and risk factors in close relatives of Utah women with early coronary death. *The Western Journal of Medicine* 145(3): 329–34.

Jorde, L.B. 1989. Inbreeding in the Utah Mormons: An evaluation of estimates based on pedigrees, isonymy, and migration matrices. *Annals of Human Genetics* 52: 339–55.

Jorde, L.B. 2001. Consanguinity and prereproductive mortality in the Utah Mormon population. *Human Heredity* 52: 61–5.

Kerber, R.A. 1995. Method for calculating the risk associated with family history of a disease. *Genetic Epidemiology* 12(3): 291–301.

Kerber, R.A., E. O'Brien, K.R. Smith, and R.M. Cawthon. 2001. Familial excess longevity in Utah genealogies. *The Journal of Gerontology: Biological Sciences* 56A(3): B130–9.

Kerber, R.A. and E. O'Brien. 2005. A cohort study of cancer risk in relation to family histories of cancer in the Utah population database. *Cancer* 103(9): 1906–15.

Langholz, B. and D.C. Thomas. 1991. Efficiency of cohort sampling designs: Some surprising results. *Biometrics* 47(4): 1563–71.

Liddell, F.D.K., J.C. McDonald, and D.C. Thomas. 1977. Methods of cohort analysis: Appraisal by application to asbestos mining. *Journal of the Royal Statistical Society* Series A 140: 469–91.

Lynch, K.A., G.P. Mineau, and D.L. Anderton. 1985. Estimates of infant mortality on the Western frontier: The use of genealogical data. *Historical Methods* 18: 155–64.

Malecot, G. 1948. *The Mathematics of Heredity*. Masson, Paris.

Mineau, G.P. 1988. Utah widowhood: a demographic profile, in A. Scadron (ed.), *On their own: Widows and widowhood in the American Southwest, 1848–1939*, University of Illinois Press, Champaign, pp. 140–65.

Mineau, G.P., K.R. Smith, and L.L. Bean. 2002. Historical trends of survival among widows and widowers. *Social Sciences and Medicine* 54: 245–54.

Mineau, G.P., K.R. Smith, and L.L. Bean. 2004. Adult mortality risks and religious affiliation: The role of social milieu in biodemographic studies. *Annales de Démographie Historique*: 85–104.

O'Brien, E., R.A. Kerber, L.B. Jorde, and A.R. Rogers. 1994. Founder effect assessment of variation in genetic contributions among founders. *Human Biology* 66: 185–204.

Smith, K.R. and G.P. Mineau. 2003. Genealogies in demographic research, in P. Demeny and G. McNicholl (eds.), *Encyclopedia of population*, Macmillan, New York, pp. 448–51.

Smith, K.R., G.P. Mineau, and L.L. Bean. 2002. Fertility and post-reproductive longevity. *Social Biology* 49(1): 55–75.

Wachter, K.W. and C.E. Finch (eds.) 1997. *Between Zeus and the Salmon: The Biodemography of Longevity*. National Academy Press, Washington, DC.

Wahlquist, W.L. 1974. *Settlement processes in the Mormon core area: 1847–1890*. Ph.D. Dissertation, University of Nebraska.

Williams, R.R. 1980. A population perspective for early and familial coronary heart disease, in J. Cairns, J.L. Lyon, and M. Skolnick (eds.), *Banbury report no. 4: Cancer incidence in defined populations*, Cold Spring Harbor Laboratory Press, Cold Spring, New York, pp. 333–50.

Williams, R.R., M. Skolnick, D. Carmelli, A.T. Maness, S.C. Hunt, S. Hasstedt, G.E. Reiber, and R.K. Jones. 1978. Utah pedigree studies: Design and preliminary data for premature male CHD deaths. Paper read at Genetic analysis of common diseases: Applications to predictive factors in coronary disease, Snowbird, Utah.

Wylie, J.E. and G.P. Mineau. 2003. Biomedical databases: Protecting privacy and promoting research. *Trends in Biotechnology* 21: 113–6.

Chapter 11
Distant Kinship and Founder Effects in the Quebec Population

Marc Tremblay[1], Hélène Vézina[1], Bertrand Desjardins[2], and Louis Houde[3]

Abstract The structure of kinship links in a given population at a given time is the result of several past demographic events that shaped the population during its evolution. Many populations display particular kinship structures due to the occurrence of specific events at some point in their history, such as founder effects. Using genealogical data retrieved from the BALSAC population register, the BALSAC-RETRO genealogical database and the Early Quebec Population Register, this study focuses on the genetic consequences of the demographic settlement and expansion experienced by the Quebec population over the last four centuries. A total of 2,223 ascending genealogies were reconstructed for the purpose of this study. These genealogies have an average depth of 9.3 generations and go back as far as the early seventeenth century. Measures of kinship show that 98 percent of all pairs of subjects share at least one distant common ancestor. Virtually all genealogies (99.2 percent) contain at least one French founder. Overall, nearly 87 percent of the current gene pool is explained by French founders who came mainly from the provinces of Normandie, Ile-de-France, Aunis, Poitou, and Perche during the seventeenth century.

Keywords Quebec population, kinship, founder effect, population register, genealogies, gene pool

1 Introduction

The structure of kinship links in a given population at a given time is the result of several past demographic events that shaped the population during its evolution. Many populations display particular kinship structures due to the occurrence of

[1] Interdisciplinary Research Group on Demography and Genetic Epidemiology, University of Quebec at Chicoutimi, Canada

[2] Interdisciplinary Research Group on Demography and Genetic Epidemiology, and Programme de recherche en démographie historique, Université de Montréal, Canada

[3] Interdisciplinary Research Group on Demography and Genetic Epidemiology, Université du Québec à Trois-Rivières, Canada

specific events at some point in their history, such as founder effects. A founder effect can be described as a long-term genetic consequence of a migration movement initiated by a relatively small number of individuals (the founders) originating from the same parent population, after which a new population was formed (Mayr 1963; O'Brien et al. 1988). The strength and impact of the founder effect at a given time will depend on a number of factors, such as the size of the initial migrant cohort and the time elapsed since their settlement, the matrimonial and reproductive behaviors of their descendants, and the subsequent relative isolation of the population. The frequency and distribution of founder genes in the population can thus vary greatly from one situation to another. In some cases, founder effects will explain, for instance, the presence of rare hereditary diseases at an elevated frequency in a given population (O'Brien et al. 1994; Peltonen, Pekkarinen, and Aaltonen 1995; Scriver 2001).

Founder effects have been described in various populations worldwide (for a recent review, see Arcos-Burgos and Muenke 2002). In a few cases, the availability of extensive demographic or genealogical data allows for an in-depth study of founder effects in the population. One notorious case is that of the Icelandic population (Árnason 2003; Helgason et al. 2000; Helgason et al. 2003a, b; Helgason et al. 2005). With a present size of about 290,000, the population of Iceland experienced a singular demographic history characterized by an initial settlement of 8,000–16,000 founders coming from Scandinavia and the British Isles during the ninth and tenth centuries, with relatively low subsequent external input (Helgason et al. 2005). Although there has been some controversy about the relative homogeneity of the Icelanders, it seems that this population is genetically more homogeneous than most European populations (Árnason 2003; Helgason et al. 2003b). This homogeneity was caused mainly by the demographic events that followed the initial founder migration, along with subsequent genetic drift (Helgason et al. 2005).

Finland is another example of a population that experienced strong founder effects (Peltonen et al. 1995; Kittles et al. 1999; Kere 2001). Although some traces of human activity dating from 7,000 years BC have been found, permanent settlement in Finland started some 2,000 years ago in the southern part of the country, with migrants originating from the south and east of the present Finnish territory (Kere 2001). The northern and eastern parts of the country were colonized later, with migrants coming from the south. The initial number of founders is not known—perhaps only a few hundred individuals—but several founding events from different groups may have taken place (Peltonen et al. 1995; Kittles et al. 1999). During the period of rapid demographic growth (eighteenth–twentieth centuries), it seems that relatively few interactions occurred between Finland and its neighboring countries, leading to an expansion of founder effects within the Finnish population (Peltonen et al. 1995; Kere 2001). Some 35 recessive diseases almost exclusively found in the Finnish population or with a frequency higher than in other populations have been identified so far (Kere 2001).

In terms of population size Finland is similar to Quebec, 1 of the 10 provinces of Canada, though somewhat smaller. The demographic history of the Quebec population shows, like those of Iceland and Finland, strong founder effects, but these effects are much more recent in the case of Quebec, where European settlement started in the seventeenth century (see details below). In a little more than 300 years, the population of Quebec increased by a factor of 500 (from approximately 15,000 people in 1690 to 7.5 million today), mainly due to high fertility levels among the descendants of the first French pioneers (Henripin and Péron 1972; Charbonneau et al. 2000). Several rare hereditary disorders are observed with an elevated frequency in the Quebec population whereas, as in Finland, other disorders are nonexistent or extremely rare (Scriver 2001).

The present study focuses on the genetic consequences of the demographic settlement and expansion experienced by the Quebec population over the last four centuries. Using extensive genealogical data, analyses of the numerous and intricate genealogical paths linking the population of Quebec and its ancestors according to their geographical origins were performed. Similar studies about the genealogical structure of the Quebec population have been published (see, for example, Bouchard and DeBraekeleer 1991; Heyer et al. 1997; Tremblay, Jomphe, and Vézina 2001), but these studies focused on the populations of one or several particular regions of the province of Quebec. This chapter is the first study of the Quebec population as a whole.

2   The Quebec Population

The province of Quebec is located in the eastern part of Canada, between Ontario and the Maritime provinces; its territory spans both shores of the Saint Lawrence River which flows from the Great Lakes to the Atlantic Ocean. Quebec is the largest of the Canadian provinces, with approximately 1.5 million km^2; most of its population (about 82 percent) is French-speaking (Statistics Canada 2006).

European peopling of the Quebec territory began with the arrival of French pioneers who settled the valley extending on either side of the Saint Lawrence River at the beginning of the seventeenth century (Charbonneau et al. 1993; Charbonneau et al. 2000). Only some 10,000 immigrants experienced a family life in the colony over the span of a century and a half of French rule, which means that the excess of births over deaths quickly became the main factor of growth. The only period of relatively high immigration was from 1663 to 1673, when the French Crown sent some 800 women, the "Filles du Roi", to alleviate the shortage of women of marrying age in the colony and to encourage the soldiers to settle (Landry 1992). This effort marked the virtual halt of female immigration; after that, foreign arrivals were few in number and predominantly male, with a small peak of military immigration at the end of the period. The great majority of immigrants came directly from France, whereas most of the others were either French people from other French North American colonies or Europeans originating from the countries bordering France. With the British takeover in the 1760s, French-speaking immigration was reduced to Acadians, French colonists of the Atlantic regions of Canada who were driven from their land and who found their way to Quebec (Dickinson 1994); other newcomers to the Saint Lawrence River Valley were from the British Isles, with the notable exception of a group of German mercenaries who settled in the 1780s (Wilhelmy 1984). It is very important to note that as the French population was Catholic and the English-speaking immigrants were Protestants, the two ethnic groups did not intermarry to any significant degree. The French population thus grew on its own, without any new arrivals from outside.

During the nineteenth century, most of the immigration movement to Quebec continued to come from the British Isles (McInnis 2000; Beaujot and Kerr 2004). Thousands of immigrants from England, Scotland, and Ireland settled in the urban areas of the province (mainly Montreal and Quebec City). Since some of these immigrants were Catholics (mainly Irish), intermarriages with the French population became a possibility, but remained limited because of the language barrier. At the beginning of the twentieth century, the origins of the immigrants became more diversified, with many newcomers from Southern and Eastern Europe. More recently, the number of immigrants from Asia, South America, and the Caribbean has overtaken the number from Europe (Duchesne 2004).

3　The BALSAC, BALSAC-RETRO, and PRDH Databases

The genealogical data used for this study were obtained through three main sources: the BALSAC population register, the BALSAC-RETRO genealogical database (both of the University of Quebec at Chicoutimi), and the Early Quebec Population Register (Programme de recherche en démographie historique (PRDH), University of Montreal). The BALSAC population register contains demographic and genealogical information on the Quebec population for the nineteenth and twentieth centuries (Bouchard et al. 1995; Bouchard 2004). Most of the original data were obtained from marriage certificates. As of June 2005, the register contained nearly 2 million records, of which 1.2 million have already been linked. The BALSAC-RETRO database was developed through the use of genealogical reconstructions for various research projects (Jomphe and Casgrain 1997; Bouchard 2004). At present, this database contains genealogical data on 350,000 individuals from all Quebec regions and goes back as far as the early seventeenth century. Most of the BALSAC-RETRO records for the nineteenth and twentieth centuries were retrieved from the BALSAC register. Data covering the seventeenth and eighteenth centuries were obtained from the Early Quebec Population Register (Légaré 1988; Desjardins 1998). This register contains approximately 700,000 records of baptisms, marriages, and burials.

4　Structure of the Genealogical Sample

A total of 2,223 ascending genealogies were reconstructed for the purpose of this study. The starting points of the genealogies (the subjects) are individuals who married in Quebec between 1945 and 1965 and whose parents were also married in Quebec.

They were chosen randomly among the available data in the BALSAC-RETRO database. All marriages are Catholic (no usable data were available for other types of marriages). The subjects' selection reflects the geographical distribution of the Quebec population around 1955. At that time, 88 percent of the Quebec population was Catholic (Henripin and Péron 1972).

Although most of the 2,223 genealogies go back to the first Quebec settlers in the early seventeenth century, some genealogical branches are limited by the available genealogical sources. Hence, all genealogical branches do not reach the same generation levels. Figure 11.1 illustrates the completeness of the genealogies, for each generation.

The completeness index (C_g), for a given generation level, is the ratio of the number of known ancestors at that generation level to the maximum possible number of ancestors at that same level:

$$C_g = A_g / (N \cdot 2^g)$$

where g is the generation level (that of the subjects' parents being the first), A_g is the number of known ancestors at level g, and N is the number of genealogies.

This measure shows the availability of the genealogical information at each generation. The maximum C_g value is 1, meaning that at generation level g, all ancestors have been identified. Figure 11.1 shows that this is the case for the first two generations (parents and grandparents), as expected from the criteria used in the sample selection process. Starting with the third generation (great-grandparents), information is missing in a few genealogies. Still, on average, the genealogies are at least 90 percent complete until the seventh generation. After the ninth generation, completeness decreases rapidly; this point corresponds to the period of the arrival of most of the seventeenth-century French immigrants. Beyond the 13th

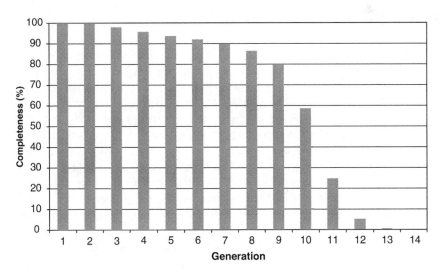

Figure 11.1 Completeness of the genealogies, per generation

Table 11.1 Basic characteristics of the genealogical sample (n = 2,223). (From BALSAC population register, BALSAC-RETRO genealogical database, and Early Quebec Population Register.)

Average genealogical depth	9.3
Maximum genealogical depth	17
Total number of ancestors mentioned in the genealogies	5,008,606
Male	2,504,303
Female	2,504,303
Number of distinct ancestors	155,363
Male	77,005
Female	78,358
Mean number of appearances per ancestor	32.2
Male	32.5
Female	32.0

generation, only a few ancestors could still be identified, with a maximum level of 17 generations (Table 11.1). The average genealogical depth, which is obtained by summing C_g through all generations, is a little more than nine generations.

In total, the genealogies contain over 5 million mentions of ancestors, but several of these mentions concern the same ancestors (i.e., many ancestors appear more than once in the genealogies). Counting each ancestor only once, the number is reduced to 155,363 distinct ancestors, with an average of 32.2 appearances per ancestor. The number of female ancestors is slightly higher than that of the males, meaning that male remarriages were more frequent in this population than female remarriages, due in part to differential mortality at adult ages during the seventeenth, eighteenth, and nineteenth centuries, and also to the fact that men could remarry and reproduce at older ages (beyond 50).

5 Kinship Levels Across Generations

Two individuals are biologically related if they have at least one common ancestor. In genetic terms, this means that these individuals will have a nonzero probability of sharing identical copies of a gene coming from that ancestor. Hence, genealogical reconstructions can help to estimate the intensity of biological kinship in a population. The greater the genealogical depths, the greater will be the probability of finding one or more common ancestors in the genealogical ascendances of any couple of individuals. The intensity of kinship between these individuals will thus depend on the number of common ancestors identified in their genealogies and on the genealogical distances (i.e., number of generations) between these ancestors and the two individuals. This intensity is measured by calculating kinship coefficients.

A kinship coefficient (Φ) can be defined as the probability that one allele (chosen at random) from a given individual (i) is identical by descent to another allele, at the same locus, from another individual (j) (Thompson 1986). It is calculated as follows:

$$\Phi i, j = \sum_A \sum_P \left(\frac{1}{2}\right)^k \left(1 + F(A)\right)$$

where A is the set of all common ancestors to i and j, P is the set of all genealogical paths between i and j through A, k is the number of individuals in P, and $F(A)$ is the inbreeding coefficient for A (i.e., A's parents' kinship coefficient).

The mean kinship coefficient for a group of individuals is calculated by dividing the sum of all coefficients by the total number of coefficients. Thus, nearly 2.5 million kinship coefficients were calculated at each generation level with the 2,223 genealogies.

Figure 11.2 shows the mean Φ value from the third to the 13th generation (before the third generation, all Φ values are null). Up to the seventh generation, the mean kinship coefficient is relatively small. At that level, 22 percent of the pairs of subjects share at least one common ancestor (Figure 11.3). Most of the kinship coefficient's

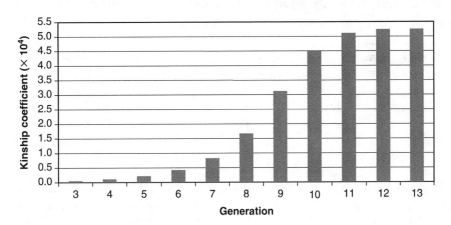

Figure 11.2 Kinship coefficients, per generation

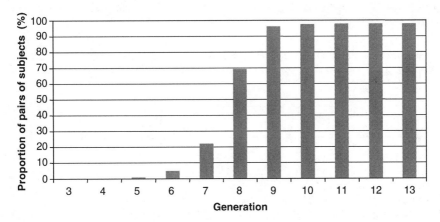

Figure 11.3 Proportion (%) of pairs of subjects having at least one common ancestor, per generation

growth occurs between the 7th ($\Phi = 0.00008$) and 10th ($\Phi = 0.00045$) generations, where nearly 98 percent of the pairs of subjects are related. After the 11th generation, the values do not change much (maximum mean Φ of 0.00052), due to the lack of genealogical information at that level. At the 13th generation, the maximum value of Φ almost reaches 0.1, but most of the coefficients are much lower. In fact, the distribution of the kinship coefficients is far from a normal distribution (nearly three quarters of the coefficients are below the mean value).

These results show the importance of distant kinship in the Quebec population. The number of common ancestors after the seventh generation reaches such proportions that every subject in the contemporary population is genetically related to almost all other subjects.

6   Distant Kinship: Frequency, Genetic Contribution, and Origins of Ancestral Founders

The genetic contribution and geographical origins of the founders of the Quebec population was investigated. These founders were defined as the most distant ancestors that could be identified in each genealogical branch. Their country of origin represents either their place of birth, marriage, or emigration.

A total of 13,119 founders were identified. The distribution of these founders according to their origin and period of marriage is given in Table 11.2. Most founders are from France, and most of these French founders were married in the seventeenth century. Less than 5 percent of all founders are from the British Isles (Great Britain or Ireland). Origin could not be determined for approximately 15 percent of the founders, most of them having married after 1765. Since French immigration almost ceased after the British Conquest, those of unknown origin are likely not French, but one must not forget that the time intervals are marriage periods. Hence, it is possible that some post-1765 founders are pre-Conquest French immigrants who married after 1765.

Table 11.2 Distribution of founders (%) according to their origin and their period of marriage (n = 13,119). (From BALSAC population register, BALSAC-RETRO genealogical database, and Early Quebec Population Register.)

Origin	Period of marriage			
	Before 1700 (n = 7,135)	1700–1765 (n = 3,583)	After 1765 (n = 2,401)	Total (n = 13,119)
France	51.6	21.0	0.7	73.4
British Isles	0.6	1.4	2.8	4.7
Germany	0.1	1.1	0.5	1.7
Other European	0.5	0.5	0.4	1.5
Acadia	0.2	0.9	0.4	1.5
Other American	0.8	0.6	0.7	2.1
Unknown	0.6	1.8	12.8	15.2
Total	54.4	27.3	18.3	100.0

Overall, more than half (54 percent) of the founders were married before 1700, and an additional 27 percent were married between 1700 and 1765. These results are in direct concordance with the degree of completeness of the genealogies.

Since the great majority of the founders came from France, we investigated in further detail the province of origin of the French founders (Figure 11.4). The three provinces with the highest proportion of founders are Normandie (16 percent), Ile-de-France (13 percent), and Poitou (11 percent). Four other provinces (Aunis, Bretagne, Saintonge, and Guyenne) have a proportion of founders between 4 and 7 percent. Hence, the most common places of origin of the French founders are in the

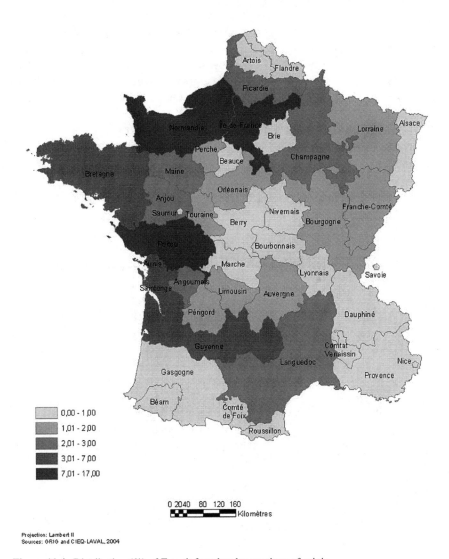

Figure 11.4 Distribution (%) of French founders by province of origin

western part of France, especially in the north. Eastern French provinces yielded few founders to the Quebec population.

As we have seen, many ancestors identified in the genealogies do not appear in only one genealogy. This is particularly true for the earliest founders. The higher the number of times a founder appears in the genealogies, the greater can its genetic contribution be to the contemporary population. Using all the links between the founders and the 2,223 subjects, the number of genealogies in which each founder appears, as well as the average number of appearances per place of origin, were calculated (Tables 11.3–11.5).

Results in Table 3 show that 77 percent of founders appear in more than one genealogy, 25 percent appear in more than 100 genealogies (i.e., 5 percent of all genealogies), and 1 percent appear in more than 1,000 genealogies. Three founders in particular appear in 2,049 genealogies, which represent 92 percent of the genealogies. Results also vary greatly according to the period of marriage: unsurprisingly, the earliest founders tend to appear in a greater number of genealogies than the more recent founders. 46 percent of founders married before 1700 appear in at least 100 genealogies; whereas most of the founders married later appear in 10 genealogies or less (only three founders married after 1700 appear in more than 100 genealogies).

Table 11.3 Distribution of founders (%) according to the number of genealogies in which they appear, by period of marriage (n = 13,119). (From BALSAC population register, BALSAC-RETRO genealogical database, and Early Quebec Population Register.)

| Number of genealogies | Period of marriage | | | |
	Before 1700 (n = 7,135)	1700–1765 (n = 3,583)	After 1765 (n = 2,401)	All periods (n = 13,119)
1	2.8	25.3	78.4	22.8
2–10	12.5	59.4	21.2	26.9
11–100	38.6	15.2	0.4	25.2
101–1000	44.1	0.1	0.0	24.0
1001–2049	1.9	0.0	0.0	1.0
Total	100.0	100.0	100.0	100.0

Table 11.4 Proportion of genealogies (%) which include at least one founder of a given origin and period of marriage (n = 2,223). (From BALSAC population register, BALSAC-RETRO genealogical database and Early Quebec Population Register.)

| Origin | Period of marriage | | | |
	Before 1700	1700–1765	After 1765	All periods
France	99.2	94.4	3.7	99.2
British Isles	96.5	18.6	11.2	97.9
Germany	10.2	8.7	4.1	21.1
Other European	94.8	11.7	1.1	95.8
Acadia	54.9	19.4	2.7	60.4
Other American	72.1	18.4	3.1	78.4
Unknown	66.8	37.2	47.2	88.2
All origins	99.2	97.2	55.4	100.0

Table 11.5 Mean proportion of genealogies (%) in which a founder appears, according to origin and period of marriage (n = 2,223). (From BALSAC population register, BALSAC-RETRO genealogical database, and Early Quebec Population Register.)

Origin	Period of marriage			
	Before 1700	1700–1765	After 1765	All periods
France	8.32	0.29	0.08	5.94
British Isles	4.31	0.21	0.07	0.63
Germany	2.11	0.12	0.08	0.20
Other European	5.85	0.34	0.05	2.25
Acadia	5.31	0.27	0.09	0.85
Other American	2.35	0.33	0.06	1.02
Unknown	3.28	0.27	0.06	0.21
All origins	8.09	0.28	0.06	4.49

Table 11.4 gives the proportion of the 2,223 Quebec genealogies that contain at least one founder of a given origin and period of marriage. Virtually all genealogies (99.2 percent) contain at least one French founder. Founders from the British Isles and other European origins are also present in most genealogies (97.9 and 95.8 percent respectively). Acadian founders appear in 60 percent of Quebec genealogies whereas German founders appear in one out of five genealogies. Again, these proportions are explained in large part by the origin of the earlier founders. Except for founders with an unknown origin, the highest proportions are those of founders married before 1700.

On average, each French founder appears in 6 percent of the 2,223 genealogies (Table 11.5). This proportion grows to a little more than 8 percent for the earliest French founders. The origin with the second highest average proportion is other European founders, with 2.3 percent (5.9 percent for those married before 1700). Early founders from Acadia (5.3 percent) and the British Isles (4.3 percent) also have a relatively high average proportion.

The frequency and generation level of the founders' appearances in the genealogies were used to calculate the founder's genetic contribution to the subjects. The genetic contribution (GC) of a given founder to a number of subjects is calculated as follows:

$$GC = \sum_{S} \sum_{P} \left(\frac{1}{2}\right)^{g}$$

where S is the set of all subjects genealogically linked with the founder, P is the set of all genealogical paths between the founder and the subject and g is the number of generations, in each path, between the founder and the subject.

This measure can be interpreted as the expected number of copies of a specific gene, among the subjects, originating from the founder (Roberts 1968; O'Brien et al. 1994; Heyer and Tremblay 1995). Thus, founders with the highest genetic contributions have the highest probabilities of having transmitted their genes to the contemporary population through their descendants.

Summing GC for all founders with the same origin and dividing the result by the number of subjects gives the proportion of the subjects' gene pool that came from that origin. This measure is useful to evaluate the importance of a source population in terms of its contribution to the settlement and expansion of another population.

Figure 11.5 shows that the individual share of each founder in the total gene pool of the Quebec population is extremely variable, with 1 percent of the founders contributing to 10 percent of the total, and half of the total genetic contribution being explained by a mere 9 percent of all founders. Conversely, 70 percent of the founders contribute collectively to less than 19 percent of the population's genes.

Genetic contribution values, stratified by the founders' origins and periods of marriage, appear in Table 11.6. Clearly, these results show the importance of the French contribution to the population of Quebec. Overall, nearly 87 percent of the gene pool is explained by French founders. British founders contribute to a little more than 2 percent whereas the contributions of German, Acadian, other European, and other American founders are only 1 percent or less. Founders who married before 1700 were responsible for about 85 percent of the genetic contribution. These results demonstrate the necessity of taking into account not only the presence of a given set of founders in the genealogies, but also the number of subjects to

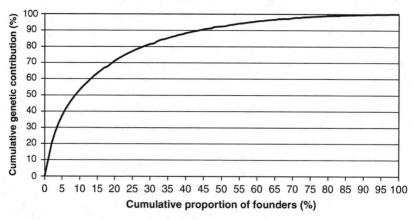

Figure 11.5 Cumulative genetic contribution of founders (%).

Table 11.6 Genetic contribution (%) of founders according to their origin and period of marriage (n = 13,119). (From BALSAC population register, BALSAC-RETRO genealogical database and Early Quebec Population Register.)

Origin	Period of marriage			
	Before 1700	1700–1765	After 1765	Total
France	81.75	4.78	0.26	86.79
British Isles	0.77	0.41	1.18	2.35
Germany	0.03	0.20	0.13	0.36
Other European	0.65	0.14	0.29	1.08
Acadia	0.33	0.34	0.15	0.81
Other American	0.51	0.17	0.29	0.98
Unknown	0.60	0.65	6.37	7.63
Total	84.63	6.69	8.68	100.00

which they are linked and the number of paths by which these links can be traced. Even though British, Acadian, German, and other non-French founders appear in a great proportion of genealogies (see Table 11.4), their relative contribution to the gene pool of the subjects is extremely small, compared to the French founders.

Figures 11.6 and 11.7 show the relative contribution of French founders in greater detail. The importance of the north-western provinces of France in the total genetic contribution of French founders to the population of Quebec is striking. The province of Normandie alone provided almost 20 percent of the French genetic contribution. Together, five provinces (Normandie, Ile-de-France, Aunis, Poitou, and Perche)

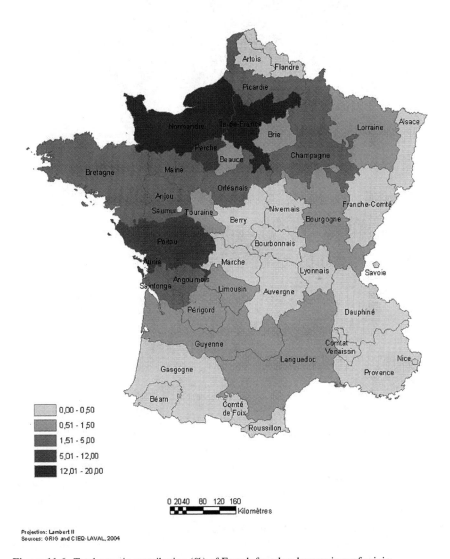

Figure 11.6 Total genetic contribution (%) of French founders by province of origin

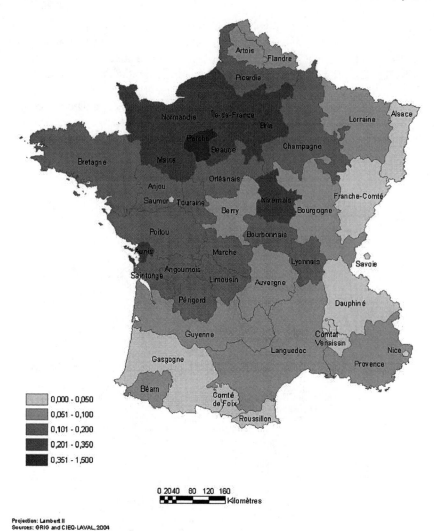

Figure 11.7 Mean genetic contribution of French founders by province of origin

account for 65 percent of the genetic contribution of all French founders. The Perche province, from which only 1.7 percent of French founders were derived, provided 9 percent of the genetic contribution. On average, the Perche founders have a genetic contribution of 1.05, which is at least three times higher than the average genetic contribution of founders from any other province (Figure 11.7). It is worth noticing that founders from Aunis, Maine, Brie, and Beauce have a slightly higher average genetic contribution than that of the more numerous founders from Normandie and Ile-de-France. Other provinces, like Languedoc and Lorraine, have much smaller average genetic contributions, their relative contribution being two to three times lower than their proportion of founders.

7 Discussion

This study of the origins and of the genealogical structure of the Quebec population has shown that early founder effects in this population are still, in many ways, strongly perceptible. Analysis of distant kinship ties shows that almost all Quebecers of French descent share at least one common ancestor. In many cases, several ancestors are common to any given pair of subjects. The most frequent common ancestors are, undoubtedly, the earliest founders of the Quebec population, born in France during the late sixteenth and early seventeenth centuries. Although many of these founders did not immigrate to Quebec, their children or grandchildren did. Hence, we think that our analysis of the founders' origins correctly reflects the origins of the actual immigrants to Quebec or, more precisely, the origins of those immigrants who still have some descendants in the contemporary population of Quebec.[1]

For comparison purposes, Table 11.7 shows the distribution of all immigrants to Quebec before 1800, based on data available in the PRDH register. The proportion of French immigrants (68 percent) is lower than the proportion of French founders in the genealogies (73 percent, see Table 11.2), despite the fact that post-1800 immigrants are not considered in Table 11.7. This difference is a consequence of the strong advantage gained by the French immigrants in their early arrivals in Quebec, which is clearly reflected by their genetic contribution to the contemporary population (Table 11.6). The high proportion of founders during the earliest period (54 percent before 1700), compared to the proportion of pre-1800 immigrants during the same period (32 percent), also reflects this strong "early founder effect". Another notable

Table 11.7 Distribution of pre-1800 immigrants (%) according to their origin and period of marriage (n = 14,743). (Early Quebec Population Register.)

	Period of marriage			
Origin	Before 1700 (n = 4,775)	1700–1765 (n = 6,929)	1766–1799 (n = 3,039)	Total (n = 14,743)
France	31.6	32.2	3.8	67.6
British Isles	0.3	2.3	3.8	6.4
Germany	0.0	0.4	2.6	3.0
Other European	0.2	0.8	0.4	1.4
Acadia	0.1	10.2	8.8	19.2
Other American	0.1	0.6	0.2	0.9
Unknown	0.0	0.4	1.0	1.5
Total	32.4	47.0	20.6	100.0

---

[1] Since our genealogical sample consists of subjects who were married in Quebec between 1945 and 1965, results that could be obtained with more recent data might show some differences, although these differences would concern mainly immigrants (or their descendants) who settled in Quebec after 1965. Also, the non-Catholics, who made up approximately 12 percent of the 1945–1965 Quebec population, were not investigated, due to lack of data: most of these individuals are probably of British descent (England, Scotland, and Wales).

difference between the proportions of founders and immigrants is that of the Acadians. In this case, it may be that a significant portion of the unknown origins in Table 11.2 is composed of Acadian founders, but the near absence of Acadian immigrants before 1700 also explains, in part, their relatively low contribution to the contemporary population.

Such founder effects are one of the main factors which can explain the presence of certain hereditary diseases in the population. Several studies have already suggested such effects are the cause of the relatively high frequencies of some rare hereditary diseases in the population of Quebec (for reviews, see Vézina 1996; Scriver 2001). In some cases, specific founders have even been identified as the probable introducers of a given mutation (Scriver 2001; Gagnon, Vézina, and Brais 2001; Vézina et al. 2005a), although in most cases, it is very difficult to pinpoint a precise founder due to the presence of several probable candidates (Heyer, Tremblay, and Desjardins 1997; Yotova et al. 2005). Simulations of gene transmission across generations have been performed in order to measure the probabilities for a given founder that one of his or her genes could reach a given frequency in the population (Heyer 1999; Austerlitz and Heyer 2000; Tremblay, Arsenault, and Heyer 2003; Heyer, Sibert, and Austerlitz 2005). Some founders were thus identified with a relatively high probability of having transmitted their genes to a proportion of the population, equivalent to the assumed carrier frequency of some recessive disorders.

The richness and the completeness of the Quebec genealogical data have helped investigators to reconsider many false or vague assumptions about the Quebec population structure and evolution. For instance, it was long believed that the population of the Saguenay-Lac-St-Jean (SLSJ) region (Northeastern Quebec) was highly inbred, or at least much more than the rest of the Quebec population, since some rare hereditary disorders were observed with an unusually high frequency in this population. Recent studies showed a different picture. Close inbreeding coefficients in the SLSJ population are in fact lower than those observed in most other regions of Quebec (Vézina, Tremblay, and Houde 2005b). Also, a recent detailed study of the SLSJ population showed that different founder effects may have taken place within the region itself, suggesting that microgeographical characterization of the population may help to better understand its genetic structure (Lavoie et al. 2005). Similar small-scale founder effects have been observed in Iceland (Helgason et al. 2005) and Finland (Kere 2001). The present study also helped to put into perspective the relative contributions of founders from various origins to the Quebec population. Popular beliefs often tend to exaggerate the importance of the contribution of founders of an "exotic" origin when these founders happen to appear somewhere in the ancestral branches. Although founders from a given origin may appear in a high proportion of genealogies, their actual genetic contribution to the population will not necessarily be very significant.

These observations strongly point to the importance and advantage of high quality population databases for the study of demographic history and genetic stratification in a given population, or even of human genetic evolution in a broader sense (Newman et al. 2001). The use of genealogical data from a population with known founder effects has long proved very helpful for the study of recessive disorders and also, more recently, of complex diseases (Wright, Carothers, and Piratsu 1999). But one must, nevertheless, still be careful when interpreting genealogical analyses since the data, in any case, are never flawless. Notwithstanding the possibility of false links (although to a relatively low degree in the case of the Quebec population databases), the number of generations reached within the genealogies and the completeness of these genealogies at each generation level are still extremely determinant. Results shown in the present study are a good example. For instance, the numerous and high kinship ties of the Quebec population would not have shown up in the same way with genealogies reaching lower generational depths. Indeed, most of the existing kinship links in the population do not appear before the seventh generation or higher. Hence, genealogical paths leading to founder effects in the population are clearly better understood with complete and deep-rooted genealogies.

Further analyses on the founders of the Quebec population should focus on determining more precisely the contribution and origins of the actual immigrants to the population; and distinction between male and female founders should be made. Comparisons of paternal (Y chromosome) and maternal (mitochondrial DNA) lines of descent in Finland and Iceland have shown quite different pictures between the origins and diversity of Y chromosome and mitochondrial DNA within each population (Kittles et al. 1999; Helgason et al. 2003). We already know that the geographical origins of the first French pioneers in Quebec show some notable differences between males and females (Charbonneau et al. 1993). Forthcoming genealogical analyses will help to identify which of the female and male founders have transmitted, up to the contemporary population, their mitochondrial and Y chromosome DNA through their female and male descendants respectively, and in what proportions.

Acknowledgments We thank our research assistants, Ève-Marie Lavoie, Lise Gobeil, Michèle Jomphe, Diane Brassard, France Néron, Frédéric Payeur, and Denis Duval for their technical support. We also thank the Social Sciences and Humanities Research Council of Canada, the Réseau de médecine génétique appliquée du Québec (RMGA-FRSQ), the Fonds québécois de recherche sur la société et la culture, ECOGENE-21, and the Canadian Institutes of Health Research for their financial assistance. An earlier version of this chapter was presented at the IUSSP Seminar "New history of kinship", held in Paris, France, 1–2 October 2004.

References

Arcos-Burgos, M. and M. Muenke. 2002. Genetics of population isolates. *Clinical Genetics* 61: 233–47.

Árnason, E. 2003. Genetic heterogeneity of Icelanders. *Annals of Human Genetics* 67: 5–16.

Austerlitz, F. and É. Heyer. 2000. Allelic association is increased by correlation of effective family size. *European Journal of Human Genetics* 8: 980–5.

Beaujot, R. and D. Kerr. 2004. *Population Change in Canada*, 2nd edition. Oxford University Press, Don Mills.

Bouchard, G. 2004. *Projet BALSAC—Rapport annuel 2003–2004*. Projet BALSAC, Université du Québec à Chicoutimi, Chicoutimi (www.balsac.uqac.ca).

Bouchard, G. and M. DeBraekeleer. 1991. *Histoire d'un génome. Population et génétique dans l'est du Québec.* Presses de l'Université du Québec, Québec.

Bouchard, G., R. Roy, B. Casgrain, and M. Hubert. 1995. Computer in human sciences: From family reconstitution to population reconstruction, in E. Nissan and K.M. Schmidt (eds.), *From information to knowledge: Conceptual and content analysis by computer*, Intellect, Oxford, pp. 201–27.

Charbonneau, H., B. Desjardins, A. Guillemette, Y. Landry, J. Légaré, and F. Nault. 1993. *The First French Canadians. Pioneers in the St. Lawrence Valley.* University of Delaware Press/ Associated University Presses, Newark/London/Toronto.

Charbonneau, H., B. Desjardins, J. Légaré, and H. Denis. 2000. The population of the St. Lawrence Valley, 1608–1760, in M.R. Haines, R.H. Steckel et al., *A population history of North America*, Cambridge University Press, Cambridge, pp. 99–142.

Desjardins, B. 1998. Le Registre de la population du Québec ancien. *Annales de démographie historique* 2: 215–26.

Dickinson, J.A. 1994. Les réfugiés acadiens au Québec, 1755–1775. *Études canadiennes/ Canadian Studies* 37: 51–61.

Duchesne, L. 2004. *La situation démographique au Québec, bilan 2004.* Les Publications du Québec, Québec.

Gagnon, A., H. Vézina, and B. Brais. 2001. Histoire démographique et génétique du Québec. *Pour la Science* 287: 62–9.

Helgason, A., B. Hrafnkelsson, J.R. Gulcher, R. Ward, and K. Stefánsson. 2003a. A population-wide coalescent analysis of Icelandic matrilineal and patrilineal genealogies: Evidence for a faster evolutionary rate of mtDNA lineages than Y chromosomes. *The American Journal of Human Genetics* 72: 1370–88.

Helgason, A., G. Nicholson, K. Stefánsson, and P. Donnelly. 2003b. A reassessment of genetic diversity in Icelanders: Strong evidence from multiple loci for relative homogeneity caused by genetic drift. *Annals of Human Genetics* 67: 281–97.

Helgason, A., S. Sigurðardóttir, J. Nicholson, B. Sykes, E.W. Hill, D.G. Bradley, V. Bosnes, J.R. Gulcher, R. Ward, and K. Stefánsson. 2000. Estimating Scandinavian and Gaelic ancestry in the male settlers of Iceland. *The American Journal of Human Genetics* 67: 697–717.

Helgason, A., B. Yngvadóttir, B. Hrafnkelsson, J. Gulcher, and K. Stefánsson. 2005. An Icelandic example of the impact of population structure on association studies. *Nature Genetics* 37(1): 90–5.

Henripin, J. and Y. Péron. 1972. The demographic transition of the Province of Quebec, in D.V. Glass and R. Revelle (eds.), *Population and social change*, Edward Arnold, London, pp. 213–31.

Heyer, É. 1999. One founder/one gene hypothesis in a new expanding population: Saguenay (Quebec, Canada). *Human Biology* 71(1): 99–109.

Heyer, É., A. Sibert, and F. Austerlitz. 2005. Cultural transmission of fitness: Genes take the fast lane. *Trends in Genetics* 21(4): 234–9.

Heyer, É. and M. Tremblay. 1995. Variability of the genetic contribution of Quebec population founders associated to some deleterious genes. *The American Journal of Human Genetics* 56: 970–8.

Heyer, É., M. Tremblay, and B. Desjardins. 1997. Seventeenth-century European origins of hereditary diseases in the Saguenay population (Quebec, Canada). *Human Biology* 69: 209–25.

Jomphe, M. and B. Casgrain. 1997. *Base de données généalogiques RETRO: Structure des données.* IREP, Programme de recherches en génétique des populations, Chicoutimi.

Kere, J. 2001. Human population genetics: Lessons from Finland. *Annual Review of Genomics and Human Genetics* 2: 103–28.

Kittles, R.A., A.W. Bergen, M. Urbanek, M.Virkkunen, M. Linnoila, D. Goldman, and J.C. Long. 1999. Autosomal, mitochondrial, and Y chromosome DNA variation in Finland: Evidence for a male-specific bottleneck. *American Journal of Physical Anthropology* 108: 381–99.

Landry, Y. 1992. *Orphelines en France, pionnières au Canada. Les Filles du roi au XVIIe siècle.* Éditions Leméac, Montréal.

Lavoie, È-M., M. Tremblay, L. Houde, and H. Vézina. 2005. Demogenetic study of three populations within a region with strong founder effects. *Community Genetics* 8: 152–60.

Légaré, J. 1988. A population register for Canada under the French regime: Context, scope, content and applications. *Canadian Studies in Population* 15: 1–16.

Mayr, E. 1963. *Animal Species and Evolution*. Harvard University Press, Cambridge, MA.

McInnis, M. 2000. The population of Canada in the nineteenth century, in M.R. Haines, R.H. Steckel et al., *A population history of North America*, Cambridge University Press, Cambridge, pp. 371–432.

Newman, D.l., M. Abney, M.S. McPeek, C. Ober, and N.J. Cox. 2001. The importance of genealogy in determining genetic associations with complex traits. *The American Journal of Human Genetics* 69: 1146–8.

O'Brien, E., L.B. Jorde, B. Rönnlöf, J.O. Fellman, and A.W. Eriksson. 1988. Founder effect and genetic disease in Sottunga, Finland. *American Journal of Physical Anthropology* 77: 335–46.

O'Brien, E., R.A. Kerber, L.B. Jorde and A.R. Rogers. 1994. Founder effect: Assessment of variation in genetic contributions among founders. *Human Biology* 66: 185–204.

Peltonen, L., P. Pekkarinen, and J. Aaltonen. 1995. Messages from an isolate: Lessons from the Finnish gene pool. *Biological Chemistry Hoppe-Seyler* 376: 697–704.

Roberts, D.F. 1968. Genetic effects of population size reduction. *Nature* 220: 1084–8.

Scriver, C. 2001. Human genetics: Lessons from Quebec populations. *Annual Review of Genomics and Human Genetics* 2: 69–101.

Statistics Canada. 2006. www.statcan.ca.

Thompson, E.A. 1986. *Pedigree Analysis in Human Genetics*. Johns Hopkins University Press, Baltimore, MD.

Tremblay, M., J. Arsenault, and É. Heyer. 2003. The transmission probabilities of founder genes in five regional populations of Quebec. *Population* 58(3): 361–80.

Tremblay, M., M. Jomphe, and H. Vézina. 2001. Comparaison de structures patronymiques et génétiques dans la population québécoise, in G. Brunet, P. Darlu, and G. Zei (eds.), *Le patronyme: Histoire, anthropologie, société*, CNRS Éditions, Paris, pp. 367–89.

Vézina, H. 1996. Démographie génétique et maladies héréditaires au Québec: L'état des recherches. *Cahiers québécois de démographie* 25(2): 293–322.

Vézina, H., F. Durocher, M. Dumont, L. Houde, C. Szabo, M. Tranchant, J. Chiquette, M. Plante, R. Laframboise, J. Lepine, H. Nevanlinna, D. Stoppa-Lyonnet, D. Goldgar, P. Bridge, J. Simard, and BCLC Haplotype Group; INHERIT BRCAs. 2005a. Molecular and genealogical characterization of the R1443X BRCA1 mutation in high-risk French-Canadian breast/ovarian cancer families. *Human Genetics* 117(2–3): 119–32.

Vézina, H., M. Tremblay, and L. Houde. 2005b. Mesures de l'apparentement biologique au Saguenay-Lac-St-Jean (Québec, Canada) à partir de reconstitutions généalogiques. *Annales de démographie historique* 2004(2): 67–84.

Wilhelmy, J.-P. 1984. *Les mercenaires allemands au Québec du XVIIIe siècle et leur apport à la population*. Maison des mots, Beloeil.

Wright, A.F., A.D. Carothers, and M. Pirastu. 1999. Population choice in mapping genes for complex diseases. *Nature Genetics* 23: 397–404.

Yotova, V., D. Labuda, E. Zietkiewicz, D. Gehl, A. Lovell, J.F. Lefebvre, S. Bourgeois, É. Lemieux-Blanchard, M. Labuda, H. Vézina, L. Houde, M. Tremblay, B. Toupance, É Heyer, T.J. Hudson, and C. Laberge. 2005. Anatomy of a founder effect: Myotonic dystrophy in Northeastern Quebec. *Human Genetics* 117(2–3): 177–87.

Index